Damage Control: Advances in Trauma Resuscitation

Editors

CHRISTOPHER HICKS
ANDREW PETROSONIAK

EMERGENCY MEDICINE CLINICS OF NORTH AMERICA

www.emed.theclinics.com

Consulting Editor
AMAL MATTU

February 2018 • Volume 36 • Number 1

ELSEVIER

1600 John F. Kennedy Boulevard ● Suite 1800 ● Philadelphia, Pennsylvania, 19103-2899

http://www.theclinics.com

EMERGENCY MEDICINE CLINICS OF NORTH AMERICA Volume 36, Number 1
February 2018 ISSN 0733-8627, ISBN-13: 978-0-323-56976-7

Editor: Colleen Dietzler
Developmental Editor: Casey Potter

Emergency Medicine Clinics of North America (ISSN 0733-8627) is published quarterly by Elsevier Inc., 360 Park Avenue South, New York, NY, 10010-1710. Months of issue are February, May, August, and November. Business and Editorial Offices: 1600 John F. Kennedy Boulevard, Suite 1800, Philadelphia, PA 19103-2899. Customer Service Office: 6277 Sea Harbor Drive, Orlando, FL 32887-4800. Periodicals postage paid at New York, NY, and additional mailing offices. Subscription prices are $100.00 per year (US students), $336.00 per year (US individuals), $644.00 per year (US institutions), $220.00 per year (international students), $455.00 per year (international individuals), $791.00 per year (international institutions), $220.00 per year (Canadian students), $405.00 per year (Canadian individuals), and $791.00 per year (Canadian institutions). International air speed delivery is included in all *Clinics'* subscription prices. All prices are subject to change without notice. **POSTMASTER:** Send address changes to *Emergency Medicine Clinics of North America*, Elsevier Periodicals Customer Service, 11830 Westline Industrial Drive, St. Louis, MO 63146. Customer Service (orders, claims, online, change of address): Elsevier Periodicals **Customer Service, 11830 Westline Industrial Drive, St. Louis, MO 63146. Tel: 1-800-654-2452 (U.S. and Canada); 314-453-7041 (outside U.S. and Canada). Fax: 314-453-5170. E-mail: journalscustomerservice-usa@elsevier.com (for print support);** **journalsonlinesupport-usa@elsevier.com (for online support).**

Reprints. For copies of 100 or more of articles in this publication, please contact the Commercial Reprints Department, Elsevier Inc., 360 Park Avenue South, New York, NY 10010-1710. Tel.: 212-633-3874; Fax: 212-633-3820; E-mail: reprints@elsevier.com.

Emergency Medicine Clinics of North America is covered in *MEDLINE/PubMed (Index Medicus), Current Contents/Clinical Medicine, EMBASE/Excerpta Medica, BIOSIS, SciSearch, CINAHL, ISI/BIOMED,* and *Research Alert.*

Contributors

CONSULTING EDITOR

AMAL MATTU, MD
Professor and Vice Chair of Education, Department of Emergency Medicine, University of Maryland School of Medicine, Baltimore, Maryland, USA

EDITORS

CHRISTOPHER HICKS, MD, MEd, FRCPC
Emergency Physician, Trauma Team Leader, St. Michael's Hospital, Assistant Professor, Department of Medicine, University of Toronto, Education Research Scientist, Li Ka Shing Knowledge Institute, International Centre for Surgical Safety, Keenan Research Centre for Biomedical Science, Toronto, Ontario, Canada

ANDREW PETROSONIAK, MD, MSc (MedEd), FRCPC
Emergency Physician, Trauma Team Leader, St. Michael's Hospital, Associate Scientist, Li Ka Shing Knowledge Institute, Assistant Professor, Department of Medicine, University of Toronto, Toronto, Ontario, Canada

AUTHORS

MEGAN BRENNER, MD, MS, RPVI, FACS
Associate Professor of Surgery, Division of Trauma/Surgical Critical Care, RA Cowley Shock Trauma Center, Division of Vascular Surgery, University of Maryland School of Medicine, Baltimore, Maryland, USA

KARIM BROHI, FRCS, FRCA
Professor of Trauma Sciences, Trauma and Neuroscience, Blizard Institute, Queen Mary University of London, London's Air Ambulance, Barts Health NHS Trust, London, United Kingdom

BRIAN BURNS, DipRTM, MSc, MD, FACEM
Greater Sydney Area HEMS, Ambulance Service of New South Wales, The University of Sydney, Sydney, New South Wales, Australia

TIM CHAPLIN, MD, FRCPC
Assistant Professor, Department of Emergency Medicine, Queen's University, Kingston, Ontario, Canada

ROSS DAVENPORT, PhD
Trauma Sciences, Blizard Institute, Queen Mary University of London, London, United Kingdom

PAUL T. ENGELS, MD, FRCSC, FACS, FCCP
Trauma, General Surgery and Critical Care, Assistant Professor, Departments of Surgery and Critical Care, McMaster University Medical Centre, Hamilton General Hospital, Hamilton, Ontario, Canada

CHRIS EVANS, MD, MSc, FRCPC
Director, Trauma Services, Assistant Professor, Department of Emergency Medicine, Kingston General Hospital, Queen's University, Kingston, Ontario, Canada

PRESTON J. FEDOR, MD, FACEP
Department of Emergency Medicine, Division of Prehospital, Austere and Disaster Medicine, The University of New Mexico, Albuquerque, New Mexico, USA

VINCENT GRANT, MD, FRCPC
Pediatric Emergency Physician, Medical Director of KidSIM: Pediatric Simulation Program, Associate Professor, Department of Pediatrics, Alberta Children's Hospital, Department of Emergency Medicine, Cumming School of Medicine, University of Calgary, Calgary, Alberta, Canada

TIM HARRIS, BM BS, BMed Sci, Dip O&G, DipIMC, FACEM, FFAEM
Professor of Emergency Medicine, Barts Health NHS Trust, Queen Mary University of London, London, United Kingdom

CHRISTOPHER HICKS, MD, MEd, FRCPC
Emergency Physician, Trauma Team Leader, St. Michael's Hospital, Assistant Professor, Department of Medicine, University of Toronto, Education Research Scientist, Li Ka Shing Knowledge Institute, International Centre for Surgical Safety, Keenan Research Centre for Biomedical Science, Toronto, Ontario, Canada

KATRIN HRUSKA, MD
Department of Emergency Medicine, Karolinska University Hospital, Huddinge, Sweden

KENJI INABA, MD, FACS, FRCSC
Associate Professor of Surgery, Emergency Medicine, and Anesthesia, Division of Trauma and Surgical Critical Care, LAC+USC Medical Center, University of Southern California, Los Angeles, California, USA

GEORGE KOVACS, MD, MHPE, FRCPC
Professor, Departments of Emergency Medicine, Anaesthesia and Medical Neurosciences, Division of Medical Education, Dalhousie University, Trauma Team Leader, Charles V. Keating Emergency & Trauma Centre, Halifax Infirmary Robie Street Entrance - QEII, Halifax, Nova Scotia, Canada

ALEX KOYFMAN, MD
Department of Emergency Medicine, The University of Texas Southwestern Medical Center, Dallas, Texas, USA

MICHAEL LAURIA, BA, NRP, FP-C
Dartmouth-Hitchcock Advanced Response Team (DHART), Dartmouth-Hitchcock Medical Center, Lebanon, New Hampshire, USA

BRIT LONG, MD
Department of Emergency Medicine, San Antonio Military Medical Center, Fort Sam Houston, Texas, USA

MATTHEW MAK, BSc, MSc, MBBS, FRCEM, FHEA
NIHR Academic Clinical Fellow and Specialty Registrar, Emergency Medicine, Barts Health NHS Trust, London, United Kingdom

ANGELO MIKROGIANAKIS, MD, FRCPC
Medical Director and Section Chief of Pediatric Emergency Medicine, Co-Director of Pediatric Critical Care Transport, Associate Professor, Department of Pediatrics, Alberta Children's Hospital, Department of Emergency Medicine, Cumming School of Medicine, University of Calgary, Calgary, Alberta, Canada

ANDREW PETROSONIAK, MD, Med, MSc (MedEd), FRCPC
Emergency Physician, Trauma Team Leader, St. Michael's Hospital, Associate Scientist, Li Ka Shing Knowledge Institute, Assistant Professor, Department of Medicine, University of Toronto, Toronto, Ontario, Canada

DAVID O. QUINLAN, MD, MSc, FRCPC
Division of Emergency Medicine, McMaster University, Emergency Physician, Hamilton Health Sciences, Hamilton General Hospital, Hamilton, Ontario, Canada

CLARE RICHMOND, FACEM, MBBS, BSci (Med Sci), Dip IMC
Greater Sydney Area HEMS, Ambulance Service of New South Wales, New South Wales, Australia; Royal Prince Alfred Hospital, Sydney, Australia

TORALPH RUGE, MD, PhD
Department of Medicine, Solna, Karolinska Institutet, Stockholm, Sweden; Department of Emergency Medicine, Karolinska University Hospital, Huddinge, Sweden

MORGAN SCHELLENBERG, MD, MPH
Trauma/Critical Care Fellow, Division of Trauma and Surgical Critical Care, LAC+USC Medical Center, University of Southern California, Los Angeles, California, USA

JONATHAN SHERBINO, MD, MEd, FRCPC, FAcadMEd
Division of Emergency Medicine, McMaster University, Emergency Physician, Hamilton General Hospital, Hamilton, Ontario, Canada

STEVEN SKITCH, MD, PhD, RDMS
Departments of Emergency Medicine and Critical Care, McMaster University, Hamilton General Hospital, Hamilton, Ontario, Canada

NICHOLAS SOWERS, MD, FRCPC
Assistant Professor, Department of Emergency Medicine, Division of Medical Education, Dalhousie University, Trauma Team Leader, Charles V. Keating Trauma & Emergency Centre, Halifax Infirmary Robie Street Entrance - QEII, Halifax, Nova Scotia, Canada

DAVID ZELT, MD, MSc, FRCSC
Associate Professor, Division Chair, Division of Vascular Surgery, Chief of Staff, Kingston General Hospital, Queen's University, Kingston, Ontario, Canada

Contents

> Resilience is built, not born, and there is no single strategy that reliably manufactures resilient performance in all circumstances. Optimizing team performance in dynamic environments involves the complex interplay of strategies that target individual preparation, team interaction, environmental optimization, and systems-level resilience engineering. To accomplish this, health care can draw influence from human factors research to inform tangible, practical, and measurable improvements in performance and outcomes, modified to suit local and domain-specific needs.

> Resuscitation of traumatic cardiac arrest is typically considered futile. Recent evidence suggests that traumatic cardiac arrest is survivable. In this article key principles in managing traumatic cardiac arrest are discussed, including the importance of rapidly seeking prognostic information, such as signs of life and point-of-care ultrasonography evidence of cardiac contractility, to inform the decision to proceed with resuscitative efforts. In addition, a rationale for deprioritizing chest compressions, steps to quickly reverse dysfunctional ventilation, techniques for temporary control of hemorrhage, and the importance of blood resuscitation are discussed. The best available evidence and the authors' collective experience inform this article.

> Trauma resuscitation is a complex and dynamic process that requires a high-performing team to optimize patient outcomes. More than 30 years ago, Advanced Trauma Life Support was developed to formalize and standardize trauma care; however, the sequential nature of the algorithm that is used can lead to ineffective prioritization. An improved understanding of shock mandates an updated approach to trauma resuscitation. This article proposes a resequenced approach that (1) addresses immediate threats

to life and (2) targets strategies for the diagnosis and management of shock causes. This updated approach emphasizes evidence-based resuscitation principles that align with physiologic priorities.

Airway management in the trauma patient presents numerous unique challenges beyond placement of an endotracheal tube, and outcomes are dependent on the provider's ability to anticipate difficulty. Airway management strategies for the care of the patient with polytrauma are reviewed, with specific considerations for those presenting with traumatic brain injury, suspected c-spine injury, the contaminated airway, the agitated trauma patient, maxillofacial trauma, and the traumatized airway. An approach to airway management that considers the potential anatomic and physiologic challenges in caring for these patients with complicated trauma is presented.

This article summarizes the evolution of trauma resuscitation from a one-size-fits-all approach to one tailored to patient physiology. The most dramatic change is in the management of actively bleeding patients, with a balanced blood product–based resuscitation approach (avoiding crystalloids) and surgery focused on hemorrhage control, not definitive care. When hemostasis has been achieved, definitive resuscitation to restore organ perfusion is initiated. This approach is associated with decreased mortality, reduced duration of stay, improved coagulation profile, and reduced crystalloid/vasopressor use. This article focuses on the tools and methods used for trauma resuscitation in the acute phase of trauma care.

Neurotrauma is a leading cause of death and is associated with many secondary injuries. A balance of mean arterial pressure (MAP) and intracranial pressure (ICP) is required to ensure adequate cerebral blood flow and cerebral perfusion pressure. Evaluation and management in the emergency department entails initial stabilization and resuscitation while assessing neurologic status. ICP management follows a tiered approach. Intubation requires consideration of preoxygenation, head of bed elevation, first-pass success, and adequate analgesia and sedation. Early consultation with neurosurgery is needed for definitive therapy. Focused evaluation and management play a significant role in optimizing patient outcomes.

Traumatic injuries to the thorax are common after both blunt and penetrating trauma. Emergency medicine physicians must be able to manage the initial resuscitation and diagnostic workup of these patients; this involves familiarity with a range of radiologic investigations and invasive bedside procedures, including resuscitative thoracotomy. This knowledge is critical to allow for rapid decision making when life-threatening injuries are encountered. This article explores the initial resuscitation and assessment of patients after thoracic trauma, discusses available imaging modalities, reviews frequently performed procedures, and provides an overview of the indications for operative intervention while emphasizing the critical decision making throughout.

A standardized approach should be used with a patient with abdominal trauma, including primary and secondary surveys, followed by additional diagnostic testing as indicated. Specific factors can make the diagnosis of serious abdominal trauma challenging, particularly in the face of multiple and severe injuries, unknown mechanism of injury, altered mental status, and impending or complete cardiac arrest. Advances in technology in diagnosis and/or treatment with ultrasound, helical computed tomography, and resuscitative endovascular balloon occlusion of the aorta (REBOA) have significantly advanced trauma care and are still the focus of current and ongoing investigations.

Severe pelvic trauma is a challenging condition. The pelvis can create multifocal hemorrhage that is not easily compressible or managed by traditional surgical methods such as tying off a blood vessel or removing an organ. Its treatment often requires reapproximation of bony structures, damage control resuscitation, assessment for associated injuries, and triage of investigations, as well as multimodal hemorrhage control (external fixation, preperitoneal packing, angioembolization, REBOA [resuscitative endovascular balloon occlusion of the aorta]) by multidisciplinary trauma specialists (general surgeons, orthopedic surgeons, endovascular surgeons, and interventional radiologists). This article explores this complex clinical problem and provides a practical approach to its management.

Vascular injuries represent a significant burden of mortality and disability. Blunt injuries to the neck vessels can present with signs of stroke either immediately or in a delayed fashion. Most injuries are detected with computed tomography angiography and managed with either antiplatelet medications or anticoagulation. In contrast, patients with penetrating injuries to the neck vessels require airway management, hemorrhage control, and damage control resuscitation before surgical repair. The keys to diagnosis and management of peripheral vascular injury include early recognition of the injury; hemorrhage control with direct pressure, packing, or tourniquets; and urgent surgical consultation.

Care of the critically injured begins well before the patient arrives at a large academic trauma center. It is important to understand the continuum of care from the point of injury in the prehospital environment, through the local hospital and retrieval, until arrival at a trauma center capable of definitive care. This article highlights the important aspects of trauma assessment and management outside of tertiary or quaternary care hospitals. Key elements of each phase of care are reviewed, including management pearls and institutional strategies to facilitate effective and efficient treatment of patients with trauma from the point of injury forward.

Old age is a risk factor for poor outcome in patients with trauma, as a result of undertriage and the presence of occult life-threatening injuries. The mechanisms of injury for geriatric trauma differ from those in younger patients, with a much higher incidence of low-impact trauma, especially falls from a low height. Frailty is a risk factor for severe injury after minor trauma, and caring for these patients requires a multidisciplinary team with both trauma and geriatric expertise. With early recognition and aggressive management, severe injuries can still be associated with good outcomes, even in very elderly patients.

Pediatric patients with trauma pose unique challenges, both practical and cognitive, to front-line care providers. The combination of anatomic, physiologic, and metabolic factors leads to unique injury patterns with different approaches and responses to treatment compared with adults. A similar traumatic mechanism can lead to slightly different internal injuries with unique management and treatment strategies between the two groups. This article is intended for community, nonpediatric trauma centers, and emergency physicians who are frequently required to assess, resuscitate, and stabilize injured children before they can be safely transferred to a pediatric trauma center for ongoing definitive care and rehabilitation.

EMERGENCY MEDICINE
CLINICS OF NORTH AMERICA

PROGRAM OBJECTIVE

The goal of *Emergency Medicine Clinics of North America* is to keep practicing emergency medicine physicians and emergency medicine residents up to date with current clinical practice in emergency medicine by providing timely articles reviewing the state of the art in patient care.

LEARNING OBJECTIVES

Upon completion of this activity, participants will be able to:
1. Review practical considerations in resuscitation of trauma patients.
2. Recognize strategies in the acute management of pelvic, hip, and abdominal traumas.
3. Discuss emergency strategies in vascular and neurotraumas.

ACCREDITATION

The Elsevier Office of Continuing Medical Education (EOCME) is accredited by the Accreditation Council for Continuing Medical Education (ACCME) to provide continuing medical education for physicians.

The EOCME designates this enduring material for a maximum of 15 *AMA PRA Category 1 Credit*(s)™. Physicians should claim only the credit commensurate with the extent of their participation in the activity.

All other healthcare professionals requesting continuing education credit for this enduring material will be issued a certificate of participation.

DISCLOSURE OF CONFLICTS OF INTEREST

The EOCME assesses conflict of interest with its instructors, faculty, planners, and other individuals who are in a position to control the content of CME activities. All relevant conflicts of interest that are identified are thoroughly vetted by EOCME for fair balance, scientific objectivity, and patient care recommendations. EOCME is committed to providing its learners with CME activities that promote improvements or quality in healthcare and not a specific proprietary business or a commercial interest.

The planning committee, staff, authors and editors listed below have identified no financial relationships or relationships to products or devices they or their spouse/life partner have with commercial interest related to the content of this CME activity:
Karim Brohi, FRCS, FRCA; Brian Burns, DipRTM, MSc, MD, FACEM; Tim Chaplin, MD, FRCPC; Paul T. Engles, MD, FRCSC, FACS, FCCP; Chris Evans, MD, MSc, FRCPC; Preston J. Fedor, MD, FACEP; Anjali Fortna; Vincent Grant, MD, FRCPC; Tim Harris, BM, BS, Bmed, Sci Dip O&G, DipIMC, FACEM, FFAEM; Christopher Hicks, MD, MEd, FRCPC; Katrin Hruska, MD; Kenji Inaba, MD, FACS, FRCSC; George Kovacs, MD, MHPE, FRCPC; Alex Koyfman, MD; Michael Lauria, BA, NRP, FP-C; Leah Logan; Brit Long, MD; Matthew Mak, Bsc, MSc, MBBS, FRCEM, FHEA; Amal Mattu, MD; Angelo Mikrogianakis, MD, FRCPC; Andrew Petrosoniak, MD, MSc (MedEd), FRCPC; Katie Pfaff; David O. Quinlan, MD, MSc, FRCPC; Clare Richmond, FACEM, MBBS, BSci (Med Sci), DipIMC; Toralph Ruge, MD, PhD; Morgan Schellenberg, MD, MPH; Jonathan Sherbino, MD, MEd, FRCPC, FAcadMEd; Steven Skitch, MD, PhD, RDMS; Nick Sowers, MD, FRCPC; Vignesh Viswanathan; David Zelt, MD, MSc, FRCSC.

The planning committee, staff, authors and editors listed below have identified financial relationships or relationships to products or devices they or their spouse/life partner have with commercial interest related to the content of this CME activity:
Megan Brenner, MD, MS, RPVI, FACS is a Clinical Advisory Board Member for Prytime Medical Devices, Inc – The REBOA Company™.
Ross Davenport, PhD is a consultant/advisor for LFB Biopharmaceuticals Limited, and has research support from LFB Biopharmaceuticals Limited.

UNAPPROVED/OFF-LABEL USE DISCLOSURE

The EOCME requires CME faculty to disclose to the participants:
1. When products or procedures being discussed are off-label, unlabelled, experimental, and/or investigational (not US Food and Drug Administration [FDA] approved); and
2. Any limitations on the information presented, such as data that are preliminary or that represent ongoing research, interim analyses, and/or unsupported opinions. Faculty may discuss information about pharmaceutical agents that is outside of FDA-approved labelling. This information is intended solely for CME and is not intended to promote off-label use of these medications. If you have any questions, contact the medical affairs department of the manufacturer for the most recent prescribing information.

TO ENROLL

To enroll in the *Emergency Medicine Clinics* Continuing Medical Education program, call customer service at 1-800-654-2452 or sign up online at http://www.theclinics.com/home/cme. The CME program is available to subscribers for an additional annual fee of $235 USD.

METHOD OF PARTICIPATION

In order to claim credit, participants must complete the following:
1. Complete enrolment as indicated above.
2. Read the activity.
3. Complete the CME Test and Evaluation. Participants must achieve a score of 70% on the test. All CME Tests and Evaluations must be completed online.

CME INQUIRIES/SPECIAL NEEDS

For all CME inquiries or special needs, please contact elsevierCME@elsevier.com.

Foreword

Damage Control: Advances in Trauma Resuscitation

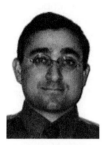

Amal Mattu, MD
Consulting Editor

When I began emergency medicine training, trauma care was considered exciting and "sexy" to my colleagues and me. There was excitement with every case, and opportunities to gain experience in procedures abounded. However, as we gained experience in trauma resuscitation, my colleagues and I discovered that trauma care was actually fairly "cookbook." Every patient was managed similarly...the A-B-Cs were employed religiously, with a low threshold for early intubation of any patient that was even mildly sick. C-spine, chest, and pelvis radiographs were obtained in nearly all patients; everybody was boarded and collared, and we routinely cut everyone's clothes off. If the patient had a penetrating wound to "the box" (torso from the pelvis to the clavicles), the patient would go to the operating room (OR), and if the patient had blunt trauma and was stable, we'd send the patient to get computerized tomography of pretty much everything...and the radiologist would give us the diagnosis. Management of these patients became somewhat boring, actually, as there was very little thought to the workup.

However, trauma care has changed markedly. The rote practice of A-B-C and the traditional Advanced Trauma Life Support course have changed, and clinical decision making is routinely incorporated into management decisions. Airway management has advanced far beyond the routine intubation of so many patients. Nonoperative management of many conditions that used to routinely go to the OR is common. Trauma has largely become a nonsurgical condition requiring more thought than ever before. Although once considered the domain of the surgeon, care of the trauma patient is now clearly recognized as a multidisciplinary responsibility, and emergency physicians are playing a leading role.

In this issue of *Emergency Medicine Clinics of North America*, Guest Editors Drs Christopher Hicks and Andrew Petrosoniak have assembled an outstanding group of emergency care providers to bring you the latest in emergency medicine knowledge regarding the care of trauma patients. A comprehensive approach is taken beginning

Emerg Med Clin N Am 36 (2018) xv–xvi
https://doi.org/10.1016/j.emc.2017.10.002
0733-8627/18/© 2017 Published by Elsevier Inc.

emed.theclinics.com

with an important discussion of how to optimize teamwork in caring for trauma patients. Traumatic arrest is discussed, including the latest evidence for thoracotomy. Next, a top-down approach to care of these patients is provided, including discussions of care of patients with brain injury, thoracic injuries, abdominal and pelvic injuries, and vascular injuries. Separate articles are provided focusing on patients at the extremes of age. Finally, a critically important article is provided that discusses care of the patient in the community, non-trauma-center setting.

This issue of *Emergency Medicine Clinics of North America* represents an important addition to the emergency medicine literature. Drs Hicks and Petrosoniak and their colleagues have provided a cutting-edge update of the current knowledge of emergency trauma care. Emergency physicians in every type of practice setting will find this issue immensely useful for the daily care of trauma patients, and it will undoubtedly improve the care of those patients. This issue also nicely exemplifies how far our specialty has progressed in trauma care beyond the basics of "A-B-C." Kudos to the contributors for an outstanding issue!

Amal Mattu, MD
Department of Emergency Medicine
University of Maryland School of Medicine
Baltimore, MD 21201, USA

E-mail address:
amalmattu@comcast.net

Preface

Seismology and Advances in Trauma Resuscitation

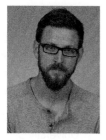 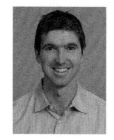

Christopher Hicks, MD, MEd, FRCPC   Andrew Petrosoniak, MD, MSc (MedEd), FRCPC
Editors

Trauma is a disease that imparts an almost unspeakable burden of illness on a global population of patients. Over the past decade, advances in the science of trauma resuscitation have changed the landscape of trauma resuscitation dramatically. Trauma is a team sport, and the science of teams has greatly advanced our ability to deliver rapid, effective multidisciplinary trauma care. Traumatic cardiac arrest, once believed to be a terminal event, is now believed to contain a population of patients with excellent survival, provided a thoughtful approach is followed. The primacy of the ABCDE approach has been called into question, prompting calls for a "resequencing" of trauma resuscitation to better align with physiologic priorities. Trauma resuscitation has moved well beyond the 2-L crystalloid challenge: trauma coagulopathy is a well-described killer, one that front-line providers can either help or hinder. Technologic and procedural advances can improve the early bedside management of the traumatic airway, facilitate neuro-resuscitation, and temporize catastrophic abdominal injuries.

The demographic of trauma is changing. Extremes of age pose unique challenges and considerations that demand thoughtful variation in practice. By 2050, the prototypical trauma patient may not be a 22-year-old healthy man, but rather a 77-year-old woman with multiple comorbid diseases and serious injuries despite a relatively "minor" mechanism.

Importantly, the bulk of the "new science" in trauma resuscitation is applicable in a broad number of practice settings, from the prehospital environment to fully equipped trauma centers, and every point in between. Much of what is known will be most useful in the hands of front-line providers rendering care within the first few minutes to hours following injury.

Prevention and public awareness will always be the cornerstones of minimizing the trauma disease burden worldwide. But while injury is pervasive, so too has resuscitation science advanced our ability to care for those injuries. This issue, in thirteen parts,

Emerg Med Clin N Am 36 (2018) xvii–xviii
https://doi.org/10.1016/j.emc.2017.10.001
0733-8627/18/© 2017 Published by Elsevier Inc.

emed.theclinics.com

will highlight the practical ways in which trauma care has evolved, and how our practice as emergency care providers should evolve along with it.

Christopher Hicks, MD, MEd, FRCPC
St. Michael's Hospital
Li Ka Shing Knowledge Institute
Department of Medicine
University of Toronto
1st Floor Bond Wing, Room 1008
30 Bond Street
Toronto, Ontario M5B 1W8
Canada

Andrew Petrosoniak, MD, MSc (MedEd), FRCPC
St. Michael's Hospital
Li Ka Shing Knowledge Institute
Department of Medicine
University of Toronto
1st Floor Bond Wing, Room 1008
30 Bond Street
Toronto, Ontario M5B 1W8
Canada

E-mail addresses:
hicksc@smh.ca (C. Hicks)
petrosoniaka@smh.ca (A. Petrosoniak)

The Human Factor
Optimizing Trauma Team Performance in Dynamic Clinical Environments

Christopher Hicks, MD, MEd, FRCPC[a],*,
Andrew Petrosoniak, MD, MSc (MedEd), FRCPC[b]

KEYWORDS

• Human factors • Patient safety • Resilience

KEY POINTS

• Equipping team members with a suite of psychological skills to manage stress, attention, and arousal
• Emphasizing specific team-based behaviors that facilitate the creation of accurate and flexible mental models, implicit communication, and adaptive coordination
• Improving awareness of environmental and equipment issues to close the gap between strategy and logistics
• Implementing systems-based initiatives aligned with Safety-II to improve system resilience in the absence of error, based on what went right

Trauma is easy; Trauma teams are hard

—Anon

Case 1. An urban emergency department receives a prehospital trauma alert: a young man with multiple gunshot wounds is en route. The team assembles beforehand, and the attending emergency physician assumes the leadership role. Team members quietly prepare for anticipated key tasks: airway, chest tube insertion, and vascular access. On arrival, the patient is unresponsive, with massive external hemorrhage from a midface gunshot wound plus 2 ballistic injuries within the cardiac box. Amid the chaos, only the recording nurse hears the paramedic's handover report: "unsuccessful intubation attempt, critical hypotension, signs of life in the field." In an attempt to optimize

The authors have no conflicts of interest to declare.
[a] Department of Emergency Medicine, St. Michael's Hospital, University of Toronto, Li Ka Shing Knowledge Institute, International Centre for Surgical Safety, Keenan Research Centre, 30 Bond Street, 1st, Floor Bond Wing, Room 1008, Toronto M5B 1W8, Canada; [b] Department of Emergency Medicine, St. Michael's Hospital, University of Toronto, 30 Bond Street, 1st Floor Bond Wing, Room 1008, Toronto M5B 1W8, Canada
* Corresponding author.
E-mail address: chrismikehicks@gmail.com

Emerg Med Clin N Am 36 (2018) 1–17
http://dx.doi.org/10.1016/j.emc.2017.08.003
0733-8627/18/© 2017 Elsevier Inc. All rights reserved.

preintubation hemodynamics, the anesthesiologist pushes phenylephrine from a vial she carries in her emergency response kit, an intervention not communicated to either team leader or recording nurse. Airway management is further complicated by mechanical trismus from the ballistic injury. This observation is made by the paramedic team and shared during sign-over, but the team leader is fixated on the cardiac ultrasound. Various individuals offer suggestions regarding next steps, prompting confusion and exasperation with the nurses. A "can't intubate, can't oxygenate" airway is declared by the anesthesiologist, who then requests a surgical airway kit. An open surgical airway tray is brought to the bedside, which is not the percutaneous set-up that the anesthesiologist prefers. Further delays occur after disagreements between the surgeon, emergency physician, and anesthesiologist about the airway approach and who should make the final decision. It is at this point that the respiratory therapist assertively declares that he cannot feel a carotid pulse.

BACKGROUND: THE TROUBLE WITH TEAMS

Trauma is a team sport. Resuscitating a severely injured patient requires the coordination of cognitive, task, and systems-based resources in a dynamic and time-dependent fashion that rapidly exceeds what an individual can bring to bear. Equally challenging is the interaction between individuals within teams during periods of ambiguity, complexity, or high coordination overhead. Trauma resuscitation poses a particular challenge: diagnosis and management occur simultaneously, in step with the ordered execution of team-based tasks and procedural interventions. Trauma teams do not operate in a bubble—the extent to which teams can effectively operationalize a resuscitation strategy is moderated in part by the clinical environment. The decision to insert a tube thoracostomy may be straightforward, yet the ambient environment, crowding, noise, lighting, and functional set-up of key equipment have a significant effect on the ability to complete the procedure quickly, safely, and successfully. A gap between strategy (the plan) and logistics (how that plan is executed) often arises from a lack of consideration for and preparation of the operational environment.[1]

At first glance, the demands of managing team-based challenges during trauma resuscitation seem daunting. Research from performance psychology, team dynamics, organizational theory and systems engineering suggest the opposite is true: the targeted integration of human factors theory can help manage complexity and improve performance in dynamic clinical environments. Standardized paradigms like crisis resource management represent a logical first step but do not help individuals and teams recognize the ambient and circumstantial factors in which implementing those skills might become problematic. For example, the team leader in case 1 was overly task focused during handover and missed important details that may have influenced management. Crisis resource management would identify this as a failure of situational awareness, but to effectively address the problem the analysis needs to go deeper. The team leader ignored task-relevant cues, a feature of hyperarousal that is known to constrain cognition and decision-making capacity.[2] The solution is not to "improve situation awareness" but to recognize the influence of acute stress on performance and apply specific strategies to moderate arousal during periods of high task load.[3] The case can be dissected further to reveal process issues (lack of standardized handover), problems with clinical logistics (availability and accessibility of surgical airway equipment), and team leadership (problematic process of shared decision-making and conflict resolution). Each of these challenges requires a specific response—marginal gains that can sum to major improvements in team performance.[4]

MANAGING COMPLEXITY: SELF, TEAM, ENVIRONMENT, AND SYSTEM

Complexity in trauma resuscitation is a function of the interplay between individuals, teams, their environment, and the system in which health care teams work.[5] Managing complexity involves improving performance at each level and the points at which they intersect. Individual team members are invariably influenced by prior experience and coping strategies, which in turn influences mental posture—the ability to remain flexible, problem-solve, and perform under acute stress. Individuals working in a team environment must employ early and effective cognitive, linguistic, and behavioral strategies to co-orient and effectively direct their efforts toward a shared sense of priorities.[6] A clinical environment that is deliberately and strategically calibrated to align with team and task priorities can facilitate the execution of common goals in a safe and efficient manner. Finally, systems require sufficient flexibility and resilience to minimize and mitigate the impact of human error and capitalize on intrinsic elements that promote and maintain safety. Specific strategies can be used at each level—self, team, environment, and system—to enhance preparation and accelerate performance. Although the behavior of individuals and teams is invariably context bound, the tools described in this article bear relevance to any team, regardless of size, composition, or extent of local resources.

Self: Psychological Skills Training for Trauma Team Members

Optimizing psychological preparation, or fitness to execute, has a profound impact on the performance of individuals and teams.[7] Elite athletes and musicians devote a significant amount of their preparatory work to the acquisition of psychological skills to manage attention and arousal. There is a level of arousal—termed, *ideal performance state*—that is associated with optimal performance: underarousal is associated with a lack of performance effort, whereas hyperarousal can produce chaotic inattention at the expense of execution.[8] The degree of arousal required for optimal performance depends on the task—complex acts can tolerate a lower degree of arousal and vice versa.[8] Few would argue that trauma resuscitation is a complex act, yet in most circumstances individuals do not take steps before, during, and after engaging in active resuscitation to manage hyperarousal to improve performance.

Stress and performance

The effects of stress on performance are determined by an individual's appraisal of task demands compared with available resources, the complexity of the task to be completed, and the relationship between the stressor and the task.[9] Elements of a clinical encounter affect individuals in different ways and to a greater or lesser extent, based on prior experience and coping strategies (both innate and acquired).[10] Stress is highly subjective and varies based on an individual's appraisal of the task at hand and the cognitive, personnel, and system-based resources available to manage it.[11] Individuals can become quickly overwhelmed when task demands outstrip perceived resources; this threat appraisal has a specific cognitive and physiologic footprint that can be identified experimentally[12]—most clinicians recognize this intuitively as a team that is falling apart (**Fig. 1**). The effect of threat appraisals on attention, memory, decision making, and teamwork are outlined in **Table 1**.

Teamwork can also be influenced by stress. As stress increases, teamwork suffers as a result of a narrowing of team perspective, which in turn correlates with impaired team performance.[13] Situations that require attention to multiple tasks and cues are more likely to suffer as a consequence of threat appraisals.[13] As attention narrows, peripheral or less relevant task cues are ignored first, followed by central or task-relevant

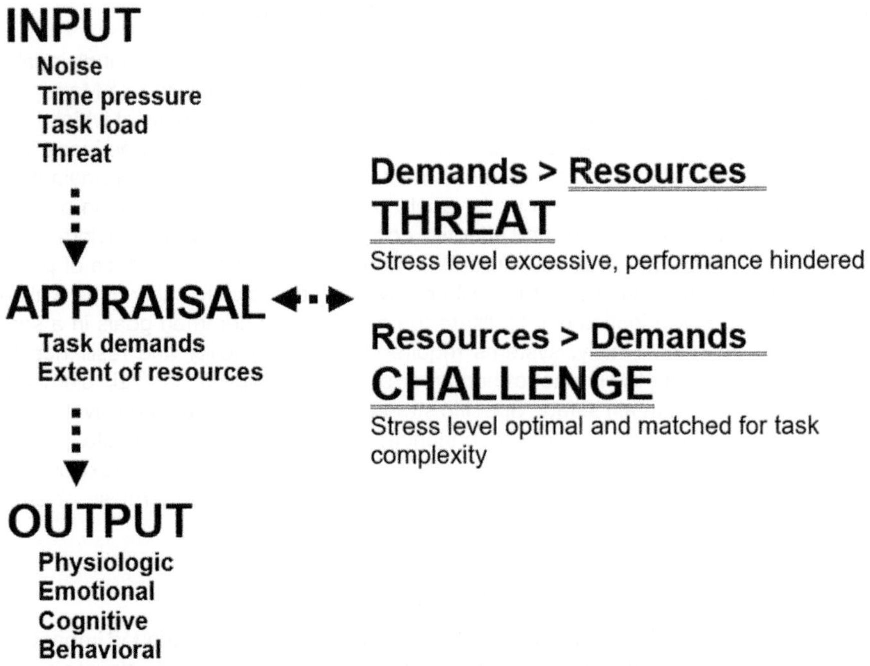

INPUT
Noise
Time pressure
Task load
Threat

APPRAISAL ◄·►
Task demands
Extent of resources

OUTPUT
Physiologic
Emotional
Cognitive
Behavioral

Demands > Resources
THREAT
Stress level excessive, performance hindered

Resources > Demands
CHALLENGE
Stress level optimal and matched for task complexity

Fig. 1. Two-step cognitive appraisal. Task demands that exceed available resources produce a threat appraisal, which has negative effects on individual and team performance. (*Adapted from* Salas E, Driskel JE, Hughes S. The study of stress and human performance. In: Driskell JE, Salas E, editors. Stress and human performance. Mahwah (NJ): Lawrence Erlbaum Associates; 1996; with permission.)

cues. Accordingly, team performance under stress can be assessed by the extent to which task-relevant cues are identified or ignored.

Specific techniques

Controlled breathing is a simple and powerful tool for managing arousal both prior to and during an acutely stressful event. A series of deep and controlled breaths, in a 4-4-4-4 pattern (4 seconds in, 4 seconds hold, 4 seconds out, and 4 seconds hold) can lower heart rate and blood pressure and attenuate the neurohormonal response associated with threat appraisals.[14] Choosing the correct timing, technique, and duration of a controlled breathing exercise is highly personal and depends on features of the individual and the task at hand. The authors recommend a series of controlled breaths, paired with visualization and self-talk, prior to engaging in a complex or high-stakes procedure and during scheduled pause and reassess moments during resuscitation.

Self-talk and cue words are used to support self-confidence and render a state of focus and clarity. Self-talk can involve brief statements of affirmation and self-reassurance ("You've got this," "You've done this before," and "Slow and steady") or relate to the specific steps in a given procedure ("I'm going to make a deep incision in the interspace just below the nipple line, all the way down toward the stretcher, as far as my hand will move"). Self-talk can also support cognitive reframing—the active act of identifying and interrupting irrational or disruptive thoughts.[15] Reframing exercises using self-talk include task chunking (breaking up a complex concept or procedure into smaller, more manageable parts) and perfection bashing (separating

Table 1
When things fall apart: impact of the threat appraisal on attention, memory, cognition, and team-based behaviors

Process	Description	Example
Attention	• Selective attention: ignoring task-relevant cues impedes situation awareness (fixation). • Tasks that require attention to multiple sources of input are particularly vulnerable.	Task fixation on an invasive airway maneuver, with subsequent failure to recognize fall in end-tidal CO_2 foreshadowing cardiac arrest
Working memory	• Working memory is constrained. • The ability to shift between multiple concepts held in working memory is impaired.	Simple drug-dose calculations are more error prone.
Decision making	• Over-reliance on heuristics—cognitive shortcuts that can produce errors in decision making • Failure of analytical systems of problem analysis—inability to shift from one hypothesis to another, even in the face of contradictory clinical information	Inability to deanchor from a presumptive diagnosis of hemorrhagic shock, even given a lack of response to blood transfusion and the suggestion of a pneumothorax on bedside ultrasound
Team	• Shift in focus from "we" to "me"—team more likely to make decisions that are based on self-preservation • Degradation of shared mental models of team process, shift toward information-seeking behaviors	Seeking to better understand an ambiguous situation, team members speak over and above one another, contributing to a cacophony of noise that further encumbers team coordination

necessary from non-necessary interventions, or prioritizing key interventions and making a deliberate decision to leave the rest). Cue words may involve a single word or short phrase that can be repeated, silently or aloud, to help the user stay in the moment when task load or complexity seems overwhelming.

Mental rehearsal (also known as psychophysical rehearsal or mental practice) can improve both the learning and performance of technical and nontechnical skills.[16–18] Similar to athletics, warming up with mental practice before a high-stakes event primes key motor/haptic and cognitive/decision-making pathways that allow for a smoother execution of complex mental and physical behaviors.[19] Mental rehearsal is also believed to help mitigate the effects of acute stress on performance and help establish and refine accurate team-based mental models.[18] To be effective, mental rehearsal exercises should be performed in real time, in as much detail as possible, and from an internal perspective, visualizing what the user would see. A scripted guide to mental rehearsal using the PETTLEP mnemonic is summarized in **Table 2**.

Stress inoculation training is a method of stress preparation that occurs in several discrete stages, in a process similar to cognitive behavioral therapy for phobia habituation.[3] In the first stage, individuals are made aware of the physiologic, emotional, and behavioral effects of acute stress. In the second stage, specific stress management skills are taught with the goal of minimizing the influence of stress on performance. Finally, those skills are applied to increasingly challenging situations to build

Table 2
The PETTLEP script for guided mental rehearsal, or mental preparation

P – Physical	Imagine all relevant physical characteristics
E – Environment	Imagine the environment in which the performance will occur
T – Task	Accurately reproduce all task steps
T – Timing	As much as possible, visualize steps in real time
L – Learning	Update visualization based on learning, experience, and changing task demands
E – Emotion	Conjure emotions that are likely to be experienced during the act itself; avoid debilitative emotions, such as fear, panic
P – Perspective	Visualize from an internal, or first-person, perspective

Adapted from Wright CJ, Smith DK. The effect of a short-term PETTLEP imagery intervention on a cognitive task. J Imagery Res Sport Phys Activ 2007;2(1):1–14.

tolerance and resilience as well as aptitude with skill application. The net effect is the conversion of *threat* appraisals to challenge appraisals, whereby individuals are functioning with a heightened sense of arousal but in a focused, controlled, and contained manner. Challenge appraisals are associated with improved performance and adaptive behavior under difficult conditions.[20] Stress inoculation training has been shown to improve team-based performance, with effects that are both lasting and generalizable.[21,22]

Overlearning involves repetition of a skill or sequence of skills beyond the point of initial mastery. The goal is to develop unconscious competence or the ability to perform with limited conscious thought.[23] As a stress preparation technique, overlearning can help shift the locus of control from external to internal, thereby maintaining a sense of influence over a series of otherwise chaotic events. This technique is well suited to accelerate competence with procedural skills, especially those carried out in complex high-stakes situations. Simulation-based training facilitates overlearning by allowing for repetition while modifying ambient conditions, context, and level of difficulty. The primary limitation of overlearning is the development of rigid mental scripts and learned motor behavior that lack adaptability and flexibility.

Team: Operationalizing Group Behaviors in Complex Scenarios

Trauma education has traditionally focused on task work—the cognitive and skills-based elements of patient care. Precious little time is devoted to the teamwork: the skills needed for an interprofessional group of experts to function as an expert team in complex and dynamic scenarios. This can be explained in part the pervasive belief that effective team behaviors develop naturally and organically over time, by way of a semirandom process of trial, error, and repetition. This faulty series of assumptions is not mirrored in other high-stakes professions, where team training is front and center in organizational safety culture.[24]

High-performance teams maintain open and flexible lines of communication, use a team structure that is adaptive to task and environment, and distribute and manage workload effectively.[25,26] Research on team performance in dynamic environments highlights the importance of shared mental models to facilitate teamwork and taskwork.[27,28] Individual team members develop a psychological map—a mental model—to "predict and explain the behavior of the world ... to recognize and remember relationships among components of the environment, and to construct expectations for what is likely to occur next."[27] The extent to which mental models are shared between team members influences their ability to execute a plan.[27,29] Mental models facilitate transactive memory—an individual's ability to draw from domain-specific knowledge and training and bring it to bear in a team setting.[30] Developing accurate shared mental models poses a specific challenge for ad hoc teams, where members are often unfamiliar with one another's baseline skills and needs. Strategies to establish flexible methods of communication, set expectations and assign roles, and provide options for team structure that are responsive to patient needs can facilitate performance by developing accurate and shared mental models.

Specific techniques

Maintain a common language The interplay between language and behavior is complex, and a full discussion is beyond the scope of this article. Several communication skills bear specific mention, because they are particularly effective tools to establish common language across a diverse group of team members.

1. Avoid mitigating language. As a subconscious nod to social hierarchies and authority gradients, team members often choose language that downplays or minimizes the meaning of what is being said.[31] This includes phrases like, "Would you be okay with intubating the patient?" or "Could someone draw up some analgesia?" which are better rephrased as the commands they are intended to be: "Please intubate." and "Mark, draw up 100 mg of ketamine." Concise and direct is not synonymous with impolite or offensive.
2. Define a resuscitation lexicon. Yamada and colleagues[32] have proposed the development of a lexicon of short words or phrases that succinctly communicate commands and requests, similar to what is used by cockpit crews. Examples include confirm ("Confirm prehospital systolic blood pressure was 70 mm Hg"), I say again ("I say again: carotid pulse is absent"), request ("Request update on volume status"), and read back ("Read back of blood products given thus far").
3. Practice closed-loop communication. Closed-loop communication has 3 steps— directing an order or request to a specific individual and having that request verbally acknowledged as both received and completed successfully. The third step is often the most challenging to implement, because *complete* is not synonymous with *completed correctly*. To ensure this requires cross-monitoring and mutual support among team members and the ability to recognize when an action or intervention does not achieve the predicted result.
4. Use graded assertiveness. The 2-challenge rule Concerned-Uncomfortable-Safety issue (C-U-S) is used to counteract authority gradients and provide a structured way to express concern about a course of action in a graded fashion.[33] The C-U-S framework begins with directly stating a concern ("I am concerned about using paralytics for this difficult airway"), which can be up-scaled to acknowledging being uncomfortable ("I am uncomfortable paralyzing this patient given the presence of severe airway trauma") if the desired response is not obtained. Finally, a safety issue is declared if the plan moves forward without adequate modification or retraction.

Set common expectations: prebriefing A significant amount of preparation—both cognitive and logistical—can occur in a short period of time using a limited amount of information prior to patient arrival. The provision of preparatory information has been shown to decrease stress and anxiety and improve performance.[34] In addition to mental preparation and planning, teams should verbalize anticipated findings and early priorities and focus preparation accordingly. This prebriefing is typically coordinated by the team leader but should be a 2-way process whereby all team members have an opportunity to provide input and propose solutions.[35] The authors use a 4-step structured prebriefing process addressing the following questions:

1. What do we know: a quick verbal summary of information available, even if rudimentary (87-year-old male driver, single vehicle collision on the driver's side, hypotensive on scene)
2. What do we expect (plan A): anticipated injuries and how to prepare for them (left-sided chest and abdomen injuries, lateral compression pelvic fracture, need for blood products, possible medical cause for collision)
3. What will we change (plan B): a defined secondary approach if the predicted initial impression is inaccurate or needs to be modified, including specific triggers for deciding when to deviate from the primary approach (hypotension that persists after pelvic binder and blood products prompts consideration for an obstructive cause for shock)
4. Roles: having identified anticipated early needs and priorities, assign specific personnel to each task in alignment with plan A (airway team, chest tube insertion, pelvic binder application, vascular access)

The European Trauma Course has published workflows for trauma resuscitation that include a structured prebriefing with early role allocation, and verbal discussion of primary (plan A) as well as secondary (plans B and C) strategies prior to patient arrival.[36] Regardless of the approach, an organized and succinct prebriefing can facilitate preparation and establish mental models prior to patient arrival. The goal should be to maintain a sense of near-field situation awareness—preparation for the first 5 minutes to 10 minutes of resuscitation, followed by a deliberate pause and reassess to update status and determine the need to move to a secondary plan of action.

Modify team structure to reflect dynamic patient needs A traditional trauma team is set up using a functional team structure—a team leader coordinating the actions of individual team members. During periods of high coordination overhead and task load, it may be beneficial for teams to move from a functional to a divisional team structure—the latter typified by the creation subteams whose responsibility is constrained to a specific task or series of interventions (**Fig. 2**).[37] In this model, the situation awareness of subteam members is deliberately restricted: they are empowered to operate semiautonomously toward a prespecified objective, such as airway management or central line insertion. This in turn offloads the team leader, freeing up cognitive resources to maintain global oversight (or far-field situation awareness), planning, and resource management. The use of subteams may also help to mitigate the impact of acute stress on performance by managing complexity: breaking down a multipronged resuscitation into smaller, more manageable components. Although subteams can function semiautonomously for short periods of time, the team periodically needs to be pulled together to maintain a shared sense of overall priorities, by way of command huddles and situation reports.

Adaptive coordination Adaptive coordination refers to a team's ability to predict and modify their behavior in response to dynamic clinical and environmental cues—in other words, this is how mental models are operationalized. In a 1999 study, Entin and Serfaty[38] examined the performance and communication strategies of 5-member naval officer teams during anti–air warfare exercises under several experimental training conditions. Teams whose leader periodically provided situation-assessment updates (Situation Reports) to summarize priorities and current situation assessment

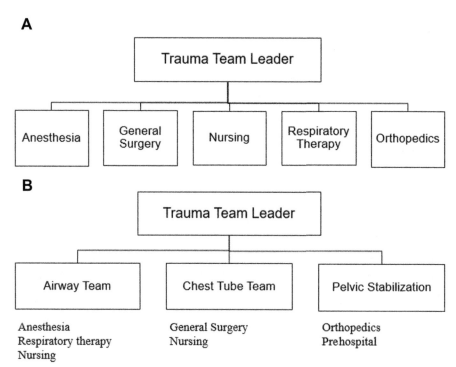

A

Trauma Team Leader

| Anesthesia | General Surgery | Nursing | Respiratory Therapy | Orthopedics |

B

Trauma Team Leader

| Airway Team | Chest Tube Team | Pelvic Stabilization |

Anesthesia
Respiratory therapy
Nursing

General Surgery
Nursing

Orthopedics
Prehospital

Fig. 2. Functional (*A*) versus divisional (*B*) trauma team structures. In a divisional structure, group members are organized into semiautonomous subteams based on clinical tasks.

demonstrated better teamwork and task completion and were more resilient to the effects of stress and task load. Furthermore, teams using sit-reps shifted from explicit to implicit modes of communication—that is, team members shared information with team members more frequently and directly, without having been asked to do so.[38] This observation is consistent with the ability to anticipate the needs of fellow team members—a key feature of shared mental models (clinicians recognize this as the "quiet code"). Translated to clinical practice, adaptive team behaviors are facilitated by team leaders who periodically pause and reassess to openly share information, summarize data, and voice specific findings, in addition to seeking team input and feedback.[39]

Environment: Optimizing Clinical Logistics and Resuscitation Ergonomics

The resuscitation environment is one of the most understudied aspects of clinical care. Poorly designed spaces lead to sequential failures—a lack of space around the head of the bed might prompt a physician to abandon the use of point-of-care ultrasound for central line placement or skip proper positioning to make up for lost time, which can in turn complicate procedures and pose risks to patients. Latent safety risks related to physical workspace are considerable: Patterson and colleagues[40] found 26 of 73 latent safety threats (LSTs) in an emergency department setting were equipment related. Participants did not identify the clinical environment as posing potential safety threats, suggesting there is a lack of awareness and understanding of clinical logistics to facilitate resuscitation goals. It may be unrealistic to expect clinical teams to invest time and energy during a dynamic resuscitation to thoughtfully organize their environment and optimize logistics—some element of environmental optimization should precede the clinical encounter.

Specific techniques

The authors propose a 3-pronged approach to optimizing the resuscitation environment that involves preparation and adjustments well before, immediately before, and in real time.

Well before Optimizing clinical logistics involves an iterative process of design, testing, and refinement. This is applicable to the clinical environment (in particular, space around the patient), equipment (location, bundling, and labeling), and processes (operationalizing a massive transfusion protocol). The authors have described a protocol to identify LSTs in trauma using in situ simulation exercises based on themes identified by a hospital's mortality and morbidity process.[41] The output from this work has been small adjustments or marginal gains that have summed to noticeable improvements in process and design.[42] This includes reorganizing the key real estate around a patient's head, neck, and thorax, adjusting the in-hospital routes used by nonclinical personnel to hasten blood product delivery, and streamlining equipment bundles by reorganizing and removing redundant tools (**Fig. 3**).

Immediately before Skilled providers should be focused on performance and execution, not fetching equipment. The authors' LST analysis has identified that nurses and physicians spend an inordinate amount of time and traverse a surprising distance to collect relevant clinical equipment (**Fig. 4**). This has a compounding effect on efficiency by delaying both the task at hand and encumbering or delaying subsequent tasks. The authors believe that lack of familiarity with the clinical environment and failure to assign roles contribute to this inefficiency. Cliff Reid argues that resuscitation should begin with a "zero point survey," whereby the team surveys and optimizes their clinical environment and assigns roles prior to engaging in the primary survey (Cliff Reid, Unpublished data , 2017). The authors believe this is an important step to include in the prebriefing element of preparation, prior to engaging in clinical care. Specifically, team members should be made aware of the location of and anticipate the need for key equipment and planned pathways for patient and team member movement. Nonclinical personnel should be assigned specific roles to support clinical logistics, including equipment gathering, layout, and patient positioning.

In real time Adjustments to the clinical environment invariably are required in response to patient needs. When possible, the authors recommend assigning a logistics and safety officer (LSO), who is responsible for optimizing the safe and efficient execution of clinical tasks. The LSO should be someone other than the trauma team leader, who remains responsible for establishing clinical priorities. The LSO role is perhaps best suited for a senior nurse working in step with the trauma team leader. The role includes crowd and noise control, patient positioning, layout and availability of equipment for procedures, safe movement of clinical personnel within the resuscitation environment, and planning for patient egress for the next phase of care. It is also the LSO's responsibility to oversee reviews of safety checklists prior to undertaking high-risk tasks like airway management or transitions in care.

System: Resilience Engineering and Safety-II

Systems capable of resilient performance are able to "adjust … functioning prior to, during, or following events (changes, disturbances, and opportunities), and thereby sustain required operations under both expected and unexpected conditions."[43] Hollnagel has defined the 4 pillars of resilient systems as

1. Ability to respond to variance, irregularities, and opportunities during both routine and nonroutine operations

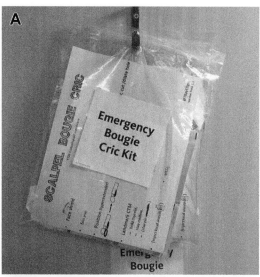

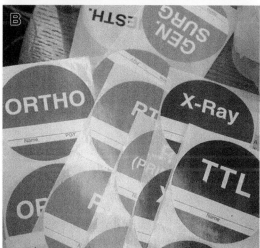

Fig. 3. Two simple trauma design hacks. (*A*) An abbreviated bougie-assisted cricothyroidotomy kit was pilot tested and refined using in situ simulation and is wall mounted in the trauma bay for quick and visible access. (*B*) Mandatory color-coded stickers (names and roles) for all team members. (*Data from* Surgical airway reference card developed by Dr Yen Chow. Available at: https://airwaynautics.com/category/surgical-airway/. Accessed March 1, 2017.)

2. Ability to monitor environmental and system-based cues, to detect safety threats
3. Ability to learn from adverse events, near misses, and successes
4. Ability to anticipate future demands, disruptions, or challenges to system function

In contemporary safety frameworks, resilience engineering is central to the notion of Safety-II—that is, a shift away from viewing safety as the absence of error and toward a model where the system's ability to succeed under varying circumstances is also analyzed.[44] The 4 pillars form the practical basis by which resilience engineering principles can be implemented to improve the performance of complex systems. By

A

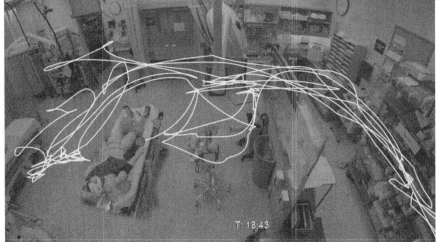

B

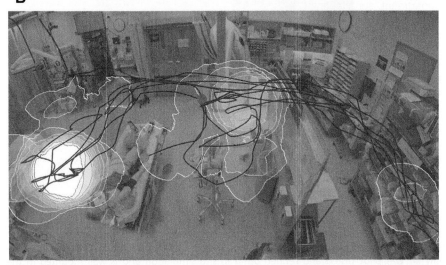

Fig. 4. Data from Trauma Resuscitation Using In-Situ Simulation Team Training (TRUST, in press) depicting clinician (*A*) and nurse (*B*) movement (*lines*) and hot zones (*spheres*) over a 12-minute period during a simulated surgical airway scenario. (*Data from* Almeida R, Pozzobon LD, Hicks C, et al. Tracking workflow during high-stakes resuscitation: the application of a novel human tracing tool during in-situ trauma simulation. In press.)

examining what goes well in addition to what went wrong, systems can identify elements of resilience and adaptation that can be applied proactively to prevent error.

Specific techniques
Ability to monitor: checklists and transitions in care Checklists can help integrate safety behaviors into both standard and nonstandard operations in situations where omissions are otherwise common, high-stakes, or both.[45] The thoughtful use of a

checklist can force-function elements of care that might otherwise be bypassed. The World Health Organization has developed a trauma care checklist that the authors have modified according to identified local needs.[46–48] The authors use the modified the World Health Organization checklist as a predeparture review before egressing from the trauma bay to summarize key tasks, seek input from team members, and ensure adequate preparations have been made to facilitate patient movement.

Transitions in care (patient handoffs or sign-overs) are high-risk periods in patient care.[49] Standardized sign-over protocols can improve data transfer and ensure a smooth transition between care teams. Key behaviors to emphasize include a hands-off, eyes-on approach, whereby team members refrain from engaging with the patient while sign-over takes place and the use of sign-over checklists to ensure data are communicated quickly and concisely.

Ability to respond: clinical care pathways for complex events Locally developed clinical care pathways to coordinate care across multiple hospital resources and teams can facilitate decision-making for complex injuries.[50] Improvised solutions can be time consuming and ineffective; decision pathways that simplify decision making can minimize the potential for conflict or competing interests to encumber clinical care. For example, a patient in hemorrhagic shock with an open book pelvic fracture and suspicion of intra-abdominal injuries requires the ordered provision of emergency department, surgical, interventional radiology, and orthopedic care in a highly time-dependent manner. An institutional protocol specifying under what circumstances a patient is transported to an operating room versus an angiography suite can assist in the efficient gathering of resources and personnel.[51] True to the concept of resilience engineering, clinical care pathways must be specific about the triggers that prompt a preferred action and flexible enough to accommodate for a range of severity and complexity.

Ability to learn and anticipate: in situ simulation and debriefing In situ simulation—simulation-based training that occurs in a team's clinical environment—incorporates elements of clinical logistics that are difficult to reproduce in a simulation laboratory.[49] At the authors' institution, trauma team members engage in regular, team-based skills development, both in a simulation laboratory and by way of in situ training in a trauma room.[41,52,53] In situ exercises paired with team-based debriefings are designed as "living morbidity and mortality rounds," whereby challenging cases identified by a hospital's safety and error tracking processes are translated into simulation scripts that form the basis for in situ training.[52] In the authors' experience, the value of regular, structured simulation-based training to improve team and environmental familiarity and identify LSTs cannot be overstated. Practical steps for developing effective in situ simulation training for emergency medicine are described in detail elsewhere.[49,54]

Debriefing is not limited to simulation—real-life trauma resuscitations provide a rich substrate for identifying LSTs and improving team performance. Debriefing after live events poses additional challenges related case complexity, unpredictability, and the physical, emotional, and cognitive availabilities of team members, requiring modifications to simulation-based approaches.[55] From a systems perspective, documentation and follow-up of issues identified during debriefings are necessary to ensure safety concerns are addressed.[55]

SUMMARY: THE FUTURE STATE OF TEAMS

Resilience is built, not born, and there is no single strategy that reliably manufactures resilient performance in all circumstances. Optimizing team performance in dynamic environments involves the complex interplay of strategies that target individual preparation, team interaction, environmental optimization, and systems-level resilience engineering. To accomplish this, health care can draw influence from human factors research to inform tangible, practical, and measurable improvements in performance and outcomes, modified to suit local and domain-specific needs.[35] Viewed with this lens, and based on the recommendations presented in this article, the future state of elite trauma teams should include

1. Equipping team members with a suite of psychological skills to manage stress, attention, and arousal
2. Emphasizing specific team-based behaviors that facilitate the creation of accurate and flexible mental models, implicit communication, and adaptive coordination
3. Improving awareness of environmental and equipment issues to close the gap between strategy and logistics
4. Implementing systems-based initiatives aligned with Safety-II to improve system resilience in the absence of error, based on what went right

Arul and colleagues[56] have described the integration of human factors and system design strategies for damage control resuscitation and surgery at the Camp Bastion combat hospital in Helmand Province, Afghanistan. They concluded that the addition of command huddles/briefings, sit-reps, trauma care checklists, and standardized sign-overs in step with improvements with environmental design and clinical care "enhanced the communication in an already good team."[56] Although improved teamwork is encouraging, future work should focus on patient-oriented quality-of-care outcomes to evaluate performance-oriented interventions.

ACKNOWLEDGMENTS

The authors wish to thank Dr Peter Brindley for his comments, edits, and keen eye for tautology.

REFERENCES

1. Weingart S. EMCrit Podcast 49 – the mind of a resus doc: logistics over strategy. EMCrit Blog 2011. Available at: https://emcrit.org/podcasts/mind-resus-doc-logistics/. Accessed April 13, 2017.
2. Tomaka J, Blascovich J, Kelsey RM, et al. Subjective, physiological, and behavioral effects of threat and challenge appraisal. J Pers Soc Psychol 1993;65(2): 248–60.
3. Miechenbaum D. Stress inoculation training: a preventative and treatment approach. In: Lehrer PM, Woolfolk RL, Sime WS, editors. Principles and practice of stress management. 3rd edition. New York: Guilford Press; 2007. p. 497–518.
4. Harrel E. How 1% performance improvements led to Olympic gold. Harvard Business Review; 2015. Available at: https://hbr.org/2015/10/how-1-performance-improvements-led-to-olympic-gold. Accessed April 10, 2017.
5. Reid C. Own the resuscitation room. EM Tutorials 2012. Available at: http://emtutorials.com/2012/11/own-the-resuscitation-room-cliff-reid/. Accessed April 10, 2017.
6. Butchibabu A, Sparano-Huiban C, Sonenberg L, et al. Implicit coordination strategies for effective team communication. Hum Factors 2016;58(4):595–610.
7. Herzog TP, Deuster PA. Performance psychology as a key component of human performance optimization. J Spec Oper Med 2014;14(4):99–105.

8. Nideffer RM. Getting in to optimal performance state. Enhanced performance systems. 2006. Available at: http://corporate.epstais.com/wp-content/articles/Getting_Into_Optimal_Performance_State.pdf. Accessed April 1, 2017.
9. Leblanc VR. The effect of acute stress on performance: Implications for health care professionals. Acad Med 2009;84(10 Suppl):S25–33.
10. Folkman S, Lazarus RS, Dunkel-Schetter C, et al. Dynamics of a stressful encounter: cognitive appraisal, coping, and encounter outcomes. J Pers Soc Psychol 1986;50(5):992–1003.
11. Tomaka J, Blascovich J, Kibler J, et al. Cognitive and physiological antecedents of threat and challenge appraisal. J Pers Soc Psychol 1997;73(1):63–72.
12. Harvey A, Nathens AB, Bandiera G, et al. Threat and challenge: cognitive appraisal and stress responses in simulated trauma resuscitations. Med Educ 2010;44(6):587–94.
13. Driskell JE, Salas E, Johnston J. Does stress lead to a loss of team perspective? Group Dyn 1999;3(4):291–302.
14. Lauria M, Gallo IA, Rush S, et al. Psychological skills to improve emergency care provider's performance under stress. Ann Emerg Med 2017. [Epub ahead of print].
15. Beck A. The past and the future of cognitive therapy. J Psychother Pract Res 1997;6:276–84.
16. Louridas M, Bonrath EM, Sinclair DA, et al. Randomized clinical trial to evaluate mental practice in enhancing advanced laparoscopic surgical performance. Br J Surg 2015;102(1):37–44.
17. Arora S, Aggarwal R, Sirimanna P, et al. Mental practice enhances surgical technical skills: a randomized controlled study. Ann Surg 2011;253(2):265–70.
18. Lorello GR, Hicks CM, Ahmed SA, et al. Mental practice: a simple tool to enhance team-based trauma resuscitation. CJEM 2016;18(2):136–42.
19. Frank C, Land WM, Popp C, et al. Mental representation and mental practice: experimental investigation on the functional links between motor memory and motor imagery. PLoS One 2014;9(4):e95175.
20. Drach-Zahavy A, Erez M. Challenge versus threat effects on the goal-performance relationship. Organ Behav Hum Decis Process 2002;88(2):667–82.
21. Saunders T, Driskell JE, Johnston JH, et al. The effect of stress inoculation training on anxiety and performance. J Occup Health Psychol 1996;1(2):170–86.
22. Driskell JE, Johnston JH, Salas E. Does stress training generalize to novel settings? Hum Factors 2001;43(1):99–110.
23. Shibata K, Sasaki Y, Bang JW, et al. Overlearning hyperstabilizes a skill by rapidly making neurochemical processing inhibitory-dominant. Nat Neurosci 2017;23(3):470–5.
24. Helmreich RL. On error management: lessons from aviation. BMJ 2000;320:781–5.
25. LaPorte TR, Consolini PM. Working in practice but not in theory: Theoretical challenges of "high-reliability organizations". J Public Adm Res Theory 1991;1(1):19–48.
26. Bogdanovic J, Perry J, Guggenheim M, et al. Adaptive coordination in surgical teams: an interview study. BMC Health Serv Res 2015;15:128.
27. Mathieu JE, Heffner TS, Goodwin GF, et al. The influence of shared mental models on team process and performance. J Appl Psychol 2000;85(2):273–83.
28. Westli KW, Johnsen BH, Eid J, et al. Teamwork skills, shared mental models, and performance in simulated trauma teams: an independent group design. Scand J Trauma Resusc Emerg Med 2010;18:47.

29. Lim BC, Klein KJ. Team mental models and team performance: A field study of the effects of team mental model similarity and accuracy. J Organ Behav 2006; 27:403–18.

30. Austin JR. Transactive memory in organizational groups: the effects of content, consensus, specialization, and accuracy on group performance. J Appl Psychol 2003;88(5):866–78.

31. Gladwell M. Outliers: the story of success. New York: Little, Brown and Company; 2008.

32. Yamada NK, Fuerch JH, Halamek LP. Impact of standardized communication techniques on errors during simulated neonatal resuscitation. Am J Perinatol 2016;33(4):385–92.

33. Pian-Smith MC, Simon R, Minehart RD, et al. Teaching residents the two-challenge rule: a simulation-based approach to improve education and patient safety. Simul Healthc 2009;4(2):84–91.

34. Inzana CM, Driskell JE, Salas E, et al. Effects of preparatory information on enhancing performance under stress. J Appl Psychol 1996;81(4):429–35.

35. Burke CS, Salas E, Wilson-Donnelly K, et al. How to turn a team of experts into an expert medical team: guidance from the aviation and military communities. Qual Saf Health Care 2004;13(Suppl 1):i96–104.

36. Workflow of an ETC Scenario. European Trauma Course. Available at: http://europeantraumacourse.com/workflow-of-an-etc-scenario/. Accessed April 10, 2017.

37. Hollenbeck JR, Moon H, Ellis AP, et al. Structural contingency theory and individual differences: examination of external and internal person-team fit. J Appl Psychol 2002;87(3):599–606.

38. Entin EE, Serfaty D. Adaptive team coordination. Hum Factors 1999;41(2): 312–25.

39. Tschan F, Semmer NK, Gautschi D, et al. Leading to recovery: group performance and coordinative activities in medical emergency driven groups. Hum Perform 2009;19(3):277–304.

40. Patterson MD, Geis GL, Falcone RA, et al. In situ simulation: detection of safety threats and teamwork training in a high risk emergency department. BMJ Qual Saf 2013;22(6):468–77.

41. Fan M, Petrosoniak A, Pinkney S, et al. Study protocol for a framework analysis using video review to identify latent safety threats: trauma resuscitation using in situ simulation team training (TRUST). BMJ Open 2016;6(11):e013683.

42. Petrosoniak A, Fan M, Trbovich P, et al. A human factors-based framework analysis for patient safety: The trauma resuscitation using in situ simulation team training (TRUST) experience. Canadian Association of Emergency Physicians Annual Meeting. Whistler (Canada), June 3–7, 2017.

43. Hollnagel E. The four cornerstones of resilience engineering. In: Nemeth C, Hollnagel E, Dekker S, editors. Resilience engineering perspectives, vol. 2, preparation and restoration. Aldershot (United Kingdom): Ashgate; 2009.

44. Hollnagel E, Wears RL, Braithwaite J. From safety-I to safety-II: a white paper. 2016. http://dx.doi.org/10.13140/RG.2.1.4051.5282.

45. Gawande A. The checklist manifesto: how to get things right. New York: Metropolitan Books; 2010.

46. Trauma care checklist. World Health Organization. Available at: http://www.who.int/emergencycare/publications/trauma-care-checklist.pdf. Accessed April 10, 2017.

47. Nolan B, Zakirova R, Bridge J, et al. Barriers to implementing the World Health Organization's Trauma Care checklist: a Canadian single-center experience. J Trauma Acute Care Surg 2014;77(5):679–83.
48. Perry S. Transitions in care: safety in dynamic environments. In: Croskerry P, Cosby KS, Schenkel S, et al, editors. Patient safety in emergency medicine. Philadelphia: Wolters Kluwer Health/Lippincott Williams & Wilkins; 2009. p. 201–8.
49. Petrosoniak A, Auerback M, Wong A, et al. In-situ simulation in emergency medicine: moving beyond the simulation lab. Emerg Med Australas 2016;29:83–8.
50. Osman A, Kumar N, Chowdhury JR. The evolution of national care pathways in spinal cord injury management. Trauma 2017;1–6. http://dx.doi.org/10.1177/1460408617701768.
51. Brohi K. Exsanguinating pelvis algorithm. Trauma.org; 2008. Available at: http://www.trauma.org/images/articles/exsanguinatingpelvisalgorithm.jpg. Accessed April 13, 2017.
52. Domouras A, Keshet I, Nathens AB, et al. Trauma Non-Technical Training (TNT-2): the development, piloting and multilevel assessment of a simulation-based, interprofessional curriculum for team-based trauma resuscitation. Can J Surg 2014; 57(5):354–5.
53. Petrosoniak A, White K, McGowan M, et al. Trauma resuscitation using in situ simulation team training (TRUST) study: bringing life to M&M rounds. Toronto: Critical Care Canada Forum; 2016.
54. Spurr J, Gatward J, Joshi N, et al. Top 10 (+1) tips to get started with in situ simulation in emergency and critical care departments. Emerg Med J 2016. http://dx.doi.org/10.1136/emermed-2015-204845.
55. Kessler DO, Cheng A, Mullan PC. Debriefing in the emergency department after clinical events: a practical guide. Ann Emerg Med 2015;65(6):690–8.
56. Arul GS, Pugh HEJ, Mercer SJ, et al. Human factors in decision making in major trauma in Camp Bastion, Afghanistan. Ann R Coll Surg Engl 2015;97:262–8.

Reanimating Patients After Traumatic Cardiac Arrest
A Practical Approach Informed by Best Evidence

 CrossMark

Chris Evans, MD, MSc, FRCPC[a], David O. Quinlan, MD, MSc, FRCPC[b],
Paul T. Engels, MD, FRCSC[c,d],
Jonathan Sherbino, MD, MEd, FRCPC, FAcadMEd[b,*]

KEYWORDS

- Trauma • Cardiac arrest • Resuscitation • Resuscitative thoracotomy
- Emergency thoracotomy

KEY POINTS

- Patients arriving at the emergency department with signs of life and/or evidence of cardiac contractility on point-of-care ultrasonography deserve aggressive resuscitative efforts.
- Chest compressions are unlikely to be effective in traumatic cardiac arrest and resources are better directed at addressing treatable causes of the cardiac arrest.
- Empiric bilateral chest decompression should be performed in all traumatic cardiac arrests, preferably via open thoracostomy.
- Simple, temporizing hemorrhage control measures to be considered in all patients include digital pressure, the use of a tourniquet, and empiric pelvic binding.
- Resuscitative thoracotomy should be considered for all patients with traumatic cardiac arrest with signs of life or point-of-care ultrasonography evidence of cardiac contractility, so long as the provider is competent in the procedure and the institution has an established protocol and the required resources.

Disclosure: None of the authors have any financial or professional conflicts of interest to declare.
[a] Trauma Services, Department of Emergency Medicine, Queen's University, Kingston General Hospital, Victory 3, 76 Stuart Street, Kingston, Ontario K7L 2V7, Canada; [b] Division of Emergency Medicine, McMaster University, Hamilton Health Sciences, Hamilton General Hospital, 2nd Floor McMaster Clinic, 237 Barton Street East, Hamilton, Ontario L8L 2X2, Canada; [c] Trauma, General Surgery and Critical Care, Department of Surgery, McMaster University, Hamilton General Hospital, 6 North Wing - Room 616, 237 Barton Street East, Hamilton, Ontario L8L 2X2, Canada; [d] Department of Critical Care, McMaster University, Hamilton General Hospital, 6 North Wing - Room 616, 237 Barton Street East, Hamilton, Ontario L8L 2X2, Canada
* Corresponding author.
E-mail address: sherbino@mcmaster.ca

Emerg Med Clin N Am 36 (2018) 19–40
http://dx.doi.org/10.1016/j.emc.2017.08.004
0733-8627/18/© 2017 Elsevier Inc. All rights reserved.

INTRODUCTION

Traumatic cardiac arrest (TCA) is not the same as cardiac arrest from coronary ischemia. Although this statement seems obvious, a clear distinction between the origins of cardiac arrest is essential to reorder and change management priorities. The 2015 International Liaison Committee on Resuscitation (ILCOR) makes this distinction.[1] However, in our experience, health care professionals who infrequently care for patients with TCA often follow standard resuscitation protocols that do not effectively address the pathophysiology of TCA. Management goals for medical cardiac arrest resulting from coronary ischemia are to support coronary perfusion to promote transition from a circulatory to electrically responsive phase to facilitate effective defibrillation.[2] In contrast, the management goals for TCA are to address massive hemorrhage and relieve obstructive causes of shock.

This article synthesizes the best available evidence to guide the management of TCA. Where the evidence is imprecise, and if appropriate, the article describe the authors' practice. This article compliments the 2015 ILCOR guidelines, providing more helpful detail and description of practice to aid health care professionals who infrequently care for patients with TCA.

This article emphasizes 5 key principles to guide management. Although these principles are arranged in a hierarchical fashion (a function of a traditional manuscript layout), the authors are not providing an algorithm. Algorithms can be helpful as memory aids in situations of high cognitive load.[3] They can also help structure learning for novices encountering complex tasks. However, algorithms are simplistic representations of patient management and do not account for the tacit knowledge required of expert trauma management. Most importantly, algorithms ignore natural decision-making processes, in which experts reorder management priorities in a dynamic fashion, responding to patient context and the unique complexity of each situation.[4] The authors encourage health care professionals to regularly consider these principles, prioritize them for action, and pause implementation when appropriate (**Fig. 1**). These principles should not be considered as a series of consecutive steps toward a linear conclusion of a trauma resuscitation.

A 54 -year-old woman was the restrained driver in a high-speed, rollover, motor vehicle collision. She is rapidly transported to the closest community hospital by

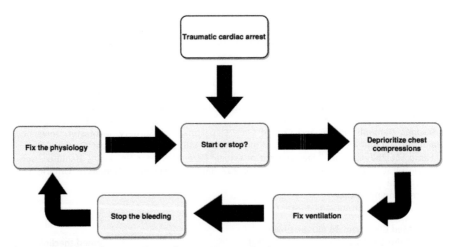

Fig. 1. Principles of traumatic cardiac arrest resuscitation.

emergency medical services (EMS) because of gross hemodynamic instability. She presents immobilized in spinal precautions, receiving supplementary oxygen. Intravenous access has not yet been established in an effort to prioritize transportation from the scene of the accident. On arrival she is obtunded. While vital signs are being determined and an initial assessment is initiated, her pulse can no longer be palpated and her respirations become erratic and gasping.

PRINCIPLE: START OR STOP?

Overall, rates of survival from traumatic arrest are low, although arguably not significantly different from the 5% to 10% range reported for out-of-hospital medical cardiac arrests.[5] A recent study including 2300 patients from North American Resuscitation Outcomes Consortium sites found a 6.3% overall rate of survival for prehospital traumatic arrest and more favorable outcomes among patients with blunt compared with penetrating mechanisms of injury.[6] Comparable rates of survival have been reported from a range of settings, including combat zones,[7] the prehospital, physician-staffed London Air Ambulance program,[8] and a systematic review examining outcomes of more than 5000 patients.[9] Thus, although rates of survival remain low, health care professionals should guard against inappropriate pessimism toward patients with TCA until further prognostic information from the initial bedside assessment is available.

There is no single variable that can be used to distinguish salvageable from unsalvageable traumatic arrest cases.[10] Overall, there are several clinical variables that have consistently been shown to be associated with a favorable prognosis following TCA (**Box 1**).[6,10–15]

Patients without at least 1 of the prognostic factors discussed earlier have an extremely poor (<1%) probability of survival. In these cases, resuscitation efforts should be considered futile. Various guidelines directing resuscitative efforts in TCA are shown in **Table 1**.

The Spectrum of Output States in Traumatic Cardiac Arrest

Patients with TCA represent a heterogeneous patient population with a spectrum of physiologic states, ranging from having no signs of life to being severely hypotensive, but with detectable electrical cardiac activity and contractility on point-of-care ultrasonography (**Table 2**). Occasionally, patients present after the return of spontaneous circulation (ROSC) physiology following prehospital resuscitative interventions.

Considering patients with TCA along this physiologic spectrum allows physicians to integrate multiple prognostic variables from the bedside assessment and does not solely rely on imprecise estimates of time since cardiac arrest. This framework also emphasizes TCA as a being a critical low-flow state",[7,18,19] in which point-of-care

---

Box 1
Favorable prognostic factors following traumatic arrest

Penetrating mechanism of injury, particularly thoracic

Vital signs at any time since first medical contact

Signs of life (any spontaneous movement, respiratory efforts, organized electrical activity on electrocardiogram, reactive pupils) at any time since first medical contact

Short duration of cardiac arrest (<10 minutes)

Cardiac contractility on point-of-care ultrasonography

Table 1
Guidelines on withholding and terminating resuscitation or performing resuscitative thoracotomy in traumatic arrest

	Context	Recommendation	Strengths and/or Limitations
National Association of EMS Physicians and American College of Surgeons Committee on Trauma[16]	Withholding resuscitation efforts	Withhold resuscitation in patients with (1) injuries incompatible with life[a]; (2) signs of prolonged cardiac arrest (dependent lividity, rigor mortis); (3) patients with blunt trauma who are apneic, pulseless, and who have no organized electrocardiographic activity; or (4) patients with penetrating trauma who are apneic, pulseless, have no organized electrocardiographic activity, and no other signs of life[b]	Extensive literature review Multidisciplinary perspective Prehospital focus
European Resuscitation Council[1]	Withholding resuscitation efforts	Consider withholding resuscitation efforts if (1) massive trauma incompatible with survival, or (2) no signs of life in the preceding 15 min	International panel Applies to prehospital and in-hospital settings Considers point-of-care-ultrasonography findings
Western Trauma Association[17]	Indication for RT	Consider RT in (1) patients with blunt trauma with <10 min of prehospital chest compressions, (2) patients with penetrating torso trauma with <15 min of chest compressions, (3) penetrating neck or extremity trauma with <5 min of prehospital chest compressions, or (4) patients with profound refractory shock	Straightforward stratification based on mechanism and time since cardiac arrest Time since cardiac arrest can be difficult to accurately estimate

	Indication for RT	
Eastern Association for the Surgery of Trauma[11]	Strong recommendation for RT in pulseless patients with signs of life[b] after penetrating thoracic trauma Conditional recommendation for RT in pulseless patients without signs of life[b] after penetrating thoracic trauma, present or absent signs of life[b] after penetrating extrathoracic injury, or present signs of life[b] after blunt injury Conditional recommendation against RT in pulseless patients without signs of life[b] following blunt trauma	Rigorous methodology More than 10,000 patients, from 72 studies, included Patient-oriented outcomes

Abbreviations: EMS, emergency medical services; RT, resuscitative thoracotomy.

[a] Decapitation, hemicorpectomy, exposed brain matter.

[b] Signs of life include reactive pupils, spontaneous movement, agonal respiratory efforts, organized electrocardiographic activity.

Table 2
Physiologic spectrum of patients with traumatic cardiac arrest

	(4) Dead	(3) PEA	(2) Pseudo-PEA	(1) Spontaneous Circulation
Cardiac Output	None	None	Very low	Variable[a]
Palpable Pulses	None	None	None	Present
Signs of Life	Absent	Absent	± Present	Present
ECG Rhythm	Asystole	Nonsinus	Nonsinus	Often sinus tachycardia
Bedside US	No contractility	No contractility	Contractility present	Contractility present (may be hyperdynamic)
End-tidal CO_2	Low/ undetectable	Low/ undetectable	Low	Low to moderate

Abbreviations: ECG, electrocardiogram; PEA, pulseless electrical activity; US, ultrasonography.
[a] Depends on a volume status, heart rate.

ultrasonography plays a critical role in differentiating patients in so-called pseudo-pulseless electrical activity from true pulseless electrical activity (PEA) states.[20] Distinguishing these two groups is important, because their prognoses are significantly different.

Patients in pseudo-PEA are in severe, end-stage shock. They have cardiac output that is not detectable by palpation of the pulse, but they may have other signs of life, including weak respiratory efforts, reactive pupils, or occasional spontaneous movement. In contrast, patients with true PEA have no cardiac output. Cardiac contractility on point-of-care ultrasonography has been reported to have 100% sensitivity for identifying survivors following TCA[12,21,22] and should be used early during resuscitation for its prognostic information.

In our practice, pulseless patients with no signs of life, asystole, and no cardiac contractility on bedside ultrasonography (group 4, dead; **Table 3**) do not receive

Table 3
Comparison of traumatic versus medical cardiac arrest

	Traumatic Cardiac Arrest	Medical Cardiac Arrest
Common causes	Hypovolemia/hemorrhage Tension pneumothorax Cardiac tamponade Hypoxia/respiratory failure Severe central nervous system injury	Dysrhythmia Myocardial infarction Pulmonary embolism Stroke/intracerebral hemorrhage Electrolyte disturbances (eg, hyperkalemia) Sepsis Drug/toxin
Effective treatments	Oxygenation/ventilation Chest decompression Blood transfusion Control of hemorrhage Resuscitative thoracotomy	Oxygenation/ventilation Electrical cardioversion Chest compressions Targeted temperature management

further resuscitative efforts. These patients do not survive. Further attempts at resuscitation would waste scarce resources (eg, blood products), divert resources from other patients, and risk exposing staff to blood-borne pathogens. It is our practice to aggressively resuscitate all other patients, particularly those in pseudo-PEA states.

The physician team leader performs a rapid assessment. The patient does not have palpable pulses. The patient has gasping irregular respirations and reactive pupils. A single point-of-care ultrasonography cardiac window reveals a hyperdynamic heart. Additional point-of-care ultrasonography information is not sought. The physician team leader indicates that the patient is in pseudo-PEA and indicates to the team that they should begin their resuscitative roles.

PRINCIPLE: DEPRIORITIZE CHEST COMPRESSIONS

It is critical for lead physicians to take a step back, reminding themselves and the other resuscitation team members that patients with TCA cannot be resuscitated using standard advanced cardiac life support (ACLS) algorithms. In most settings, especially outside the emergency department or trauma suite (eg, in the prehospital setting), chest compressions are considered standard of care regardless of the cause of the cardiac arrest.[23] Although current ACLS algorithms that prioritize chest compressions are important in medical cardiac arrest, they can impede timely interventions to correct blood loss and alleviate obstructive causes of shock in TCA. Deprioritizing chest compression early in TCA resuscitation is key.[19,24,25] Later in the resuscitation, chest compressions may be beneficial to support cerebral and cardiac perfusion, while intravascular blood resuscitation is ongoing.

A comparison of the causes and treatments of traumatic versus medical cardiac arrest is provided in **Table 3**.

There are several physiologic as well as logistical reasons to consider withholding chest compressions, at least initially, in the resuscitation of patients with TCA. First, unlike patients in medical cardiac arrest, who are presumed to be euvolemic, most patients with TCA are profoundly hypovolemic because of severe hemorrhage or functionally hypovolemic because of impaired preload from either a tension pneumothorax or cardiac tamponade. Although well-performed external chest compressions may be able to deliver close to a third of the normal cardiac output in the euvolemic state, in animal models with tamponade or hypovolemia this is not true.[23] In animal models with tamponade physiology, chest compressions seem to increase intrapericardial pressures and worsen cardiac output.[23] Meanwhile, in severe hypovolemic states, external chest compressions do not increase output.[23] Establishing intravascular blood volume and relieving any obstruction to cardiac filling must take precedence over chest compressions.

In our experience, team members are often more comfortable withholding chest compressions when the physician team leader is able to articulate to the team why chest compressions do not work in TCA and why they might be harmful. Most often, performing chest compressions impedes the team from performing the procedures that address the cause of TCA. Other downsides to chest compressions potentially include iatrogenic injuries to thoracic and abdominal organs, worsening existing injuries, and slowing the flow of blood via rapid infuser devices.[19]

Of special note, if the patient's presentation and mechanism of injury do not fit with a primary traumatic arrest but are more consistent with a primary medical arrest followed by a trauma (eg, elderly patient with minor trauma, single-vehicle collisions, ventricular fibrillation or ventricular tachycardia as the presenting rhythm, paucity of physical findings of trauma on the patient), the resuscitation is best approached using standard ACLS strategies.[1]

With EMS prehospital notification, the physician team leader has assembled and briefed the health care team on their roles. Included in the team are a respiratory therapist, 2 experienced emergency nurses, and a second emergency physician. The blood bank has been informed about the need for blood. Anticipating the potential for TCA, the physician team leader has reminded the team that cardiopulmonary resuscitation (CPR) is not the first priority. CPR is not performed and the members quickly prepare to perform other, time-sensitive, procedures.

PRINCIPLE: FIX VENTILATION

All patients with traumatic arrest require early airway control to relieve airway obstruction, deliver oxygen, optimize ventilation, and prevent aspiration.[24] Airway obstruction may be managed temporarily with oral or nasal airways and bag-mask ventilation, but ventilation through a bag-mask device may prove difficult in patients with facial trauma, especially with midface fractures and significant bleeding. The need for a definitive airway should be anticipated.

Airway Management

The authors suggest initially providing 100% oxygen through a bag-mask device to ensure adequate oxygenation. If ROSC is obtained, oxygen levels should be titrated to avoid hyperoxemia, which may worsen traumatic brain injury.[26,27]

A cuffed endotracheal tube in the trachea remains the gold standard for airway management, because it allows precise titration of oxygen, protection from aspiration, and controlled ventilation. Most patients with TCA do not require any sedation or paralysis for laryngoscopy and intubation. However, some patients with minimal cardiac output (group 2, pseudo-PEA; see **Table 2**) may retain muscle tone and protective airway reflexes, requiring a dose of a short-acting paralytic. The low cardiac output state requires a doubling of the standard paralytic dose. Sedation is not necessary in this clinical context. Confirmation of endotracheal placement with an end-tidal carbon dioxide detector is standard of care.

Intubation may be difficult in patients with traumatic arrest for several reasons, including facial trauma, blood or emesis obscuring laryngoscopy, and the need to maintain cervical spine precautions. If difficulties are encountered or there are not adequate personnel to intubate the patient and perform other time-sensitive procedures, a supraglottic airway device can be placed. Multiple intubation attempts have the potential to distract the team from other important tasks that need to be performed simultaneously. A supraglottic device provides adequate oxygenation and ventilation for the duration of the resuscitation. With ROSC, conversion of a supraglottic device to an endotracheal tube should be prioritized based on other tasks to be performed and the complexity of airway injury.

Chest Decompression

Tension pneumothorax is notoriously difficult to diagnose in patients with blunt traumatic arrest. The authors agree with existing guidelines suggesting that empiric bilateral chest decompression be performed on all patients with blunt and penetrating thoracic TCA to avoid missing a tension pneumothorax.[19,24,25,28] In addition, tension physiology may develop during the course of resuscitating a patient with blunt chest trauma and bilateral chest decompression also prevents this complication.

Our practice is to perform open thoracostomies (ie, sharp and blunt dissection of the chest wall at the anterior axillary line, fourth to fifth intercostal space, to facilitate internal palpation of the hemithorax)[29] rather than needle thoracostomies for chest decompression. The rationale for this approach is that it ensures that a potential tension pneumothorax is fully decompressed (the clinician can palpate the lung). The second advantage of the open thoracostomy is in diagnosing massive hemothorax as a cause of the arrest. The open thoracostomy can be converted to a chest tube once the patient has stabilized.

If the physician performs a needle thoracostomy, the authors recommend placement in the anterior axillary line at the fourth to fifth intercostal space (where the chest wall is thin). Data from a meta-analysis suggests a 13% failure rate at this site, compared with a 38% failure rate at the traditional landmark of the second intercostal space in the midclavicular line when using a 4-cm (1.5-inch) needle.[30] Use of a 6.44-cm (2.5-inch) needle will penetrate the chest wall and decompress the pleura in 95% of the population.[31]

The physician team leader directs the respiratory therapist to insert a supraglottic airway and ventilate the patient by hand using 100% oxygen. An excessively rapid ventilation rate that impedes venous blood return to the heart is avoided, as is an excessively slow ventilation rate that does not correct hypoxia or respiratory and metabolic acidosis. The plan is to intubate the patient after the initial set of procedures is performed. The second physician performs bilateral open thoracostomies using a clean technique (ie, sterile gloves, rapid skin cleaning, and the use of a sterile towel for local draping). No air or blood returns from the right hemithorax, whereas on the left side there is a large return of air and ongoing, oozing blood loss.

PRINCIPLE: STOP THE BLEEDING

Control of hemorrhage can be divided into temporizing and definitive procedures. In TCA caused by massive hemorrhage, the clinician must identify and provide temporizing control of hemorrhage while the patient's intravascular volume is simultaneously restored via blood transfusion. To this end, there are several potential options to achieve temporary hemorrhage control, including use of manual pressure and topical hemostatic agents for external hemorrhage, tourniquets for peripheral vascular hemorrhage, pelvic ring closure for pelvic hemorrhage, and thoracotomy for control of cardiac or major vascular hemorrhage. These options are all bridges to definitive hemorrhage control, which occurs in an operating theatre, angiography suite, or a hybrid operating theater that combines both capabilities. Institutional processes for accessing local or regional resources must be developed and not spontaneously developed in an ad hoc fashion.

Manual Pressure and Topical Hemostatic Agents

Manual pressure is the basis for control of all surgical bleeding. The ability to occlude a bleeding source is reliant on the ability to effective apply pressure to it (ie, can it be pinched between fingers or compressed against something firm like a bony structure?) and on the size of the area of hemorrhage (ie, is it a vessel or the entire surface of an organ?).

Topical hemostatic agents can be divided into mechanical hemostats, active hemostats, flowable hemostats, and fibrin sealants. They are often used in combination.[32] External topical hemostatic agents include gauze bandages impregnated with a hemostatic agent. These bandages can be applied to the surface of a bleeding area in combination with pressure or potentially packed into bleeding open wounds. Long used in the military, hemostatic bandages, such as HemoCon, Quikclot, are now being deployed for civilian trauma as part of a national American effort to optimize care provided by immediate responders (ie, the public) (http://www.bleedingcontrol.org). The application of manual pressure using gauze or hemostatic gauze to any bleeding site is the first maneuver to obtain temporary hemorrhage control.[33]

Tourniquets for Peripheral Vascular Hemorrhage

The use of tourniquets has waxed and waned for decades but, based on valuable experience from recent military conflicts[34,35] and in civilian trauma,[36–38] the use of tourniquets is now standard care.[39] Tourniquets are indicated for significant extremity hemorrhage if direct pressure is ineffective or impractical. Commercially produced windlass, pneumatic, or ratcheting devices that occlude arterial flow are preferred, whereas the use of narrow, elastic, or bungee-type devices is not recommended. Preferred tourniquets include the Combat Application Tourniquet and the pneumatic tourniquet. Although some junctional hemorrhage devices have been developed to control bleeding from the groin (the so-called Black Hawk Down injury) or axilla, they are not typically available outside of the military setting and their application is not straightforward.[40] The application of an improvised tourniquet should only be considered if a commercial device is unavailable. Tourniquets placed in the prehospital setting should not be released until the patient has reached definitive care.[33] The time of placement of a tourniquet should be recorded, preferably on the patient or tourniquet.

Pelvic Binders for Pelvic Hemorrhage

Bleeding from pelvic fractures continues to be a leading cause of preventable traumatic death in major trauma centers.[41] The bleeding from pelvic fractures is often multifocal (ie, arterial, venous, and bony hemorrhage), diffuse, and difficult to compress. Minimizing pelvic bleeding requires reapproximation of the bony pelvic architecture to prevent further injury to the myriad of pelvic vessels.[42] Our practice is to use a folded sheet positioned over the greater trochanters and anterior iliac spines and held snug with a simple square knot or pair of large, straight, Kelly hemostats. In our experience, this approach is preferable to commercially available devices for both fiscal reasons and more readily accessible groin access (by cutting a hole in the sheet without releasing the pelvic binder) if subsequent angiography or resuscitative endovascular balloon occlusion of the aorta (REBOA) is required. Our practice is to empirically apply a pelvic binder to patients with TCA with blunt abdominal or pelvic injury. It is a fast and simple procedure with insignificant side effects, whereas the physical examination of a mechanically unstable pelvis can be unreliable.

Another maneuver to control pelvic hemorrhage is preperitoneal packing.[43] However, such a procedure requires a skilled operator, typically a trauma surgeon or orthopedic trauma surgeon, as well as the necessary surgical equipment. This maneuver is typically performed in the operating theater, sometimes concurrently with abdominal exploration. This maneuver is not our standard practice in blunt TCA.

Thoracotomy for Control of Intrathoracic Cardiac or Vascular Hemorrhage

Resuscitative thoracotomy (RT) is the ultimate invasive procedure to attempt reanimation of patients with TCA. This procedure is controversial, especially when accounting for the risks of infectious disease exposure to health care providers and the futility of the procedure when applied without appropriate patient selection.[13,44] There are consensus guidelines on indications to perform an RT (see **Table 1**). The best outcomes occur when RT is performed for patients with thoracic stab injuries who arrive with signs of life in the emergency department.[10]

The primary goals of RT are to release pericardial tamponade and to control intrathoracic bleeding. Evacuation of bronchovenous air embolism, elimination of a bronchopleural fistula, performing open cardiac massage, and temporary occlusion of the descending thoracic aorta to optimize brain and cardiac perfusion or control abdominal or pelvic hemorrhage are also indications for RT.[45,46] However, these are rarely indications for performing an RT in a center without significant experience and appropriate surgical support.

Historical indications for RT have changed because comparisons of open cardiac massage with closed-chest compressions for superior hemodynamics[47,48] have failed to show improved patient-oriented outcomes.[49,50] Patients requiring occlusion of the descending thoracic aorta to restore perfusion of the brain and heart have shown mortalities greater than 90% in some studies.[51]

RT is, at best, a temporizing maneuver.[52] To have any chance of a successful outcome, the patient needs to be rapidly transported to a well-equipped and staffed operating theater with a surgeon immediately available who is capable of repairing the underlying injury.[52] Regardless of clinical discipline,[53,54] the physician performing the RT must be competent in the procedure with the ability to successfully address the cause of the patient's TCA. The hospital must identify a priori a process to perform an RT and to provide definitive care if the patient is reanimated.

The steps to performing an RT are well described elsewhere.[45] Although typically started as a left anterolateral thoracotomy, extension across the sternum into a bilateral thoracotomy or clamshell incision may be required for adequate exposure to the heart, superior mediastinum, or right pulmonary hilum.[55] Cadaver-based experiments suggest that access time may be equivalent for these incisions, but time to control of a cardiac injury may be shorter for the clamshell incision.[56]

A primary objective of an RT is releasing pericardial tamponade by opening the pericardium. Any bleeding from a ventricular injury may be temporized with judicious finger pressure by the pads of the finger, which move with the beating of the heart. Larger defects not controlled by finger pressure may be closed using a skin stapler and/or occluded via the inflated balloon of a Foley catheter. Of note, a novel device has recently been described that provides temporary hemorrhage control for ventricular injuries without the negative effects on cardiac function that Foley balloon catheters often create.[57] Atrial ruptures are best controlled with application of a clamp to close the defect. Although suturing of cardiac injuries is required for definitive control, this requires a skilled operator and equipment not typically available in the emergency department. It is best accomplished in the operating theater. However, cardiac tamponade secondary to trauma is poorly treated by percutaneous pericardiocentesis, although it may be used as a temporizing measure in centers without the ability to perform an RT.[58]

The second goal of controlling intrathoracic hemorrhage can be accomplished by inspecting for bleeding sources. Chest wall bleeding can be packed and focal bleeding from the lung or major vessels can be controlled with focal pressure. If this is ineffective, clamping of the pulmonary hilum or a pulmonary hilar twist may also be used for severe bleeding, although the latter maneuver requires division of the inferior pulmonary ligament.[59] Occlusion of the hilum with a clamp or external compression is simpler to perform than a hilar twist. If significant blood loss is present from a right-sided open thoracostomy, a bilateral thoracotomy is necessary to identify and control the source of bleeding.

Our practice is to perform an RT if a physician competent in the procedure is present, the patient in TCA has signs of life in the emergency department, or there is cardiac contractility on point-of-care ultrasonography. Our practice is to perform a left anterolateral thoracotomy, only extending to a clamshell incision if initial decompression of the right hemithorax reveals significant blood loss. If ROSC is achieved, our practice is to cover the incision with dry, sterile surgical towels in anticipation of rapid transportation of the patient to an operating theater. The open thoracostomy of the right hemithorax is then converted to a right-sided chest tube. Our practice is to continue the resuscitation until all reversible causes of TCA have been treated.[1]

Resuscitative Endovascular Balloon Occlusion of the Aorta for Control of Abdominal or Pelvic Hemorrhage

The use of REBOA, although first described in the Korean War, is being rapidly adopted in the care of civilian patients with trauma.[60–62] The greatest utility of REBOA is as an alternative to RT for the occlusion of the thoracic descending aorta to stop abdominal or pelvic hemorrhage.[63] Its use is covered in more detail in Steven Skitch and colleagues' article, "Acute Management of the Traumatically Injured Pelvis"; and Megan Brenner and Christopher Hicks's article, "Major Abdominal Trauma: Critical Decisions and New Frontiers in Management," in this issue. Our current practice does not include REBOA in the management of TCA.

Other Direct Pressure Maneuvers

A few specific scenarios worth mentioning include penetrating injuries to zone 1 of the neck. Severe hemorrhage from such wounds often originates from the subclavian vessels or from intrathoracic vessels, both of which are difficult to compress externally. The placement of a Foley catheter into the wound with subsequent inflation may be considered[64] (See Angelo Mikrogianakis and Vincent Grant's article, "The Kids are Alright: Pediatric Trauma Pearls," in this issue).

Penetrating injuries to the face or facial smashes can create severe bleeding that may require facial packing. However, with complete disruption of the bony architecture there is no ability to obtain tamponade, because there is nothing to pack against. In such scenarios, consideration for external bolstering by completely wrapping the face and head circumferentially may be considered.[65]

As a principle, hemorrhage control in patients with TCA must be obtained, at least in a temporizing manner, in order to have any possibility of ROSC. **Table 4** lists temporizing measures to use as appropriate.

Table 4 Temporizing hemorrhage control measures	
Source of Hemorrhage	**Intervention**
Severe scalp laceration	• Closure of wound with skin stapler, clamp, or rapid whipstitch suture
Open soft tissue wounds	• Direct pressure • Packing with hemostatic gauze • Closure of wound with skin stapler, clamp, or rapid whipstitch suture
Mechanically unstable pelvis	• Pelvic binder
Open extremity injury or amputation	• Reduce fracture • Direct pressure • Pack wound • Tourniquet application
Junctional zone (eg, groin, axilla)	• Direct pressure
Zone 1 penetrating neck wound	• Direct pressure • Foley balloon tamponade
Severe facial smash	• Nasopharyngeal packing • Consider circumferential bolster of the head
Massive hemothorax	• Resuscitative thoracotomy
Pericardial tamponade	• Resuscitative thoracotomy

The patient has a partial amputation of the left ankle. Direct pressure with gauze and realignment of the bony anatomy is performed by one of the nurses. Oozing from the wound is ongoing with blood pooling on the floor. The nurse applies a pneumatic tourniquet and blood flow stops. Simultaneously, the pelvis is bound using a folded sheet that was placed on the resuscitation bed with the initial EMS activation. The physician with the most point-of-care ultrasonography experience (the second physician) attempts to identify a pericardial effusion. Significant thoracic injury prevents obtaining a good cardiac view. The physician team leader makes the decision to perform a left anterolateral thoracotomy. The operating room is informed and the thoracic surgeon and on-call anesthetist is paged to the emergency department. The physician team leader begins to prep the chest for a clean procedure (ie, sterile gloves, rapid skin cleaning, local draping with sterile towels). A clamshell incision is not planned, because the right-sided open thoracostomy did not reveal any major bleeding. However, sterile prep includes the right side of the chest. In anticipation of the thoracotomy, the respiratory therapist and second physician intubate the patient. Sedation and paralytic agents are not required. An orogastric tube is also placed to assist in identifying the esophagus from the aorta if compression of the aorta is required.

PRINCIPLE: FIX THE PHYSIOLOGY
Warm the Patient and Keep the Patient Warm

Environmental exposure, blood loss, and resuscitation with hypothermic fluids all contribute to heat loss in patients with TCA. Unlike patients with medical cardiac arrest, who have been shown to benefit from postarrest hypothermia, patients with hypothermic trauma have been shown to have greater complication rates and higher mortality.[66] Hypothermia contributes to worsening coagulopathy in patients with hemorrhaging trauma[66] as a result of reduced enzyme activity, platelet dysfunction, and reduced clotting factor activity.[67] In addition, hypothermia and acidosis compound coagulopathy.[68]

Maintaining normothermia during resuscitation is best achieved through a combination of passive and active warming. Wet clothing must be removed. The ambient temperature of the trauma suite should be increased whenever possible. Although exposure and injury identification are priorities during the physical examination, warm blankets or forced air warming blankets should be placed on the patient after the physical examination is complete.

All resuscitative fluids should be delivered warm and under pressure (with the exception of platelets) via a rapid infuser (Level 1 Rapid Infusor). Rapid infusion devices are capable of warming fluids to 36°C to 40°C depending on the delivery rate. Maximum in vivo delivery rates are listed at 1100 mL/min and vary depending on fluid type, catheter size, and catheter length (Smith Medical).

Intravenous Access

The initial fluid resuscitation in a TCA should be done through multiple large-bore peripheral intravenous catheters (14–18 gauge) secured in the upper limbs. Intravenous access above the diaphragm is necessary because of the possibility of venous obstruction or extravasation from injured venous structures inferior to the right heart. In the event of penetrating injury to the upper extremity, axilla, or lateral neck, peripheral access should be secured on the side contralateral to the injury.

If attempts for peripheral catheterization are unsuccessful, expedient placement of intraosseus catheters in the proximal humerus should be the next step in management. The proximal humerus is the preferred intraosseus location because it is both located above the diaphragm and has been shown to have comparable flow rates with other intraosseus locations in human studies.[69–71] Sternal placement has been described; however, the authors do not recommend this site because it is more challenging given the thinner cortical bone of the sternum and the risk for mediastinal injury. Sternal catheter location may also interfere with ongoing management and intrathoracic procedures. Intraosseus access has been shown to be faster and to have a greater first-attempt success rate than central venous access in critically ill patients.[72] Intraosseus catheters have also been endorsed for use in TCA.[73]

Attempts to secure central venous access should not be made in the immediate care of arrested patients in whom intravenous or intraosseus access has been established. It may eventually be required, if peripheral or intraosseus access cannot be secured, or to aid in a large-volume fluid resuscitation. In these cases, catheter selection should be limited to 8-French to 9-French percutaneous introducer sheaths. The flow rate from the 16-gauge distal port of a triple-lumen central catheter (15-cm length) has been shown to be approximately 3 times slower than that of a 14-gauge, 5-cm peripheral catheter.[74] These multiple-lumen central venous catheters should not be used.

The subclavian vein is the optimal site for central venous access if required. A rigid cervical collar will invariably be in place in patients with blunt trauma and prevents internal jugular vein access. Femoral vein access is less desirable given that it is below the diaphragm.

Intravascular Resuscitation

Over the past 2 decades, advancements in the resuscitation of patients with trauma have focused on damage control resuscitation. The principles include minimizing the use of crystalloid fluids, transfusing balanced ratios of blood products, permissive hypotension, and damage control surgery (ie, rapid, temporary repair of injuries without definitive surgical correction to minimize physiologic insult during the operation).

Large-volume resuscitation with crystalloid fluid leads to coagulopathy through the dilution of clotting factors, fibrinogen, platelets, and calcium. Crystalloids can worsen acidemia given that Ringer lactate solution (pH 6.5) and normal saline (pH 5.5) are both acidic fluids. In addition, the chloride load in normal saline can precipitate hyperchloremic metabolic acidosis.

The use of crystalloid fluid should mainly be limited to the delivery of medications. Judicious use may be considered in the initial resuscitation of the intravascular space only until blood products become available. It should be recognized that most patients with trauma presenting in shock have likely received a significant volume of crystalloid in the prehospital environment. The amount of unintended crystalloid fluid delivered to the patient in the trauma suite can be significant.

The optimal fluid for the initial resuscitation of the intravascular space in patients with TCA is whole blood (or the components that constitute it). In patients whose primary mechanism of arrest is profound hemorrhagic shock rather than obstructive shock, the anticipated blood volume deficit is likely to require a significant transfusion volume. Almost all of these patients will have assessment of blood consumption (ABC) scores totaling 2 or greater, which has shown to be both a reasonably sensitive and specific prediction score for the need for massive transfusion (MT).[75,76]

The authors recommend the initiation of an institutionally coordinated MT protocol in patients with TCA once a decision to resuscitate the patient is made. Such protocols have been shown to aid in communication and speed of delivery of blood products.[77] Early and frequent communication with the blood bank is necessary for the expedited release and delivery of blood products, as well as conservation of blood bank resources.

Military[78] and civilian[79–81] trauma studies have shown the benefits of equal ratios of fresh frozen plasma and platelets to packed blood cells in order to best approximate the components of whole blood. There is no current consensus on the most beneficial component ratio. It is our practice to approximate an ongoing resuscitation ratio of 1:1:1 (red blood cells (RBCs)/fresh frozen plasma/platelets) once a decision to initiate MT is made.

A nurse attempts intravenous access in the left antecubital fossa. On completion of endotracheal intubation of the patient, the second physician places an intraosseus cannula in the right humerus. The hospital does not have an MT protocol. However, the blood blank has provided 4 units of packed RBCs. These units are infused under pressure and warmed. Fresh frozen plasma and platelets are being made available. The physician team leader performs a left anterolateral thoracotomy. The pericardium is opened and the heart delivered. A small clot is removed. No large cardiac lacerations are identified. There is significant oozing from the left lung, which stops with direct pressure applied by a nurse. Open cardiac massage is performed using a hinged, clapping motion of 2 cupped hands to avoid fingertip pressure on the heart. With the administration of blood, a carotid pulse is palpated as the heart spontaneously beings to beat.

PRINCIPLE: FIX THE PHYSIOLOGY (AFTER RETURN OF SPONTANEOUS CIRCULATION)

Once ROSC is achieved, monitoring for the complications commonly seen during an MT is important. Hypocalcemia is of particular importance because calcium is a cofactor for several stages of the clotting cascade and plays a role in vascular tone and myocardial contractility. Hypocalcemia results from hemodilution as well as chelation with the citrate contained in stored RBCs.

Addressing Coagulopathy

The ongoing need for component transfusion should also be considered. Additional factor-specific replacement can be considered based on International Normalized Ratio, prothrombin time, platelet count, and fibrinogen. Although not universally available, transfusion may be guided by thromboelastography or rotational thromboelastometry. In addition, it is our practice to administer tranexamic acid to patients with TCA who experience ROSC based on extrapolation of evidence of benefit in bleeding, nonarrested patients with trauma.[82]

Addressing Anticoagulation

Patients treated with antiplatelet agents or anticoagulants (vitamin K antagonists, anti-IIa agents, anti-Xa agents) before trauma provide an additional challenge with hemorrhage control. Reversal of these agents should occur early after ROSC (**Table 5**). Consultation with a hematologist may be helpful, particularly with direct oral anticoagulants, for which empiric reversal therapies have limited evidence.

Blood Pressure Management

After a pulse is restored, the primary goal in resuscitation is to maintain end-organ perfusion while managing injures. The authors recommend the early placement of an arterial catheter for real-time blood pressure monitoring. Automated cuff pressure can be unreliable[83] and rapid changes in blood pressure may be missed by interval measurements.

Table 5
Antiplatelet and anticoagulant reversal therapies

Medication	Treatment
Antiplatelet agents (ASA, clopidogrel, dipyridamole)	Platelet transfusion ddAVP
Anti–vitamin K agents (warfarin)	Vitamin K and Prothrombin complex concentrate
Anti–factor IIa agents (dabigatran)[a]	Idarucizumab or Prothrombin complex concentrate
Anti–factor Xa agents (apixaban, rivaroxaban, edoxaban)[a,b]	Prothrombin complex concentrate

Abbreviations: ASA, acetylsalicylic acid; ddAVP, desamino-D-arginine vasopressin (desmopressin).
[a] Recombinant factor VIIa can be considered in the treatment of refractory bleeding in consultation with a hematologist.
[b] Novel reversal agents for these medications are in development at the time of publication.
Data from Hogg K, Panag A, Worster A, et al. Direct oral anticoagulants: a practical guide for the emergency physician. Eur J Emerg Med 2016;23(5):330–6.

The concept of permissive hypotension (or just-adequate normotension) is intended to preserve end-organ perfusion without disruption of clot formation via increasing intravascular pressure and loss of vasoconstriction. However, the evidence for this practice is not widely generalizable to the emergency department resuscitation of patients with TCA.[84]

The authors suggest that the patient's comorbidities, injury pattern, and clinical response to therapy should be considered in targeting a specific blood pressure. Our recommendations are for a mean arterial pressure goal of approximately 65 mm Hg. Permissive hypotension has not been thoroughly studied in closed head injuries and should not be used in these patients.[85]

Vasopressors should not be routinely used in the resuscitation of patients with trauma. Ongoing shock in the absence of a neurogenic cause (eg, cervical or high thoracic spinal cord injury) should prompt a repeated examination to rule out evolving or a previously missed obstructive cause, continued blood resuscitation, and an aggressive plan to control bleeding. The authors agree with the European Guideline on the Management of Major Bleeding in Trauma parameters for use of a vasoactive medication to support perfusion. Vasopressors should only be used when severe hypotension not responsive to blood product therapy and efforts to control hemorrhage are present.[86] In this context, norepinephrine is a typical first-line agent, unless there is evidence of cardiac dysfunction on point-of-care ultrasonography that may best respond to epinephrine.

Cardiac Dysfunction/Dysrhythmia

Ventricular dysrhythmia in patients after TCA should be treated with electrical cardioversion or defibrillation. Negative chronotropy, negative ionotropy, and vasodilatory properties common to many antiarrhythmic medications are likely harmful in the post-TCA period. Supraventricular tachycardias should not be treated initially, given the likelihood that they maybe a physiologic response.

Sedation and Analgesia

Analgesia and sedation are important to relieve pain and anxiety secondary to traumatic injuries and painful procedures, as well as to aid in the ventilation of intubated post-ROSC patients with TCA. All commonly used pharmacologic agents for induction of anesthesia and sedation can cause precipitous hypotension by decreasing sympathetic tone. The authors recommend using 25% to 50% of a standard dose and closely monitoring patient response. No consensus exists with respect to the safest sedation and analgesia protocol in the critically ill patients with trauma.

The authors use ketamine as a single agent or with the addition of a short-acting opioid such as fentanyl.[87] Historic concerns for increased intracranial pressure associated with the use of ketamine in brain-injured patients have been reconsidered.[88] Despite the common belief that ketamine is a hemodynamically neutral agent, hypotension is frequently observed in critically ill patients.[89] Etomidate is also a reasonable sedative agent if available. However, guidelines have recommended against etomidate for prolonged sedation via infusion in patients with trauma.[90] The authors recommend against the use of propofol or benzodiazepines as sedative agents in the patients after TCA.

Within 20 minutes the anesthetist and thoracic surgeon arrive in the emergency department and make arrangements to bring the patient immediately to the operating theater. The thoracotomy incision is covered with dry, sterile surgical towels. The right open thoracostomy is converted to a chest tube. Forced air warming blankets cover the patient. An arterial catheter is placed to monitor blood pressure. Spinal immobilization is maintained. Blood products, as available, are infused one at a time, aiming for equal administration of RBC, plasma, and platelets, to maintain a mean arterial pressure of 65 mm Hg. Ketamine boluses of 25 mg are titrated to patient effect. Blood work is sent to guide ongoing resuscitation. A point-of-care ultrasonography scan suggests intra-abdominal free fluid. A pelvic radiograph does not show any fracture. The regional trauma center (15 minutes away by ambulance) is contacted to assist in guiding further management, including timing of imaging the brain. The preliminary plan is to surgically control thoracic bleeding, perform a laparotomy and pack the abdomen, and continue blood resuscitation. Arrangements for transfer of the patient postoperatively to the trauma center are being made.

SUMMARY

TCA is a survivable condition. Recognition and management of TCA as a distinct pathophysiologic process from medical cardiac arrest is essential. Principles of resuscitation include making a rapid decision to proceed with resuscitation based on prognostic information available at the bedside (signs of life and point-of-care ultrasonography evidence of cardiac contractility), deprioritizing chest compressions, correcting dysfunctional ventilation, temporarily controlling ongoing hemorrhage, and initiating a balanced ratio of blood product transfusion as the first step in addressing physiologic derangement. Health care professionals, who appreciate the complexity and nuance of trauma care, prioritize for action these principles, pause implementation when appropriate, and do not assume that an algorithm is a preferred approach in TCA.

REFERENCES

1. Truhlář A, Deakin CD, Soar J, et al. European Resuscitation Council guidelines: cardiac arrest in special circumstances. Resuscitation 2015;95:148–201.
2. Weisfeldt ML, Becker LB. Resuscitation after cardiac arrest: a 3-phase time-sensitive model. JAMA 2002;288(23):3035–8.
3. Young JQ, Van Merrienboer J, Durning S, et al. Cognitive load theory: implications for medical education: AMEE guide no. 86. Med Teach 2014;36(5):371–84.

4. Klein G. Naturalistic decision making. Hum Factors 2008;50(3):456–60.
5. Go AS, Mozaffarian D, Roger VL, et al. Heart disease and stroke statistics–2014 update: a report from the American Heart Association. Circulation 2014;129(3): e28.
6. Evans CC, Petersen A, Meier EN, et al. Prehospital traumatic cardiac arrest: Management and outcomes from the resuscitation outcomes consortium Epistry-Trauma and PROPHET registries. J Trauma Acute Care Surg 2016;81(2):285–93.
7. Tarmey NT, Park CL, Bartels OJ, et al. Outcomes following military traumatic cardiorespiratory arrest: a prospective observational study. Resuscitation 2011; 82(9):1194–7.
8. Lockey D, Crewdson K, Davies G. Traumatic cardiac arrest: who are the survivors? Ann Emerg Med 2006;48(3):240–4.
9. Zwingmann J, Mehlhorn AT, Hammer T, et al. Survival and neurologic outcome after traumatic out-of-hospital cardiopulmonary arrest in a pediatric and adult population: a systematic review. Crit Care 2012;16(4):R117.
10. Rhee PM, Acosta J, Bridgeman A, et al. Survival after emergency department thoracotomy: review of published data from the past 25 years. J Am Coll Surg 2000;190(3):288–98.
11. Seamon MJ, Haut ER, Van Arendonk K, et al. An evidence-based approach to patient selection for emergency department thoracotomy: a practice management guideline from the Eastern Association for the Surgery of Trauma. J Trauma Acute Care Surg 2015;79(1):159–73.
12. Inaba K, Chouliaras K, Zakaluzny S, et al. FAST ultrasound examination as a predictor of outcomes after resuscitative thoracotomy: a prospective evaluation. Ann Surg 2015;262(3):512–8.
13. Slessor D, Hunter S. To be blunt: are we wasting our time? emergency department thoracotomy following blunt trauma: a systematic review and meta-analysis. Ann Emerg Med 2015;65(3):297.
14. Duron V, Burke RV, Bliss D, et al. Survival of pediatric blunt trauma patients presenting with no signs of life in the field. J Trauma Acute Care Surg 2014;77(3): 422–6.
15. National Association of EMS Physicians and American College of Surgeons Committee on Trauma. Termination of resuscitation for adult traumatic cardiopulmonary arrest. Prehosp Emerg Care 2012;16(4):571.
16. Millin MG, Galvagno SM, Khandker SR, et al. Withholding and termination of resuscitation of adult cardiopulmonary arrest secondary to trauma: resource document to the joint NAEMSP-ACSCOT position statements. J Trauma Acute Care Surg 2013;75(3):459–67.
17. Burlew CC, Moore EE, Moore FA, et al. Western Trauma Association critical decisions in trauma: resuscitative thoracotomy. J Trauma Acute Care Surg 2012;73(6): 1359–63.
18. Smith JE, Le Clerc S, Hunt PA. Challenging the dogma of traumatic cardiac arrest management: a military perspective. Emerg Med J 2015;32(12):955–6.
19. Smith JE, Rickard A, Wise D. Traumatic cardiac arrest. J R Soc Med 2015;108(1): 11–6.
20. Soar J, Nolan JP, Böttiger BW, et al. European Resuscitation Council guidelines: adult advanced life support. Resuscitation 2015;95:100–47.
21. Cureton EL, Yeung LY, Kwan RO, et al. The heart of the matter: utility of ultrasound of cardiac activity during traumatic arrest. J Trauma Acute Care Surg 2012;73(1): 102–10.

22. Schuster KM, Lofthouse R, Moore C, et al. Pulseless electrical activity, focused abdominal sonography for trauma, and cardiac contractile activity as predictors of survival after trauma. J Trauma 2009;67(6):1154–7.
23. Luna GK, Pavlin EG, Kirkman T, et al. Hemodynamic effects of external cardiac massage in trauma shock. J Trauma 1989;29(10):1430–3.
24. Sherren PB, Reid C, Habig K, et al. Algorithm for the resuscitation of traumatic cardiac arrest patients in a physician-staffed helicopter emergency medical service. Crit Care 2013;17(2):308.
25. Lockey DJ, Lyon RM, Davies GE. Development of a simple algorithm to guide the effective management of traumatic cardiac arrest. Resuscitation 2013;84(6): 738–42.
26. Brenner M, Stein D, Hu P, et al. Association between early hyperoxia and worse outcomes after traumatic brain injury. Arch Surg 2012;147(11):1042–6.
27. Damiani E, Adrario E, Girardis M, et al. Arterial hyperoxia and mortality in critically ill patients: a systematic review and meta-analysis. Crit Care 2014;18(6):711.
28. Harris T, Masud S, Lamond A, et al. Traumatic cardiac arrest: a unique approach. Eur J Emerg Med 2015;22(2):72–8.
29. Deakin CD, Davies G, Wilson A. Simple thoracostomy avoids chest drain insertion in prehospital trauma. J Trauma 1995;39(2):373–4.
30. Laan DV, Vu TD, Thiels CA, et al. Chest wall thickness and decompression failure: A systematic review and meta-analysis comparing anatomic locations in needle thoracostomy. Injury 2016;47(4):797–804.
31. Clemency BM, Tanski CT, Rosenberg M, et al. Sufficient catheter length for pneumothorax needle decompression: a meta-analysis. Prehosp Disaster Med 2015; 30(3):249–53.
32. Schreiber MA, Neveleff DJ. Achieving hemostasis with topical hemostats: making clinically and economically appropriate decisions in the surgical and trauma settings. AORN J 2011;94(5):S1–20.
33. Bulger EM, Snyder D, Schoelles K, et al. An evidence-based prehospital guideline for external hemorrhage control: American College of Surgeons Committee on Trauma. Prehosp Emerg Care 2014;18(2):163–73.
34. Bellamy RF. The causes of death in conventional land warfare: implications for combat casualty care research. Mil Med 1984;149(2):55–62.
35. Bellamy RF, Maningas PA, Vayer JS. Epidemiology of trauma: military experience. Ann Emerg Med 1986;15(12):1384–8.
36. Dorlac WC, DeBakey ME, Holcomb JB, et al. Mortality from isolated civilian penetrating extremity injury. J Trauma 2005;59(1):217–22.
37. Schroll R, Smith A, McSwain NE Jr, et al. A multi-institutional analysis of prehospital tourniquet use. J Trauma Acute Care Surg 2015;79(1):10–4 [discussion: 4].
38. Passos E, Dingley B, Smith A, et al. Tourniquet use for peripheral vascular injuries in the civilian setting. Injury 2014;45(3):573–7.
39. Inaba K, Siboni S, Resnick S, et al. Tourniquet use for civilian extremity trauma. J Trauma Acute Care Surg 2015;79(2):232–7 [quiz: 332–3].
40. Lyon M, Johnson D, Gordon R. Use of a novel abdominal aortic and junctional tourniquet to reduce or eliminate flow in the brachial and popliteal arteries in human subjects. Prehosp Emerg Care 2015;19(3):405–8.
41. Tien HC, Spencer F, Tremblay LN, et al. Preventable deaths from hemorrhage at a level I Canadian trauma center. J Trauma 2007;62(1):142–6.
42. Tran TL, Brasel KJ, Karmy-Jones R, et al. Western Trauma Association critical decisions in trauma: management of pelvic fracture with hemodynamic instability-2016 updates. J Trauma Acute Care Surg 2016;81(6):1171–4.

43. Burlew CC, Moore EE, Stahel PF, et al. Preperitoneal pelvic packing reduces mortality in patients with life-threatening hemorrhage due to unstable pelvic fractures. J Trauma Acute Care Surg 2017;82(2):233–42.

44. Passos EM, Engels PT, Doyle JD, et al. Societal costs of inappropriate emergency department thoracotomy. J Am Coll Surg 2012;214(1):18–25.

45. Mejia JC, Stewart RM, Cohn SM. Emergency department thoracotomy. Semin Thorac Cardiovasc Surg 2008;20(1):13–8.

46. Seamon MJ, Pathak AS, Bradley KM, et al. Emergency department thoracotomy: still useful after abdominal exsanguination? J Trauma 2008;64(1):1–7 [discussion: 8].

47. Alzaga-Fernandez AG, Varon J. Open-chest cardiopulmonary resuscitation: past, present and future. Resuscitation 2005;64(2):149–56.

48. Boczar ME, Howard MA, Rivers EP, et al. A technique revisited: hemodynamic comparison of closed- and open-chest cardiac massage during human cardiopulmonary resuscitation. Crit Care Med 1995;23(3):498–503.

49. Bradley MJ, Bonds BW, Chang L, et al. Open chest cardiac massage offers no benefit over closed chest compressions in patients with traumatic cardiac arrest. J Trauma Acute Care Surg 2016;81(5):849–54.

50. Suzuki K, Inoue S, Morita S, et al. Comparative effectiveness of emergency resuscitative thoracotomy versus closed chest compressions among patients with critical blunt trauma: a nationwide cohort study in Japan. PLoS One 2016;11(1): e0145963.

51. Asensio JA, Murray J, Demetriades D, et al. Penetrating cardiac injuries: a prospective study of variables predicting outcomes. J Am Coll Surg 1998;186(1): 24–34.

52. Civil I. Emergency room thoracotomy: has availability triumphed over advisability in the care of trauma patients in Australasia? Emerg Med Australas 2010;22(4): 257–9.

53. Strumwasser A, Grabo D, Inaba K, et al. Is your graduating general surgery resident qualified to take trauma call? A 15-year appraisal of the changes in general surgery education for trauma. J Trauma Acute Care Surg 2017;82(3):470–80.

54. Fitzgerald M, Tan G, Gruen R, et al. Emergency physician credentialing for resuscitative thoracotomy for trauma. Emerg Med Australas 2010;22(4):332–6.

55. Meredith JW, Hoth JJ. Thoracic trauma: when and how to intervene. Surg Clin North Am 2007;87(1):95–118, vii.

56. Flaris AN, Simms ER, Prat N, et al. Clamshell incision versus left anterolateral thoracotomy. Which one is faster when performing a resuscitative thoracotomy? The tortoise and the hare revisited. World J Surg 2015;39(5):1306–11.

57. Rezende-Neto JB, Leong-Poi H, Rizoli S, et al. New device for temporary hemorrhage control in penetrating injuries to the ventricles. Trauma Surgery and Acute Care Open (TASCO) 2016;1:1–5.

58. Lee TH, Ouellet JF, Cook M, et al. Pericardiocentesis in trauma: a systematic review. J Trauma Acute Care Surg 2013;75(4):543–9.

59. Wilson A, Wall MJ Jr, Maxson R, et al. The pulmonary hilum twist as a thoracic damage control procedure. Am J Surg 2003;186(1):49–52.

60. Brenner ML, Moore LJ, DuBose JJ, et al. A clinical series of resuscitative endovascular balloon occlusion of the aorta for hemorrhage control and resuscitation. J Trauma Acute Care Surg 2013;75(3):506–11.

61. Martinelli T, Thony F, Declety P, et al. Intra-aortic balloon occlusion to salvage patients with life-threatening hemorrhagic shocks from pelvic fractures. J Trauma 2010;68(4):942–8.

62. Norii T, Crandall C, Terasaka Y. Survival of severe blunt trauma patients treated with resuscitative endovascular balloon occlusion of the aorta compared with propensity score-adjusted untreated patients. J Trauma Acute Care Surg 2015; 78(4):721–8.

63. DuBose JJ, Scalea TM, Brenner M, et al. The AAST prospective Aortic Occlusion for Resuscitation in Trauma and Acute Care Surgery (AORTA) registry: data on contemporary utilization and outcomes of aortic occlusion and resuscitative balloon occlusion of the aorta (REBOA). J Trauma Acute Care Surg 2016;81(3): 409–19.

64. Weppner J. Improved mortality from penetrating neck and maxillofacial trauma using Foley catheter balloon tamponade in combat. J Trauma Acute Care Surg 2013;75(2):220–4.

65. Naimer SA, Nash M, Niv A, et al. Control of massive bleeding from facial gunshot wound with a compact elastic adhesive compression dressing. Am J Emerg Med 2004;22(7):586–8.

66. Ferrara A, MacArthur JD, Wright HK, et al. Hypothermia and acidosis worsen coagulopathy in the patient requiring massive transfusion. Am J Surg 1990;160(5): 515–8.

67. Watts DD, Trask A, Soeken K, et al. Hypothermic coagulopathy in trauma: effect of varying levels of hypothermia on enzyme speed, platelet function, and fibrinolytic activity. J Trauma 1998;44(5):846–54.

68. Martin RS, Kilgo PD, Miller PR, et al. Injury-associated hypothermia: an analysis of the 2004 National Trauma Data Bank. Shock 2005;24(2):114–8.

69. Hammer N, Mobius R, Gries A, et al. Comparison of the fluid resuscitation rate with and without external pressure using two intraosseous infusion systems for adult emergencies, the CITRIN (Comparison of InTRaosseous infusion systems in emergency medicINe)-study. PLoS One 2015;10(12):e0143726.

70. Ngo AS, Oh JJ, Chen Y, et al. Intraosseous vascular access in adults using the EZ-IO in an emergency department. Int J Emerg Med 2009;2(3):155–60.

71. Ong ME, Chan YH, Oh JJ, et al. An observational, prospective study comparing tibial and humeral intraosseous access using the EZ-IO. Am J Emerg Med 2009; 27(1).8–15.

72. Leidel BA, Kirchhoff C, Bogner V, et al. Comparison of intraosseous versus central venous vascular access in adults under resuscitation in the emergency department with inaccessible peripheral veins. Resuscitation 2012;83(1):40–5.

73. Engels PT, Erdogan M, Widder SL, et al. Use of intraosseous devices in trauma: a survey of trauma practitioners in Canada, Australia and New Zealand. Can J Surg 2016;59(6):374–82.

74. Reddick AD, Ronald J, Morrison WG. Intravenous fluid resuscitation: was Poiseuille right? Emerg Med J 2011;28(3):201–2.

75. Cotton BA, Dossett LA, Haut ER, et al. Multicenter validation of a simplified score to predict massive transfusion in trauma. J Trauma 2010;69(Suppl 1):S33–9.

76. Nunez TC, Voskresensky IV, Dossett LA, et al. Early prediction of massive transfusion in trauma: simple as ABC (assessment of blood consumption)? J Trauma 2009;66(2):346–52.

77. Riskin DJ, Tsai TC, Riskin L, et al. Massive transfusion protocols: the role of aggressive resuscitation versus product ratio in mortality reduction. J Am Coll Surg 2009;209(2):198–205.

78. Borgman MA, Spinella PC, Perkins JG, et al. The ratio of blood products transfused affects mortality in patients receiving massive transfusions at a combat support hospital. J Trauma 2007;63(4):805–13.

79. Holcomb JB, Wade CE, Michalek JE, et al. Increased plasma and platelet to red blood cell ratios improves outcome in 466 massively transfused civilian trauma patients. Ann Surg 2008;248(3):447–58.

80. Holcomb JB, Tilley BC, Baraniuk S, et al. Transfusion of plasma, platelets, and red blood cells in a 1:1:1 vs a 1:1:2 ratio and mortality in patients with severe trauma: the PROPPR randomized clinical trial. JAMA 2015;313(5):471–82.

81. Shaz BH, Dente CJ, Nicholas J, et al. Increased number of coagulation products in relationship to red blood cell products transfused improves mortality in trauma patients. Transfusion 2010;50(2):493–500.

82. Shakur H, Roberts I, Bautista R, et al. Effects of tranexamic acid on death, vascular occlusive events, and blood transfusion in trauma patients with significant haemorrhage (CRASH-2): a randomised, placebo-controlled trial. Lancet 2010;376(9734):23–32.

83. Davis JW, Davis IC, Bennink LD, et al. Are automated blood pressure measurements accurate in trauma patients? J Trauma 2003;55(5):860–3.

84. Bickell WH, Wall MJ Jr, Pepe PE, et al. Immediate versus delayed fluid resuscitation for hypotensive patients with penetrating torso injuries. N Engl J Med 1994; 331(17):1105–9.

85. Carney N, Totten AM, O'Reilly C, et al. Guidelines for the management of severe traumatic brain injury, fourth edition. Neurosurgery 2016;80(1):6–15.

86. Rossaint R, Bouillon B, Cerny V, et al. The European guideline on management of major bleeding and coagulopathy following trauma: fourth edition. Crit Care 2016;20:100.

87. Upchurch CP, Grijalva CG, Russ S, et al. Comparison of etomidate and ketamine for induction during rapid sequence intubation of adult trauma patients. Ann Emerg Med 2017;69(1):24–33.e2.

88. Himmelseher S, Durieux ME. Revising a dogma: ketamine for patients with neurological injury? Anesth Analg 2005;101(2):524–34.

89. Miller M, Kruit N, Heldreich C, et al. Hemodynamic response after rapid sequence induction with ketamine in out-of-hospital patients at risk of shock as defined by the shock index. Ann Emerg Med 2016;68:181–8.e2.

90. Bernhard M, Matthes G, Kanz KG, et al. Emergency anesthesia, airway management and ventilation in major trauma. Background and key messages of the interdisciplinary S3 guidelines for major trauma patients. Anaesthesist 2011;60(11): 1027–40 [in German].

Resuscitation Resequenced

A Rational Approach to Patients with Trauma in Shock

Andrew Petrosoniak, MD, MSc (MedEd), FRCPC*,
Christopher Hicks, MD, MEd, FRCPC

KEYWORDS

- Trauma • Resuscitation • Shock • Shock index • ATLS

KEY POINTS

- Apply evidence-based clinical measures to identify shocked patients with trauma, such as Shock Index (SI) greater than or equal to 1.0, prehospital systolic blood pressure (sBP) less than 90 mm Hg, or sustained sBP less than 110 mm Hg.
- Critical hypoxemia or dynamic airway in patients with trauma represents the rare circumstance for immediate definitive airway management on emergency department arrival.
- Among most patients with trauma in shock, a resequenced approach to trauma care is preferable, emphasizing physiologic optimization before intubation.
- A reduction of 25% to 50% of the usual rapid sequence intubation induction agent dose is recommended in patients with SI greater than or equal to 1.0 or other evidence of shock.

CASE 1.1: ADVANCED TRAUMA LIFE SUPPORT APPROACH

A 63-year-old female pedestrian is struck by a car. Her Glasgow Coma Scale (GCS) score in the field is 13. In the emergency department (ED), evaluation proceeds according to the Advanced Trauma Life Support (ATLS) protocol. Her vitals are as follows: respiratory rate (RR) 26 breaths/min, O_2 saturation 90% on 100% oxygen, heart rate (HR) 105 beats/min (bpm), blood pressure (BP) 103/80 mm Hg, and temperature 36.0°C. Her airway is assessed to be patent, and air entry is decreased in the right chest. A focused assessment with sonography in trauma (FAST) examination is positive for free fluid in the right upper quadrant. Her pelvis is mechanically stable. Her peripheral neurologic examination is normal. She has no past medical history, takes no medications, and has no drug allergies.

Disclosures: The authors have no conflicts of interest or funding sources to declare.
Department of Emergency Medicine, St. Michael's Hospital, 1-008c Shuter Wing, 30 Bond street, Toronto, Ontario M5B 1W8, Canada
* Corresponding author.
E-mail address: petro82@gmail.com

Emerg Med Clin N Am 36 (2018) 41–60
http://dx.doi.org/10.1016/j.emc.2017.08.005
0733-8627/18/© 2017 Elsevier Inc. All rights reserved.

emed.theclinics.com

Following the A-B-C-D-E (airway-breathing-circulation-disability-exposure) heuristic, the team identifies her management priorities as (1) need for intubation based on projected clinical course, (2) chest tube placement, (3) blood product administration, (4) axial imaging (panscan). According to the ATLS shock classification, the patient is in class II shock (estimated blood loss, 750–1500 mL). Two units of uncrossmatched packed red blood cells (PRBCs) are requested and 1 L of crystalloid is given as an initial bolus.

A rapid sequence intubation (RSI) with 120 mg (2 mg/kg) of ketamine and 120 mg (2 mg/kg) succinylcholine is performed without difficulty. Five minutes after intubation, the patient becomes profoundly hypotensive, with a BP of 53/30 mm Hg. Suspecting a tension pneumothorax, the team quickly decompresses the right chest with a needle thoracostomy in the second intercostal space, midclavicular line, and an additional 1 L of crystalloid is given before blood products. A massive transfusion protocol (MTP) is activated, and tranexamic acid (TXA) is administered. Following chest tube placement, the patient's BP improves to 75/40 mm Hg; however, she remains hypotensive for an additional 30 minutes until 3 units of PRBCs are administered. Her hemodynamics stabilize, and she is transported to the computed tomography (CT) suite, where her systolic BP once again decreases to less than 70 mm Hg, requiring further blood products. She is found to have a small subdural hematoma, a right-sided pneumothorax, and a grade 3 liver laceration.

INTRODUCTION

Trauma resuscitation is a complex and dynamic process that is best managed by experienced, highly trained teams. Until the development of ATLS, patients received heterogeneous care by physicians lacking formal trauma resuscitation training.[1] The development of ATLS brought a much needed standardized approach to the care of critically injured patients. It facilitated a common language among care providers, highlighting the importance of a team approach and introduced the A-B-C-D-E sequence to trauma care.[2]

Using this simplified algorithm, teams are directed to assess injuries during a primary trauma survey in a predictable and sequential manner (ie, address A before moving on to B, and so on). The premise is to move in a stepwise and ordered fashion, particularly when multiple injuries may exist, in order to, for example, not miss the subtle tension pneumothorax by fixating on the obvious limb amputation. This paradigm is based primarily on experience rather than carefully conducted trials.

The sequence of priorities in ATLS until recently aligned similarly with the Advanced Cardiac Life Support (ACLS) approach of airway-breathing-circulation (A-B-C). Updated guidelines, based on new evidence, introduced a radical reordering of ACLS priorities to C-A-B in an effort to emphasize chest compressions.[3] High-quality chest compressions are linked to improved survival in medical cardiac arrest, and interruptions to cardiopulmonary resuscitation for any reason is associated with increased mortality.[3]

In major trauma, the value of strict and rigid adherence to the A-B-C-D-E sequence is also questionable.[1] Specifically, the ATLS approach overemphasizes the need to immediately secure a definitive airway and undervalues the importance of shock identification and preintubation resuscitation. The primacy of the airway often comes at the expense of more critical interventions related to supporting circulation and preventing hemodynamic collapse.

This article outlines an evidence-based update for the initial resuscitation of critically injured patients on arrival in the ED. It presents an algorithm (**Fig. 1**) that focuses first

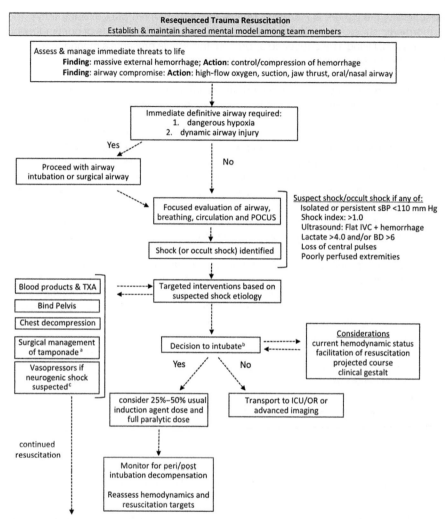

Fig. 1. A resequenced approach to trauma resuscitation. [a] Consider delaying RSI/definitive airway until arrival in operating room. [b] RSI preferred in most instances. [c] Vasopressors are typically avoided in favor of blood product administration, except in neurogenic shock. BD, base deficit; IVC, inferior vena cava; ICU, intensive care unit; OR, operating room; POCUS, point of care ultrasound; sBP, systolic BP.

on immediate threats to life followed by the identification and targeted management of shock and occult shock causes. In this resequenced approach, intubation should occur after the resuscitation has been initiated, unless critical hypoxia or a dynamic airway injury is present. Where evidence is lacking, a preferred approach is explicitly provided, based on our experience.

CASE 1.2: RESEQUENCED APPROACH

The case presented at the beginning of this article highlights the potential issues that can arise by strictly adhering to the A-B-C-D-E sequence outlined by ATLS.

Specifically, the patient is intubated before the management of both obstructive and hemorrhagic shock, prompting a dangerous but predictable episode of postintubation hypotension. Using a resequenced approach, this article presents a management plan to mitigate these risks by way of targeted interventions to manage a shock state before RSI.

In trauma resuscitation resequenced, the team addresses key management priorities, as outlined in **Fig. 1**. The patient requires intubation urgently but not immediately, given she is self-ventilating with an oxygen saturation of 90% and is protecting her airway. With a positive FAST and Shock Index (SI) greater than 1.0, the team leader chooses to focus on hemodynamic optimization before RSI, specifically a presumed right-sided tension pneumothorax and intra-abdominal injury. The SI, defined as the HR divided by systolic BP, is an important clue to the presence of shock and occult shock, and is sensitive for predicting critical bleeding, the need for blood products, and incidence of postintubation hypotension.[4–6] The team leader fosters a shared mental model (SMM) with the team members by verbally outlining management priorities in the following sequence: (1) blood product administration and MTP activation, (2) right chest decompression with finger thoracostomy, and (3) RSI using a reduced dose of ketamine. The team performs regular airway and neurologic evaluations to monitor for clinical deterioration that may warrant more rapid airway intervention. Following finger thoracostomy, the patient's oxygen saturation improves to 95%. Two units of PRBCs are administered, HR decreases to 85 bpm, and the BP remains 105/50 mm Hg. An uncomplicated RSI is performed using a reduced dose of ketamine (0.5 mg/kg). There is no postintubation hypotension. The patient is given postintubation analgesia and sedation, and remains hemodynamically appropriate during transport to, from, and during CT imaging. In case 1.1, the clinicians doggedly followed the ATLS algorithm. As a result, the patient experienced prolonged hypotension with a risk of postintubation cardiac arrest, which increased her risk for a poor neurologic outcome related to prolonged hypoperfusion in the setting of a significant head injury. In contrast, the team in case 1.2 optimized the patient's hemodynamic status before intubation, resulting in more consistent hemodynamics following intubation.

THE RESEQUENCED APPROACH TO TRAUMA RESUSCITATION: A SHARED MENTAL MODEL

According to SMM theory, team performance is optimized when team members have a common understanding of the team and task requirements without the need for explicit discussion.[7] The algorithmic features of ATLS may help to foster an SMM among team members.[8] A resequenced plan for trauma resuscitation requires that all team members understand how and when priorities should deviate from the A-B-C-D-E approach. Preferably, regular team training exercises and/or prebriefings before patient arrival should be used to establish a workable SMM of team-based and task-based processes, particularly when it differs from the standard ATLS approach.[9,10] The importance of resequencing SMMs cannot be overstated, because the resequenced approach to trauma resuscitation needs to be operationalized with careful consideration to each team member's understanding of process and order of care.

WHERE DOES AIRWAY FIT WITHIN TRAUMA RESUSCITATION?

As outlined in **Fig. 1**, airway evaluation is necessary immediately on patient arrival as part of the primary survey. Whether definitive airway management must always occur before interventions related to breathing or circulation is questionable, particularly when phys-iologic considerations instead support the prioritization of obstructive or hemorrhagic shock causes.[11] In our experience, most patients with trauma do not immediately require a definitive airway (eg, within the initial 10 minutes of arrival). Instead, the airway can be managed temporarily with supportive maneuvers while an airway plan is devised and physiologic risks for postintubation hypotension are addressed.

Intubation causes an increase in intrathoracic pressure, resulting in a decrease in right atrial pressure.[11] The reversal in intrathoracic physiology following intubation (compared with spontaneous respirations) has a significant impact on the shock states that are common among patients with trauma. In hemorrhagic shock, an already low venous return can decrease further with positive pressure ventilation.[11] Although not studied exclusively in trauma, preintubation hypotension is a significant risk factor for postintubation cardiac arrest, highlighting the importance of adequate volume resuscitation before intubation.[12] In obstructive shock states (eg, tension pneumothorax, cardiac tamponade), decreased venous return and may also be wors-ened by positive pressure ventilation. Focused interventions to relieve obstructive causes should be considered before intubation in order to optimize hemodynamics and establish safer peri-intubation and postintubation conditions.

There are several situations in which definitive airway management must be the im-mediate priority of the trauma team:

1. Critical hypoxemia, despite high-flow oxygen and supportive airway maneuvers
2. Dynamic airway: blunt, penetrating, or burn injuries to the head, neck, or oropharynx that may compromise oxygenation, ventilation, or airway management, and that are suspected to worsen on a very short time course

Even when airway is the immediate priority, concurrent management of shock states can occur to a greater or lesser extent, depending on team size and structure. A single physician working with a respiratory therapist and nurse may elect to perform a needle decompression and request blood products in line with intubation efforts, whereas a larger team may be able to address multiple priorities concurrent with airway management.

In summary, a small minority of patients with trauma (those with critical hypoxia or dynamic airway injuries) require definitive airway management immediately on arrival in the ED. Instead, most patients benefit from aggressive resuscitation before intuba-tion. Interventions include those that stay hemorrhage, optimize perfusion, and relieve obstructive shock causes. Once these interventions are initiated or completed, then definitive airway management can proceed.

IDENTIFICATION OF SHOCK AND OCCULT SHOCK IN PATIENTS WITH TRAUMA

Shock is a clinical state defined by circulatory failure resulting in insufficient cellular ox-ygen use, and manifests with clinical and hemodynamic derangements.[13] Occult shock can exist if these obvious clinical disturbances are subtle or absent despite un-derlying hypoperfusion.[14] In an effort to identify occult shock, several strategies have been proposed using biomarkers (lactate, base deficit [BD]), vital signs (BP, HR), or SI, each of which have specific benefits and limitations.[15–17]

Early shock identification is critical in order to prevent clinical deterioration and refrac-tory shock states.[18–20] Furthermore, airway management that precedes resuscitation can worsen hemodynamics. Several studies show that an SI greater than or equal to 0.9 and preintubation systolic BP (sBP) less than 90 mm Hg are independent predictors for postintubation cardiac arrest.[12,21] Hypotension, hypoxemia, and pH/acidosis (the

HOP killers) are physiologic disturbances that can result in poor outcomes among critically ill ED patients undergoing emergency airway management.[22] Although not unique to patients with trauma, they should be considered and corrected in line with, and ideally before, active airway management for patients in whom shock or occult shock is suspected. Delays in the identification and management of shock and occult shock among patients with trauma is associated with poor outcomes, such as multiorgan failure, increased intensive care unit (ICU) length of stay, and ultimately death.[14,15] The imperative to identify patients with shock is clear, particularly because early damage control surgery results in substantial benefits.[23] The early identification of occult shock is equally important because under-recognition is associated with worse patient outcomes.[24]

Challenges exist in the early identification of shock in patients with trauma.[25] Variable pathophysiologic and compensatory mechanisms produce a range of hemodynamic presentations that complicate assessment.[26] Traditionally, ED physicians have applied the ATLS shock classification to predict the amount of blood loss, a system comprising 4 shock classes using vital signs and mental status. The widespread application of this system occurred without formal study or validation and recently the accuracy of these classifications has been called into question.[27] ATLS underestimates the prevalence of bradycardia in hemorrhagic shock and fails to consider the complex pathophysiology related to blood loss and tissue injury.[26] A study of a German trauma registry showed that only 9.3% of patients with trauma can be properly categorized according to ATLS shock classification.[28] In an audit of the United Kingdom Trauma Registry from 1989 to 2007, patients progressing to stage 4 shock (>2 L of blood loss) increased HR from 82 to 95 bpm, while showing no significant changes in GCS, respiratory rate, or sBP.[27] The ATLS shock categories are inaccurate in geriatric patients with trauma, because of decreased physiologic reserve, comorbid disease, restricted vascular elasticity, and concurrent use of cardiovascular medications.[29,30] The traditional shock categories also do not account for other causes of shock (obstructive, neurogenic) or mixed shock causes.

Over the past decade, clinicians and researchers have sought simple and more accurate methods for identifying and quantifying shock in patients with trauma. In general, these techniques are best studied in hemorrhagic shock, with the exception of bedside ultrasonography, which can be used to identify hemorrhagic and some forms of obstructive shock. During the initial resuscitation period, indices for shock identification can be organized into 2 broad categories:

1. Clinical indicators: obtained exclusively at the bedside
2. Laboratory indicators: additional laboratory testing required

The role of each indicator as a potential alternative to the traditional ATLS approach is discussed here, highlighting their utility during the prehospital phase and initial resuscitation period (time spent in the ED before transport to imaging or definitive care). There is no perfect indicator to reliably and accurately identify shock in all cases; each has benefits and pitfalls, with applicability related to local resources and clinician preference. Our approach to using each indicator is summarized in **Table 1**.

CLINICAL INDICATORS
Vital Signs

Despite their limitations, vital signs are still a central element of the trauma primary survey.[27,28] Vital signs are obtained immediately on patient arrival and repeated frequently; trends in vital signs can often be more informative than a single, static measurement.

Table 1
Application of clinical and laboratory indicators in patients with trauma with suspected shock

Indicator	How It Is Applied to Practice
Clinical Indicators	
Vital signs	Prehospital
	Recognize abnormal vital signs and communicate to ED team before arrival
	Standardized EMS sign-over that incorporates lowest prehospital sBP
	In hospital
	Team training that teaches not to rely on traditional ATLS shock classification
	Explicitly communicate concern for shock (±hemorrhage) to team members if sBP <110 mm Hg
	Liberal request for blood products following isolated prehospital or sustained ED sBP <110 mm Hg
	Strongly consider blood products following repeated/sustained sBP <90 mm Hg
SI	Calculate SI for all patients with trauma
	SI ≥1.0: communicate to all team members about concern for shock
	SI ≥1.0 + suspected hemorrhage: TXA and blood product administration
	In geriatric patients, consider shock if SI ≥1.0 despite otherwise normal vital signs
	Dose reduction for RSI induction agents if SI ≥1.0
Ultrasonography	eFAST examination for all patients with trauma
	Pericardial fluid on eFAST should prompt cautious approach to intubation, preferably in operating room with surgeon prepped for intervention
	eFAST before intubation to rule out clinically significant pneumothorax
	Serial eFAST examinations if persistent hemodynamic compromise without initial signs of hemorrhage
	Pneumothorax visualized on ultrasonography and hemodynamic instability warrants immediate chest decompression
	Rare application of IVC examination
Laboratory Indicators	
BD	Patients with a BD >6 require aggressive resuscitation and risk hypotension during/after intubation
	BD >6 requires significant diagnostic effort to identify source of hemorrhage and/or shock cause
	Integrate in decision making for those at risk of crumping after departure from trauma bay
	Preferential reliance in patients with suspected shock and concomitant alcohol intoxication
Lactate	Complements BD and often used interchangeably
	Levels >4.0 warrant increased suspicion for occult shock, in combination with other indicators
Viscoelastic assays (ROTEM or TEG)	Acknowledge limited evidence for use
	Reasonable predictor of MTP
	Integrate abnormal findings into decision for targeted blood product administration (eg, evidence of hyperfibrinolysis, consider second dose of TXA)

Abbreviations: eFAST, Extended Focused Assessment with Sonography for Trauma; EMS, emergency medical services; ROTEM, rotational thromboelastometry; TEG, thromboelastography.

Hypotension is defined by ATLS as sBP less than or equal to 90 mm Hg, but this cutoff is debatable.[31] A sustained sBP less than or equal to 90 mm Hg is associated with a 60% mortality and BD values of greater than 20, suggesting that this cutoff may capture only the sickest of patients.[32] Several studies have proposed that an sBP of less than 105 or less than 110 mm Hg may be more appropriate estimates of hypoperfusion.[31–34] In one study, patients with trauma with an sBP of 90 to 109 mm Hg had a significantly increased risk of death (5% vs 1%) compared with those with an sBP greater than 109 mm Hg.[33] The investigators concluded that an sBP of 90 to 109 mm Hg warrants aggressive resuscitation and surgical evaluation. Even a single, isolated decrease in sBP to less than 105 mm Hg is associated with a 12-fold increase in the need for immediate therapeutic intervention.[16]

The importance of prehospital hypotension that normalizes without intervention should not be underestimated. Multiple studies have shown an association between isolated prehospital hypotension and an increased risk for serious injury, surgical intervention, and mortality.[35–37] Repeat episodes of hypotension in the ED confer an even greater risk of serious morbidity and death.[38,39]

The predictive value of vital signs among geriatric patients remains uncertain. In one study, 20% of patients more than 65 years old had normal vital signs (defined as sBP >90 mm Hg and HR <120 bpm) despite laboratory measures suggesting hypoperfusion.[30] These data align with other studies to support the need to redefine normal in the geriatric population.[15,34,40] In a separate study, HR did not predict massive transfusion among geriatric patients.[29] In contrast, sBP, pulse pressure, and diastolic BP all proved to be strongly predictive of more than 5 units of PRBCs within 24 hours of arrival to hospital.

In addition, physical examination findings can provide additional evidence of shock. Poorly perfused extremities or loss of central pulses are important findings in profound shock; however, their reliability and accuracy have not been well studied. BP as assessed by the presence or absence of peripheral or central pulses tends to underestimate the degree of hypotension.[41] Used together, our experience is that combining an assessment of trends in vital signs, adequacy of peripheral perfusion, and physical examination findings can yield a more accurate estimate of the presence and degree of shock during the primary survey, compared with BP or HR alone.

Shock Index

The SI, defined as HR/sBP, is a simple and reliable method for estimating degree of shock and predicting clinical outcomes in a variety of settings, including trauma resuscitation.[6,42,43] The SI is useful in trauma because of its simplicity, strong inter-rater reliability, and accuracy as a predictor of blood loss.[44,45] Although there is no precise cutoff for an abnormal SI, a value of greater than or equal to 1.0 is associated with significant increases in transfusion requirements, injury severity, and mortality.[4,46,47] Estimating an SI of greater than or equal to 1.0 is also straightforward and requires no formal calculation (HR > sBP), which is important during periods of high cognitive and task load.

Notably, the SI is predictably unreliable in the following circumstances[6]:

1. Altered physiologic compensation (eg, geriatrics)
2. Presence of underlying medical conditions (eg, undertreated hypertension)
3. Medication-related disturbances (eg, β-blockers)

Importantly, geriatric patients with trauma often have 1 or more of these circumstances. Although the best available evidence strongly supports the utility of SI in trauma as a predictor of clinical outcomes, the results are less definitive among geriatric patients. In one study of more than 200,000 patients with trauma, SI was the strongest predictor of mortality among patients 65 years of age and older.[48] In contrast, a smaller study of 1987 patients did not find that SI was an independent predictor of mortality.[29] This difference highlights the complexity of geriatric physiology following critical injuries and the challenges that face clinicians in detecting shock among elderly patients.

The delta SI (d-SI) has been proposed as a way to overcome the underlying hypertension and impaired tachycardic responses that are prevalent among geriatric patients with trauma. The d-SI is defined as the change in SI from the prehospital setting to arrival in the ED. A difference of greater than 0.1 is considered significant, and suggests the presence of shock or occult shock. A recent retrospective study found that mortalities were significantly higher among those with d-SI exceeded 0.1 (16.6% vs 9.5%).[49] Although these data are preliminary, they may prove useful once confirmed in prospective studies.

In our practice, the authors use an SI of greater than 1 or d-SI of greater than 0.1 in conjunction with the presence of isolated hypotensive episodes to identify patients at risk for worse outcome.

Ultrasonography

The FAST is a standard part of the evaluation of patients with trauma.[2] The presence of abdominal free fluid directs clinicians to consider intra-abdominal organ injury as a source of hemorrhage, and in the presence of hypotension supports emergent operative intervention. In contrast, a negative FAST study despite hypotension should generate a search for extra-abdominal causes of hemorrhage and other shock causes.[50,51] Pericardial fluid is also rapidly identified during the FAST examination, and, when present, prompts consideration for tamponade physiology as a cause for shock. Notably, the evidence is limited for improved patient outcomes with the integration of a FAST examination.[52] Several investigators have questioned the role of the FAST examination in hemodynamically stable patients.[53,54] Despite these limitations, given the minimal impact on team efficiency and acquisition of potentially useful data, the authors follow the published guidelines applying a FAST examination for patients with all blunt mechanisms and most patients with penetrating mechanisms of trauma.

The extended FAST (eFAST) includes an evaluation of thoracic structures for pneumothorax and hemothorax. There is growing evidence that eFAST is a superior diagnostic modality to supine chest radiograph (CXR) for detecting pneumothorax.[55–57] Compared with supine CXR, emergency physician (EP)–performed lung ultrasonography shows superior sensitivity (86%–98% vs 28%–75%) and equal specificity (98%–100% vs 100%).[58] Whether this translates to improved patient-oriented outcomes remains to be seen. These studies support our current diagnostic approach in the trauma bay with eFAST integration during the primary survey, followed by CT when stability permits.

The utility and accuracy of bedside ultrasonography to assess the inferior vena cava (IVC) has not been systematically studied. In critical care, the utility may only exist at extremes of measurements, but this remains a matter of much debate.[59–61] In our experience, when ultrasonography shows findings suggestive of shock, assessing the IVC to estimate size, collapse, and respiratory variation rarely adds to our clinical impression.

LABORATORY INDICATORS
Base Deficit

The BD is defined as the number of base units required to return the pH of whole blood to 7.4, assuming a normal Pco_2.[62] In trauma, BD correlates closely with transfusion requirements, injury severity, and mortality.[63] It is particularly valuable during the initial phases of resuscitation, because an increased BD can help identify patients who will crump, a term used to describe acute and unexpected physiologic deterioration. In severely injured patients with prehospital hypotension who are normotensive in the ED, a BD of greater than 6 was predictive of both recurrent hypotension and death (5-fold mortality increase) compared with those with a BD less than 6.[38] Specifically, a BD greater than 6 detected patients with transient hypotension who were likely to crump again. These findings were confirmed in a recent systematic review that concluded that BD greater than 6 is useful for prognostication and to guide resuscitation in patients with trauma.[64]

Lactate

Lactate may also be used as a surrogate predictor of blood loss. Why cellular lactate production increases is a subject of debate; it is postulated to increase either as a byproduct of anaerobic cellular metabolism or in response to metabolic stress endogenous epinephrine release.[65,66] In either case, an increased lactate level measured shortly after injury is widely accepted as a predictor of shock and mortality in patients with trauma.[66–68] The utility of following lactate clearance is less certain, with a recent study showing no difference in predictive value between a single initial value and lactate clearance over time.[69]

Gale and colleagues[70] concluded that initial lactate level is a superior prognostic marker for in-hospital mortality. Using a slightly different outcome, Caputo and colleagues[17] found that lactate and BD had similar test characteristics for predicting shock, defined as the need for operative intervention or massive transfusion.[70] Based on the best available data, EPs should recognize that both an increased lactate level and the presence of a BD (>6) are reasonable surrogate predictors of injury severity. An abnormality of either test supports the diagnosis of shock (or occult shock) and warrants attention, an approach supported by recent guidelines.[71] Lactate level may also increase in patients who have consumed significant amounts of alcohol, making it of questionable utility in this population.[71] It may be reasonable in cases of intoxication to rely on BD instead, which remains unaffected. In summary, these markers may be the only indicators that the patient is physiologically compromised and should be integrated into resuscitation decision making.

Viscoelastic Assays

On arrival in the ED, 25% to 30% of severely injured patients are coagulopathic, and fail to form adequate clots in response to hemorrhage.[72] This early trauma coagulopathy (acute coagulopathy of trauma and shock [ACoTS]) is associated with a 4-fold increase in mortality and high rates of organ failure, highlighting the importance of early identification.[73] Standard coagulation tests are inadequate to identify ACoTS because they only identify early phases of clot formation.[74] Two point-of-care viscoelastic assays have emerged as promising alternatives for early coagulopathy detection in trauma: thromboelastography (TEG) and rotational thromboelastometry (ROTEM).[74] Existing data remain insufficient to recommend a preferred assay.[71] A recent systematic review identified that several abnormal clotting parameters detected by ROTEM (fibrin-based extrinsically activated test with tissue factor (FIBTEM) and extrinsically-activated test with tissue factor (EXTEM) are consistently associated with early coagulopathy, higher rates of massive transfusion, and overall increased mortality.[74] FIBTEM represents a state of hypofibrinogenemia, and EXTEM relates to dysfunction within the extrinsic clotting pathway. European guidelines for hemorrhage in trauma make a grade 1 recommendation that viscoelastic assays be used to characterize coagulopathy and guide hemostatic therapy despite a low level of supporting evidence.[71] Clinicians should remain cautious in their application of viscoelastic tests given the lack of high-quality evidence and unclear cutoffs for each parameter.[75]

CLINICAL INDICATORS: SUMMARY

There is no single indicator that can reliably predict both the presence and degree of shock for all patients with trauma. The authors suggest that a combination of indicators be integrated into clinical decision making in a systematic and measured fashion. Practically, this begins with clinical indicators that may be adjusted based on metabolic assessment with lactate or BD.

HOW CAN TRAUMA RESUSCITATION BE RESEQUENCED TO ALIGN WITH PHYSIOLOGIC PRIORITIES?

The traditional A-B-C-D-E sequence advocated by ATLS may not be appropriate for every trauma patient. Our resequenced approach represents a rational shift away from a highly scripted and algorithmic paradigm, toward a trauma resuscitation that is based on physiologic priorities.

In **Fig. 1**, invasive airway management is recommended after other priorities have been addressed, unless dangerous hypoxia or a dynamic airway is present. This rationale stems from the recognized risks associated with postintubation hypotension and cardiac arrest, and the problematic manner in which the primacy of airway management diverts attention away from more immediately life-threatening priorities. Instead, trauma teams should focus on the identification of shock, using a combination of strategies outlined earlier (see **Table 1**). Recently, airway management in critical illness was reframed as resuscitative sequence intubation, in an attempt to minimize the rapid manner in which many RSIs take place.[76] Although not specific to patients with trauma, the concept emphasizes physiologic optimization before intubation, which the authors have found to be of crucial importance for patients with trauma in shock.

During the initial stages of resuscitation it is often not possible to confirm the precise cause of shock. Instead, diagnosis and management occur simultaneously, often erring toward active management when faced with diagnostic uncertainty and critical illness. This management may include blood product and TXA administration with persistent hypotension without an identifiable source of hemorrhage; a pelvic binder placed before pelvis radiographs in patients with a high suspicion of injury; or finger thoracostomy when either physical examination, ultrasonography, or CXR suggest pneumothorax in the presence of shock. Importantly, the authors argue that each of these steps should precede intubation in most shocked patients with trauma, especially those without life-threatening hypoxia or airway compromise.

Two causes of shock warrant specific attention because of nuances in their management: cardiac tamponade and neurogenic shock.

In cardiac tamponade, the hemopericardium impedes adequate ventricular filling and impairs venous return. Intubation and positive pressure ventilation result in increased intrathoracic pressure, further compromising venous return. The end result is worsening hypotension or cardiac arrest after intubation. There are no large human studies to validate these concerns; however, the deleterious physiologic effects are apparent in both animal studies and human case series.[77–79] Identification of a pericardial effusion in trauma should prompt clinicians to use a significantly higher threshold for intubation. Ho and colleagues[79] propose that, in patients with a "palpable central pulse, irrespective of the degree of neurological impairment, intubation should be delayed" until surgical relief of tamponade can be achieved. Whether a thoracotomy is performed in the ED or in the operating room (OR) should be based on institution-specific resources. If intubation must be performed before thoracotomy, judicious use of anesthetic induction agents followed by ventilation with low pressures is recommended.[79]

The diagnosis of neurogenic shock can pose a significant management dilemma because these patients have different hemodynamic targets than bleeding patients. The former may ultimately require vasopressor support to achieve a target mean arterial pressure greater than 80 mm Hg, in an attempt to optimize spinal cord perfusion.[80] In our practice, we resuscitate hypotensive patients with blood products while searching for hemorrhage and other obstructive causes for shock. Once addressed or excluded, and neurogenic shock is suspected, we administer vasopressor support. Although the data are poor, norepinephrine is recommended unless there is profound bradycardia, in which case epinephrine may be preferred.[81]

THE DECISION TO INTUBATE: YES. PREPARE AND PROCEED

The decision to intubate during a trauma resuscitation is both complex and multifactorial. A complete overview of the considerations, strategies, and techniques is covered elsewhere in this issue. An overview is provided here of the decision making and practical considerations for definitive airway management in patients with shock or occult shock trauma. More specifically, these are patients deemed appropriate for sedation and paralysis to facilitate airway management.

The decision to intubate a patient with trauma in shock is based on several factors, including:

- Current hemodynamic status: will the patient tolerate a further delay to intubation in an effort to optimize hemodynamics (eg, blood product administration)?
- Facilitation of resuscitation: is the patient unable to safely tolerate further procedures (eg, bag mask ventilation, pelvic binder, venous access) without intubation?
- Projected course: are there indicators that delaying airway interventions will complicate the procedure later during the resuscitation?
- Clinical gestalt: the clinician's experience should not be underestimated. In certain instances, there may be a combination of multiple factors that, individually, may not be sufficient to warrant intubation but together necessitate definitive airway control.

If intubation is not required, then the trauma team can proceed with their plan toward definitive care (eg, transfer to OR, ICU, or CT suite). A plan to defer airway management still mandates an ongoing evaluation of the patient's clinical status and targeted resuscitation based on injuries and hemodynamics.

Drug and Dose Selection

In general, RSI is the recommended approach for intubation in patients with trauma.[82] More situation-specific strategies can be found in this issue's article on trauma airway management (see George Kovacs and Nick Sowers article, "Airway Management in Trauma," in this issue).

In our practice, the induction agent and dose selection for RSI follow an appraisal of the patient's hemodynamic status. A key decision point is whether shock is present, either apparent or occult. In general, we take a multipronged, evidence-guided approach to induction agent and dose selection using all available information, including:

- Prehospital hypotension (either episodic or sustained)
- SI

- Response to resuscitation
- Age and comorbidities
- Documented and suspected injuries
- Clinical course prehospital and in the ED

A standardized approach to RSI in trauma has been shown to be both safe and effective.[83,84] Using a standard agent and dosing regimen facilitates drug administration and may reduce dosing errors. In one study of severely injured patients (injury severity score = 24), patient outcomes were compared before and after the implementation of a ketamine-based RSI protocol (using 2 mg/kg). The investigators concluded that a standardized medication protocol simplifies RSI and allows efficient airway management in trauma without any significant difference in hypotensive events.[83] Another study compared etomidate with fentanyl and ketamine.[84] Although overall hemodynamics were preserved in both groups, a hypotensive response was more likely (1% vs 6%; $P = .05$) in the ketamine group. This finding may be attributed to the combination of both fentanyl and ketamine or the possible negative inotropic effects of ketamine in a shock state.[85,86] There are clear benefits to a standardized RSI protocol; however, caution is needed with standardized dose selection in patients with hemodynamic compromise. Mechanisms to facilitate clinician-guided dose reductions when clinically indicated should be applied.

Multiple agents are used for RSI induction, including fentanyl, midazolam, etomidate, ketamine, and propofol. Etomidate and ketamine are often viewed as hemodynamically neutral, having little or no impact on BP. In the absence of shock, both etomidate and ketamine are rarely associated with hypotension; however, a critical pitfall is extrapolating this to shocked patients.[87] All induction agents may contribute to hypotension in shock states, including etomidate and ketamine.[88,89] A recent prehospital study evaluated the effect of ketamine during RSI on patients with trauma with low and high SIs (defined as SI <0.9 and SI >0.9, respectively).[5] Patients with a high SI were significantly more likely to experience hypotension than those with a low SI (26% vs 2%). This study corroborates previous data suggesting that, in catecholamine-depleted states, ketamine has negative inotropic effects.[85,90]

It is clear that there is no perfect agent; however, the authors' preferred RSI induction agent is ketamine given its overall favorable safety profile and breadth of data supporting its use in trauma. The typical dose of 1.5 to 2 mg/kg, administered to patients with obvious or occult shock, may still result in hemodynamic compromise.[5,88] We therefore recommend a dose reduction of 25% to 50% in patients with an SI greater than 1.0 or a clinical status suggestive of shock.

Should an alternative induction agent be selected (eg, etomidate) in a patient with an SI greater than or equal to 1.0, the authors advocate similar dose reductions (25%–50% of the typical induction dose) to minimize the risk of postintubation hypotension. In these circumstances, the dose is far more important than the drug. Of note, this does not apply to paralytic drug dosing; an adequate dose should be administered to overcome reduced peripheral perfusion (2 mg/kg of succinylcholine or 1.2–1.6 mg/kg of rocuronium).[91,92]

WHAT PITFALLS EXIST IN THE RESUSCITATION OF PATIENTS WITH TRAUMA IN THE EMERGENCY DEPARTMENT?

Combining both our experience and available evidence, **Table 2** summarizes a list of pitfalls and mitigation strategies during the resuscitation of critically injured patients.

Table 2
Pitfalls and mitigation strategies for trauma care in the emergency department

Pitfall	Mitigation Strategy
Reliance on ATLS shock classification in resuscitation decision making	Apply evidence-based indicators to identify shock and occult shock (eg, SI)
Unrecognized signs of shock	Integrate key clinical manifestations into EMS/ED handover process and in team communications (eg, isolated/repeated hypotension, sustained sBP <110 mm Hg)
Strict application of A-B-C paradigm in trauma management	Resequenced approach to address physiologic priorities: (1) manage immediate threats to life, (2) targeted management for identified shock causes
Intubation before resuscitation in patients with trauma with evidence of shock	Unless critical hypoxia or dynamic airway is identified, defer difficult airway (instead provide temporary airway support) until resuscitation is underway or complete. This strategy may reduce risk of postintubation hypotension/cardiac arrest
Intubation before obstructive shock causes are diagnosed and treated	Before all trauma intubations, common causes for obstructive shock should be diagnosed and managed when appropriate (tension pneumothorax). In cardiac tamponade, strongly consider deferral of definitive airway until pericardial blood evacuation can be performed
Use standard dose for RSI induction agent regardless of preintubation hemodynamics	If shock or occult shock is identified, decrease induction agent by 25%–50% of standard dose regardless of agent (even ketamine). Administer full paralytic dose
Expect similar hemodynamic manifestations of shock in geriatric patients	Shock is a complex entity in geriatric patients. Suspect shock if SI $\geq$1.0, delta SI $\geq$0.1, sBP <110 mm Hg, or abnormal laboratory indicators (lactate, BD, ROTEM)

SUMMARY

The identification and resuscitation of the shocked patients with trauma is a complex and dynamic process. Using the traditional, sequential approach formalized by ATLS can at times lead to ineffective prioritization of critical injuries in favor of less urgent interventions. This article proposes the application of evidence-based methods for shock identification combined with trauma resuscitation guided by physiologic priorities. A resequenced trauma resuscitation represents an important paradigm shift in trauma care toward physiologic optimization before intubation. This resequenced approach first addresses immediate threats to life followed by targeted management strategies for the diagnosis and management of shock causes. This approach is both practical and feasible across a variety of settings in which trauma care is provided. Improved resuscitation strategies will inevitably optimize outcomes for patients with trauma.

ACKNOWLEDGMENTS

The authors wish to thank Dr Reuben Strayer for his valuable feedback during the writing of this article.

REFERENCES

1. Wiles MD. ATLS: archaic trauma life support? Anaesthesia 2015;70(8):893–7.
2. Committee on Trauma, American College of Surgeons. Advanced trauma life support for doctors. Chicago: American College of Surgeons; 2013.
3. Field JM, Hazinski MF, Sayre MR, et al. Part 1: executive summary: 2010 American Heart Association guidelines for cardiopulmonary resuscitation and emergency cardiovascular care. Circulation 2010;122(18 Suppl 3):S640–56.
4. Mutschler M, Nienaber U, Munzberg M, et al. The shock index revisited - a fast guide to transfusion requirement? A retrospective analysis on 21,853 patients derived from the Trauma Register DGU. Crit Care 2013;17(4):R172.
5. Miller M, Kruit N, Heldreich C, et al. Hemodynamic response after rapid sequence induction with ketamine in out-of-hospital patients at risk of shock as defined by the shock index. Ann Emerg Med 2016;68(2):181–8.e2.
6. Olaussen A, Blackburn T, Mitra B, et al. Review article: shock index for prediction of critical bleeding post-trauma: a systematic review. Emerg Med Australas 2014; 26(3):223–8.
7. Mathieu J, Goodwin G, Heffner T, et al. The influence of shared mental models on team process and performance. J Appl Psychol 2000;85(2):273–83.
8. Mohammad A, Branicki F, Abu-Zidan FM. Educational and clinical impact of Advanced Trauma Life Support (ATLS) courses: a systematic review. World J Surg 2014;38(2):322–9.
9. Miller D, Crandall C, Washington C 3rd, et al. Improving teamwork and communication in trauma care through in situ simulations. Acad Emerg Med 2012;19(5): 608–12.
10. Berkenstadt H, Ben-Menachem E, Simon D, et al. Training in trauma management: the role of simulation-based medical education. Anesthesiol Clin 2013; 31(1):167–77.
11. Mosier JM, Joshi R, Hypes C, et al. The physiologically difficult airway. West J Emerg Med 2015;16(7):1109–17.

12. Kim WY, Kwak MK, Ko BS, et al. Factors associated with the occurrence of cardiac arrest after emergency tracheal intubation in the emergency department. PLoS One 2014;9(11):e112779.

13. Vincent JL, De Backer D. Circulatory shock. N Engl J Med 2013;369(18): 1726–34.

14. Blow O, Magliore L, Claridge JA, et al. The golden hour and the silver day: detection and correction of occult hypoperfusion within 24 hours improves outcome from major trauma. J Trauma 1999;47(5):964–9.

15. Martin JT, Alkhoury F, O'Connor JA, et al. 'Normal' vital signs belie occult hypoperfusion in geriatric trauma patients. Am Surg 2010;76(1):65–9.

16. Seamon MJ, Feather C, Smith BP, et al. Just one drop: the significance of a single hypotensive blood pressure reading during trauma resuscitations. J Trauma 2010;68(6):1289–94 [discussion: 1294–5].

17. Caputo ND, Kanter M, Fraser R, et al. Comparing biomarkers of traumatic shock: the utility of anion gap, base excess, and serum lactate in the ED. Am J Emerg Med 2015;33(9):1134–9.

18. Alarhayem AQ, Myers JG, Dent D, et al. Time is the enemy: mortality in trauma patients with hemorrhage from torso injury occurs long before the "golden hour". Am J Surg 2016;212(6):1101–5.

19. Harris T, Davenport R, Hurst T, et al. Improving outcome in severe trauma: what's new in ABC? Imaging, bleeding and brain injury. Postgrad Med J 2012;88(1044): 595–603.

20. Meizoso JP, Ray JJ, Karcutskie CA 4th, et al. Effect of time to operation on mortality for hypotensive patients with gunshot wounds to the torso: the golden 10 minutes. J Trauma Acute Care Surg 2016;81(4):685–91.

21. Heffner AC, Swords DS, Neale MN, et al. Incidence and factors associated with cardiac arrest complicating emergency airway management. Resuscitation 2013; 84(11):1500–4.

22. Weingart S. The HOP mnemonic and AirwayWorld.com. 2012; Available at: https://emcrit.org/blogpost/hop-mnemonic/. Accessed February 12, 2017.

23. Shapiro MB, Jenkins DH, Schwab CW, et al. Damage control: collective review. J Trauma 2000;49(5):969–78.

24. Rogers A, Rogers F, Bradburn E, et al. Old and undertriaged: a lethal combination. Am Surg 2012;78(6):711–5.

25. Gruen RL, Brohi K, Schreiber M, et al. Haemorrhage control in severely injured patients. Lancet 2012;380(9847):1099–108.

26. Kirkman E, Watts S. Haemodynamic changes in trauma. Br J Anaesth 2014; 113(2):266–75.

27. Guly HR, Bouamra O, Spiers M, et al. Vital signs and estimated blood loss in patients with major trauma: testing the validity of the ATLS classification of hypovolaemic shock. Resuscitation 2011;82(5):556–9.

28. Mutschler M, Nienaber U, Brockamp T, et al. A critical reappraisal of the ATLS classification of hypovolaemic shock: does it really reflect clinical reality? Resuscitation 2013;84(3):309–13.

29. Fligor SC, Hamill ME, Love KM, et al. Vital signs strongly predict massive transfusion need in geriatric trauma patients. Am Surg 2016;82(7):632–6.

30. Salottolo KM, Mains CW, Offner PJ, et al. A retrospective analysis of geriatric trauma patients: venous lactate is a better predictor of mortality than traditional vital signs. Scand J Trauma Resusc Emerg Med 2013;21:7.

31. Eastridge BJ, Salinas J, McManus JG, et al. Hypotension begins at 110 mm Hg: redefining "hypotension" with data. J Trauma 2007;63(2):291–7 [discussion: 297–9].
32. Parks JK, Elliott AC, Gentilello LM, et al. Systemic hypotension is a late marker of shock after trauma: a validation study of Advanced Trauma Life Support principles in a large national sample. Am J Surg 2006;192(6):727–31.
33. Edelman DA, White MT, Tyburski JG, et al. Post-traumatic hypotension: should systolic blood pressure of 90-109 mmHg be included? Shock 2007;27(2):134–8.
34. Edwards M, Ley E, Mirocha J, et al. Defining hypotension in moderate to severely injured trauma patients: raising the bar for the elderly. Am Surg 2010;76(10): 1035–8.
35. Codner P, Obaid A, Porral D, et al. Is field hypotension a reliable indicator of significant injury in trauma patients who are normotensive on arrival to the emergency department? Am Surg 2005;71(9):768–71.
36. Lipsky AM, Gausche-Hill M, Henneman PL, et al. Prehospital hypotension is a predictor of the need for an emergent, therapeutic operation in trauma patients with normal systolic blood pressure in the emergency department. J Trauma 2006;61(5):1228–33.
37. Shapiro NI, Kociszewski C, Harrison T, et al. Isolated prehospital hypotension after traumatic injuries: a predictor of mortality? J Emerg Med 2003;25(2):175–9.
38. Bilello JF, Davis JW, Lemaster D, et al. Prehospital hypotension in blunt trauma: identifying the "crump factor". J Trauma 2011;70(5):1038–42.
39. Franklin GA, Boaz PW, Spain DA, et al. Prehospital hypotension as a valid indicator of trauma team activation. J Trauma 2000;48(6):1034–7 [discussion: 1037–9].
40. Oyetunji TA, Chang DC, Crompton JG, et al. Redefining hypotension in the elderly: normotension is not reassuring. Arch Surg 2011;146(7):865–9.
41. Deakin CD, Low JL. Accuracy of the advanced trauma life support guidelines for predicting systolic blood pressure using carotid, femoral, and radial pulses: observational study. BMJ 2000;321(7262):673–4.
42. Tseng J, Nugent K. Utility of the shock index in patients with sepsis. Am J Med Sci 2015;349(6):531–5.
43. Reinstadler SJ, Fuernau G, Eitol C, et al. Shock index as a predictor of myocardial damage and clinical outcome in ST-elevation myocardial infarction. Circ J 2016; 80(4):924–30.
44. Pacagnella RC, Souza JP, Durocher J, et al. A systematic review of the relationship between blood loss and clinical signs. PLoS One 2013;8(3):e57594.
45. Mitra B, Fitzgerald M, Chan J. The utility of a shock index ≥ 1 as an indication for pre-hospital oxygen carrier administration in major trauma. Injury 2014;45(1): 61–5.
46. King RW, Plewa MC, Buderer NM, et al. Shock index as a marker for significant injury in trauma patients. Acad Emerg Med 1996;3(11):1041–5.
47. Vandromme MJ, Griffin RL, Kerby JD, et al. Identifying risk for massive transfusion in the relatively normotensive patient: utility of the prehospital shock index. J Trauma 2011;70(2):384–8 [discussion: 388–90].
48. Pandit V, Rhee P, Hashmi A, et al. Shock index predicts mortality in geriatric trauma patients: an analysis of the National Trauma Data Bank. J Trauma Acute Care Surg 2014;76(4):1111–5.
49. Joseph B, Haider A, Ibraheem K, et al. Revitalizing vital signs: the role of delta shock index. Shock 2016;46(3 Suppl 1):50–4.
50. Quinn AC, Sinert R. What is the utility of the focused assessment with sonography in trauma (FAST) exam in penetrating torso trauma? Injury 2011;42(5):482–7.

51. Farahmand N, Sirlin CB, Brown MA, et al. Hypotensive patients with blunt abdominal trauma: performance of screening US. Radiology 2005;235(2):436–43.
52. Stengel D, Rademacher G, Ekkernkamp A, et al. Emergency ultrasound-based algorithms for diagnosing blunt abdominal trauma. Cochrane Database Syst Rev 2015;(9):CD004446.
53. Natarajan B, Gupta PK, Cemaj S, et al. FAST scan: is it worth doing in hemodynamically stable blunt trauma patients? Surgery 2010;148(4):695–700 [discussion: 700–1].
54. Smith J. Focused assessment with sonography in trauma (FAST): should its role be reconsidered? Postgrad Med J 2010;86(1015):285–91.
55. Abdulrahman Y, Musthafa S, Hakim SY, et al. Utility of extended FAST in blunt chest trauma: is it the time to be used in the ATLS algorithm? World J Surg 2015;39(1):172–8.
56. Soult MC, Weireter LJ, Britt RC, et al. Can routine trauma bay chest x-ray be bypassed with an extended focused assessment with sonography for trauma examination? Am Surg 2015;81(4):336–40.
57. Hamada SR, Delhaye N, Kerever S, et al. Integrating eFAST in the initial management of stable trauma patients: the end of plain film radiography. Ann Intensive Care 2016;6(1):62.
58. Wilkerson RG, Stone MB. Sensitivity of bedside ultrasound and supine anteroposterior chest radiographs for the identification of pneumothorax after blunt trauma. Acad Emerg Med 2010;17(1):11–7.
59. Juhl-Olsen P, Vistisen ST, Christiansen LK, et al. Ultrasound of the inferior vena cava does not predict hemodynamic response to early hemorrhage. J Emerg Med 2013;45(4):592–7.
60. Zhang Z, Xu X, Ye S, et al. Ultrasonographic measurement of the respiratory variation in the inferior vena cava diameter is predictive of fluid responsiveness in critically ill patients: systematic review and meta-analysis. Ultrasound Med Biol 2014;40(5):845–53.
61. Sefidbakht S, Assadsangabi R, Abbasi HR, et al. Sonographic measurement of the inferior vena cava as a predictor of shock in trauma patients. Emerg Radiol 2007;14(3):181–5.
62. Schiraldi F, Guiotto G. Base excess, strong ion difference, and expected compensations: as simple as it is. Eur J Emerg Med 2014;21(6):403–8.
63. Juern J, Khatri V, Weigelt J. Base excess: a review. J Trauma Acute Care Surg 2012;73(1):27–32.
64. Ibrahim I, Chor WP, Chue KM, et al. Is arterial base deficit still a useful prognostic marker in trauma? A systematic review. Am J Emerg Med 2016;34(3):626–35.
65. Nguyen HB, Rivers EP, Knoblich BP, et al. Early lactate clearance is associated with improved outcome in severe sepsis and septic shock. Crit Care Med 2004;32(8):1637–42.
66. Marik P, Bellomo R. Lactate clearance as a target of therapy in sepsis: a flawed paradigm. OA Critical Care 2013;1(1):3.
67. Ouellet JF, Roberts DJ, Tiruta C, et al. Admission base deficit and lactate levels in Canadian patients with blunt trauma: are they useful markers of mortality? J Trauma Acute Care Surg 2012;72(6):1532–5.
68. Neville AL, Nemtsev D, Manasrah R, et al. Mortality risk stratification in elderly trauma patients based on initial arterial lactate and base deficit levels. Am Surg 2011;77(10):1337–41.

69. Dekker SE, de Vries HM, Lubbers WD, et al. Lactate clearance metrics are not superior to initial lactate in predicting mortality in trauma. Eur J Trauma Emerg Surg 2016. [Epub ahead of print].

70. Gale SC, Kocik JF, Creath R, et al. A comparison of initial lactate and initial base deficit as predictors of mortality after severe blunt trauma. J Surg Res 2016; 205(2):446–55.

71. Spahn DR, Bouillon B, Cerny V, et al. Management of bleeding and coagulopathy following major trauma: an updated European guideline. Crit Care 2013;17(2): R76.

72. Brohi K, Singh J, Heron M, et al. Acute traumatic coagulopathy. J Trauma 2003; 54(6):1127–30.

73. Frith D, Brohi K. The acute coagulopathy of trauma shock: clinical relevance. Surgeon 2010;8(3):159–63.

74. Veigas PV, Callum J, Rizoli S, et al. A systematic review on the rotational thrombelastometry (ROTEM®) values for the diagnosis of coagulopathy, prediction and guidance of blood transfusion and prediction of mortality in trauma patients. Scand J Trauma Resusc Emerg Med 2016;24(1):114.

75. Hunt H, Stanworth S, Curry N, et al. Thromboelastography (TEG) and rotational thromboelastometry (ROTEM) for trauma induced coagulopathy in adult trauma patients with bleeding. Cochrane Database Syst Rev 2015;(2):CD010438.

76. Levitan R. Timing resuscitation sequence intubation for critically ill patients. 2015. Available at: http://www.acepnow.com/article/timing-resuscitation-sequence-intubation-for-critically-ill-patients/. Accessed February 20, 2017.

77. Moller CT, Schoonbee CG, Rosendorff C. Haemodynamics of cardiac tamponade during various modes of ventilation. Br J Anaesth 1979;51(5):409–15.

78. Faehnrich JA, Noone RB Jr, White WD, et al. Effects of positive-pressure ventilation, pericardial effusion, and cardiac tamponade on respiratory variation in transmitral flow velocities. J Cardiothorac Vasc Anesth 2003;17(1):45–50.

79. Ho AM, Graham CA, Ng CS, et al. Timing of tracheal intubation in traumatic cardiac tamponade: a word of caution. Resuscitation 2009;80(2):272–4.

80. Ploumis A, Yadlapalli N, Fehlings MG, et al. A systematic review of the evidence supporting a role for vasopressor support in acute SCI. Spinal Cord 2010;48(5): 356–62.

81. Stein DM, Pineda JA, Roddy V, et al. Emergency neurological life support: traumatic spine injury. Neurocrit Care 2015;23(Suppl 2):S155–64.

82. Cook TM, Woodall N, Harper J, et al, Fourth National Audit Project. Major complications of airway management in the UK: results of the Fourth National Audit Project of the Royal College of Anaesthetists and the Difficult Airway Society. Part 2: intensive care and emergency departments. Br J Anaesth 2011;106(5):632–42.

83. Ballow SL, Kaups KL, Anderson S, et al. A standardized rapid sequence intubation protocol facilitates airway management in critically injured patients. J Trauma Acute Care Surg 2012;73(6):1401–5.

84. Lyon RM, Perkins ZB, Chatterjee D, et al. Significant modification of traditional rapid sequence induction improves safety and effectiveness of pre-hospital trauma anaesthesia. Crit Care 2015;19:134.

85. Waxman K, Shoemaker WC, Lippmann M. Cardiovascular effects of anesthetic induction with ketamine. Anesth Analg 1980;59(5):355–8.

86. Gelissen HP, Epema AH, Henning RH, et al. Inotropic effects of propofol, thiopental, midazolam, etomidate, and ketamine on isolated human atrial muscle. Anesthesiology 1996;84(2):397–403.

87. Sikorski RA, Koerner AK, Fouche-Weber LY, et al. Choice of general anesthetics for trauma patients. Curr Anesthesiology Rep 2014;4(3):225–32. Available at: https://link.springer.com/article/10.1007/s40140-014-0066-5. Accessed October 26, 2017.
88. Dewhirst E, Frazier WJ, Leder M, et al. Cardiac arrest following ketamine administration for rapid sequence intubation. J Intensive Care Med 2013;28(6):375–9.
89. Heffner AC, Swords DS, Nussbaum ML, et al. Predictors of the complication of postintubation hypotension during emergency airway management. J Crit Care 2012;27(6):587–93.
90. Lippmann M, Appel PL, Mok MS, et al. Sequential cardiorespiratory patterns of anesthetic induction with ketamine in critically ill patients. Crit Care Med 1983; 11(9):730–4.
91. Patanwala AE, Erstad BL, Roe DJ, et al. Succinylcholine is associated with increased mortality when used for rapid sequence intubation of severely brain injured patients in the emergency department. Pharmacotherapy 2016;36(1): 57–63.
92. Welch JL, Seupaul RA. Update: does rocuronium create better intubating conditions than succinylcholine for rapid sequence intubation? Ann Emerg Med 2017; 69(5):e55–6.

Airway Management in Trauma

George Kovacs, MD, MHPE, FRCPC[a,b,c,d],*, Nicholas Sowers, MD, FRCPC[a,d]

KEYWORDS

- Airway • Trauma • Airway management

KEY POINTS

- Airway management in trauma presents numerous unique challenges.
- A safe approach to airway management in trauma requires recognition of these anatomic and physiologic challenges.
- An approach to airway management for these complicated patients is presented based on an assessment of anatomic challenges and optimizing physiologic parameters.

INTRODUCTION

The "ABCs" of trauma resuscitation were born from the assumption that correcting hypoxemia and hypotension reduces morbidity and mortality. Definitive care for severely injured or polytrauma patients includes the ability to provide advanced airway management in a variety of settings: in the emergency department, 20% to 30% intubations are for trauma.[1,2] Airway management in the trauma patient presents numerous unique challenges beyond placement of an endotracheal tube (ETT), with outcomes dependent on the provider's ability to predict and anticipate difficulty and have a safe and executable plan.

DOES EARLY DEFINITIVE TRAUMA AIRWAY MANAGEMENT SAVE LIVES?

Despite significant advances in prehospital care, injury prevention, and the development of trauma systems, early mortality from trauma has essentially remained

Disclosure Statement: The authors have nothing to disclose.
[a] Department of Emergency Medicine, Division of Medical Education, Dalhousie University, 3rd Floor, HI Site, Suite 355, Room 364D, Halifax, Nova Scotia B3H 3A7, Canada; [b] Department of Anaesthesia, Division of Medical Education, Dalhousie University, 3rd Floor, HI Site, Suite 355, Room 364D, Halifax, Nova Scotia B3H 3A7, Canada; [c] Department of Medical Neurosciences, Division of Medical Education, Dalhousie University, 3rd Floor, HI Site, Suite 355, Room 364D, Halifax, Nova Scotia B3H 3A7, Canada; [d] Charles V. Keating Trauma & Emergency Centre, QEII Health Sciences Centre, 1799 Robie Street, Halifax, Nova Scotia B3H 3G1, Canada
* Corresponding author. Charles V. Keating Emergency & Trauma Centre, QEII Health Sciences Centre, 1799 Robie Street, Halifax, Nova Scotia B3H 3G1, Canada.
E-mail address: gkovacs@dal.ca

Emerg Med Clin N Am 36 (2018) 61–84
https://doi.org/10.1016/j.emc.2017.08.006   emed.theclinics.com
0733-8627/18/© 2017 The Authors. Published by Elsevier Inc. This is an open access article under the CC BY-NC-ND license (http://creativecommons.org/licenses/by-nc-nd/4.0/).

unchanged.[3] R. Adams Cowley, founder of Baltimore's Shock Trauma Institute, defined the "golden hour" as a window to arrest the physiologic consequences of severe injury by rapidly transporting trauma patients to definitive care.[4,5] The "stay and play" versus "scoop and run" approach to prehospital trauma care has been a topic of debate since the early 1980s.[6,7] Specific to airway management, there is evidence to support the argument that advanced airway management can be performed in the prehospital setting without delaying transfer to a trauma center.[8,9] More recent data suggest that when performed by skilled emergency medical services (EMS) providers, advanced airway management is associated with a significant decrease in mortality.[9,10] In the hospital setting, delayed intubation is associated with increased mortality in noncritically injured trauma patients.[11]

Conversely, there is a growing body of evidence that prehospital advanced airway management may increase mortality for trauma patients in some circumstances.[8,12–14] How does one reconcile this seemingly conflicting data? Is endotracheal intubation (ETI) for prehospital trauma patients harmful? The answer is, "it depends." The Eastern Association for the Surgery of Trauma (EAST) practice guidelines on ETI immediately following trauma acknowledged the conflicting prehospital data, stating the following:

"No conclusion could be reached regarding prehospital intubation for patients with traumatic brain injury, with or without RSI [rapid sequence intubation]. *Diversity of patient population, differing airway algorithms, various experience among emergency medical service personnel in ETI, and differing reporting make consensus difficult."*[15]

It may be that the technical, procedure-focused management imperative of "getting the tube" is diverting attention away from the physiologic principles of oxygen delivery. Translated physiologically, the ABC priorities of trauma resuscitation are "stop the bleeding, maintain perfusion and oxygenate." Lifesaving oxygenation maneuvers may include a jaw thrust, temporary bag-mask ventilation (BMV), placement of a supraglottic airway device, or ETI. Advanced does not necessarily mean better.

TRAUMA AND THE DIFFICULT AIRWAY

A "difficult airway" is defined as difficulty with laryngoscopy and intubation, BMV, supraglottic device ventilation, and/or front of neck airway (FONA) access.[16,17] Anatomic markers are in general poor predictors of difficulty with airway management, with 90% of difficult intubations unanticipated, prompting debate about the value of trying to predict what is usually unpredictable.[18–21] The pathophysiology of trauma adds an additional layer of complexity and difficulty (**Table 1**).

The "physiologically difficult airway" is used to describe nonanatomic patient factors that can influence the outcome of airway management. Uncorrected hypoxemia, hypocapnia, and hypotension can have devastating consequences in the periintubation period. All trauma patients should have both anatomic and physiologic factors considered, planned for, and ideally corrected as part of their airway plan.[22]

In patients in whom both ETI and rescue oxygenation (bag-mask or supraglottic airway ventilation) are anticipated to be difficult, most existing airway algorithms recommend an "awake" intubation approach, in which the patient maintains spontaneous respiration throughout the procedure. There are a variety of reasons why awake intubation is uncommonly used for the trauma airway, and these are discussed later in this text.

Although the difficult airway is defined with reference to an experienced airway provider with an array of available recourses, other context-related challenges, including human factors, environment, clinician experience, and skill will invariably influence

Table 1
Predictors of difficult airway management in trauma

Difficult Airway	Trauma Related Difficulty	Approach
Difficult laryngoscopy and intubation		
Limited mouth opening/ jaw displacement	Collar/improper MILS Trismus	Open collar/ear-muff MILS
Inability to position	MILS	ELM/bougie/VL
Blood/vomitus	Facial injuries/full stomach, delayed gastric emptying	2 suctions/SALAD approach FONA
Penetrating or blunt neck trauma	Disrupted or distorted airway	Awake primary FIE; if not feasible RSI VL-assisted FIE
Difficult BVM		
Limited jaw thrust	Mandibular fractures	Early SGA use
Poor seal	Facial injuries with swelling, disruption	Early SGA use
Blood/vomitus	Facial injuries/full stomach, delayed gastric emptying	2 suctions/SALAD approach FONA
Penetrating or blunt neck trauma	Distorting subcutaneous emphysema, disrupted airway	Passive oxygen delivery/ minimize PPV
Difficult SGA use		
Blood/vomitus	Facial injuries/full stomach, delayed gastric emptying	2 suctions/SALAD approach FONA
Penetrating or blunt neck trauma	Distorted/disrupted airway	Direct visualization FIE/FONA, low tracheotomy
FONA		
Penetrating or blunt neck trauma	Distorted/disrupted airway CTM not accessible or injury at or below CTM	Low tracheotomy

Abbreviations: BVM, bag-valve-mask; CTM, cricothyroid membrane; ELM, external laryngeal manipulation; FIE, flexible intubating endoscope; FONA, front of neck airway; MILS, manual inline stabilization; PPV, partial-pressure ventilation; RSI, rapid sequence intubation; SALAD, suction-assisted laryngoscopy airway decontamination; SGA, supraglottic airway; VL, video laryngoscopy.

outcomes. Understanding when and why trauma patients may encounter difficulty in airway management can help guide the logistical and mental exercise of developing specific mitigating strategies and contingency planning. A call for help should always be viewed as a patient-focused measure, not a sign of provider weakness.

AIRWAY MANAGEMENT TRAUMA SCENARIOS
The Head-Injured Patient

Traumatic brain injury (TBI) is the most common cause of mortality in trauma patients. Airway management in this cohort of patients is often performed for airway protection. Given the relatively high incidence of peri-intubation desaturation, hypocapnea, and hypotension in emergency intubations, the benefit of ETI for airway protection to prevent aspiration must be weighed against the risk of the occurrence of physiologic adverse events known to increase morbidity and mortality in TBI patients.[23–26] If intubating for the purpose of airway protection, it is usually less time sensitive and should not be rushed. Every precaution should be taken to adequately preoxygenate and resuscitate first.

Apnea resulting from head injury requires immediate intervention. There are 3 mechanisms by which apnea may occur in TBI:

1. Severe or catastrophic brain injury
2. Impact brain apnea (IBA)
3. Loss of consciousness with resultant functional airway obstruction

Severe or catastrophic brain injury is usually nonsurvivable, and associated with early death. Predictions of outcome are usually not made until the patient has undergone a full trauma resuscitation, which often includes ETI. Contrastingly, IBA and functional airway obstruction may be correctable with simple airway opening maneuvers, with or without brief ventilation support. IBA from head trauma results in a primary respiratory arrest without significant parenchymal injury to the brain.[27] In contrast to patients with head injury with functional airway obstruction, patients with IBA do not respond to simple airway opening maneuvers alone, and may require brief ventilation support to prevent secondary hypoxic insult. With appropriate treatment, prognosis is generally good.

Head-injured patients with a decreased level of consciousness frequently receive prehospital advanced airway management.[10] In one series, 30% to 40% of patients are assessed as having partial or complete airway obstruction on EMS arrival.[10] A proportion of these patients will respond to basic maneuvers, and those who do not usually have more severe, less survivable injuries. This observation in part explains the comparatively poor survival rates for trauma patients who are intubated in the prehospital setting.

Management pearls for the patient with traumatic brain injury (TBI)

- Hypoxemia and hypotension during airway management significantly worsens outcomes in patients with TBI.
- Airway management for airway protection should proceed only after adequate measures have been taken to prevent intubation related physiologic disturbances.
- Postintubation hypocapnia is also associated with poor outcomes in patients with TBI and often the result of adrenaline induced overzealous postintubation ventilation.
- Postinjury apnea requiring ventilation support does not necessarily predict poor outcome.

Airway Management in Patients with Suspected Cervical Spine Injuries

Trauma resuscitations typically proceed under the assumption that the patient has an unstable cervical spine (c-spine) injury until proven otherwise. In the prehospital environment, trauma patients are often placed in a cervical spine collar and secured to a rigid backboard with blocks. Although a long-standing tradition in emergency medicine and trauma care, there is very limited published evidence to support the notion that cervical spine collars and immobilization prevent secondary spinal cord injury.[28,29] Although the incidence of c-spine injuries is relatively low (occurring in approximately 2% in the general trauma population and 6%–8% in patients with head and facial trauma), practitioners often operate with deep concern that intubation may cause secondary spinal cord injury, making it one of the most frequently encountered reasons for difficulty in trauma airway management.[30–33]

A frequently studied outcome is the amount of translational or angular movement of the cervical spine caused by airway manipulation. Although it appears that spinal movement occurs to a variable degree depending on the airway technique used, it is unclear whether or not this results in any important differences in clinical outcomes.[34] In cadaveric studies of unstable c-spine injuries, movement occurring with both direct laryngoscopy (DL) and indirect laryngoscopy do not significantly exceed the physiologic values observed with intact spines.[35,36] Despite the need to be cautious, even in patients with known cervical spine injuries, secondary neurologic deterioration is rare, with a reported incidence of 0.03%.[33,37–39]

Trauma patients with suspected spinal injury are typically fully supine, inhibiting the practitioner's ability to optimally position the patient for DL. Manual inline stabilization (MILS) worsens the view obtained with DL in up to 50% of cases.[40] Minimizing challenges with laryngoscopy and intubation mandates proper application of MILS, whereby the provider tasked with this role immobilizes the head and neck without immobilizing the mandible (**Fig. 1**). C-spine collars and improperly applied MILS will restrict mouth opening and tongue and mandibular displacement required for optimal laryngoscopy. Despite properly applied MILS, the provider should still expect a higher occurrence of a poor view with DL, longer intubation times, and more frequent failed intubation attempts.[40] This scenario is often easily managed by applying external laryngeal manipulation or use of a bougie.

Another theoretic concern is that application of MILS results in the need for an increased applied force during laryngoscopy, which paradoxically may lead to more movement during intubation than occurs without MILS.[40,41] Recognizing our inability to correct the fundamental geometric challenge of DL, the provider may opt to use a "look-around-the-corner" indirect device, such as a video laryngoscope with a hyperangulated blade. The 3 classes of video laryngoscopes are described in **Box 1**.[42]

Box 1
Classes of video laryngoscopes

1. Macintosh video laryngoscopy (VL; also known as standard geometry blade) for example, C-MAC (Mac Blade; Karl Storz, Tuttlingen, Germany), McGrath Mac (Mac blade; Medtronic, Minneapolis, MN), GlideScope Titanium Mac (GlideScope, Verathon, WA), Venner APA (Mac blade; Venner Medical, Singapore, Republic of Singapore).

2. Hyperangulated VL (also known as indirect VL), for example, C-MAC (D-Blade), McGrath Mac (X blade) standard GlideScope, KingVision (nonchanneled blade; Ambu, Ballerup, Denmark).

3. Channeled blade VL, for example, King Vision, Pentax AWS (Pentax, Tokyo, Japan), Airtraq (Teleflex Medical, Wayne, PA).

Data from Kovacs G, Law JA. Lights camera action: redirecting videolaryngoscopy. EMCrit. 2016. Available at: https://emcrit.org/blogpost/redirecting-videolaryngoscopy/. Accessed February 25, 2017.

It would seem intuitive that because indirect hyperangulated video laryngoscopy (VL) consistently provides an improved glottic view and that c-spine immobilization consistently impairs the glottic view with DL, that VL is the better choice for trauma patients.[43–45] However, having a good view with VL does not mean that easy ETI will follow.[46] When using a hyperangulated video laryngoscope, a deliberate restricted view may be desired to facilitate the often seemingly frustrating paradox of having a great view of the glottis but not being able to deliver the ETT.[42,46,47]

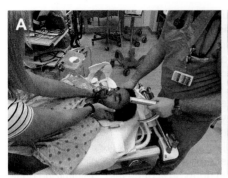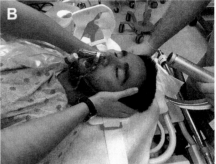

Fig. 1. (*A*) MILS applied incorrectly limiting mandibular range of motion (ROM). (*B*) MILS applied correctly with hands over the ears (ear-muff approach) not limiting mandibular ROM.

Literature comparing intubation devices in c-spine immobilized patients has yielded inconsistent findings, and no consensus as to the optimal approach.[38,44,45,48,49] A recent meta-analysis by Suppan and colleagues[45] reported more failed intubations for DL compared with several alternative intubating devices in patients with c-spine immobilization. Although the investigators acknowledge the weaknesses of available literature, they note there was no statistically significant difference in first-attempt success between the more commonly used VL devices (GlideScope, C-MAC) and DL.[45] It is less likely that there is a "the right device" for the unstable c-spine and more important is the right experienced practitioner, using a device with which he or she is the most comfortable.[50,51]

Airway management in the patient with a possible c-spine injury must strike a balance between minimizing movement and the need to quickly and successfully intubate on first attempt, thereby minimizing the harm of hypoxemia that may be associated with multiple attempts at intubation.[52] It seems reasonable to consider that if the patient's spinal cord has survived the massive forces of the crash, as well as repositioning during extrication and immobilization, that the chances that movement occurring during *controlled* airway management will result in cord injury is extremely low. As suggested by Aprahamian and colleagues,[33,53] the primary benefit of a rigid cervical collar is to serve as a reminder about the potential existence of an unstable c-spine injury.

Management pearls for patients with unstable cervical spine injuries

- Imaging should not delay airway management and assume all trauma patients have unstable cervical spines.
- The provider should optimally use the intubation device he or she is most experienced with.
- Be prepared for a poor view with direct laryngoscopy (DL) and always have a bougie ready for use.
- Rigid cervical collars must be opened or removed and replaced by properly applied manual inline stabilization (MILS).
- Properly applied MILS should avoid immobilization of the mandible.
- If using a hyperangulated video laryngoscope, a deliberate restricted glottic view may facilitate difficult ETT advancement.

The Contaminated Airway

The presence of airway contamination with either blood or vomitus has been shown to decrease the rate of first-attempt intubation success, regardless of the device used.[54] Blood and vomit in the airway can lead to early and late complications related to difficult airway management and/or aspiration. The bloody airway is not uncommon in trauma patients with injuries to the face and/or neck and may range in severity from scant bleeding, which is easily managed, to significant hemorrhage. The combination of altered levels of consciousness, diminished protective airway reflexes, delayed gastric emptying, and full stomachs place trauma patients at high risk of vomiting and aspiration during airway management. Management of contaminated airway must begin with the expectation that the degree of blood, vomit, and secretions appreciated externally represents only a fraction of what may be encountered on initiation of an RSI. As such, providers must ensure that adequate suction is available (at least 2 large rigid suction catheters). Consideration must be given to positioning, placing the patient in reverse Trendelenburg or, if safe to do so, seated upright or even leaning forward to allow drainage of blood and secretions. For c-spine immobilized patients, suction must be immediately within reach, and restraints securing the patient to the bed should be avoided. During the preoxygenation phase, positive-pressure ventilation (PPV) should be used only if necessary balanced against the patient's oxygenation status, as ventilatory pressures of 20 cm H2O or more are likely to ventilate the stomach, increasing the risk of regurgitation and aspiration.

When blood or vomitus is overwhelming suction capabilities, the provider may place either one rigid suction or an ETT in the upper esophagus to divert the offending contaminants. The ETT or rigid suction may then be stabilized to the left of the laryngoscope and the second suction used during laryngoscopy in search of the epiglottis (**Fig. 2**). Often the epiglottis may be "lifted" (more easily accomplished in a reverse Trendelenburg) out of the contaminant during laryngoscopy, providing an anatomic reference for placing a bougie.

Most of the literature comparing DL with VL in the bloody or vomitus-filled airway is simulation-based, and concern exists about the vulnerability of VL camera lens in the contaminated airway.[55,56] Recently, Sakles and colleagues[54] retrospectively reviewed

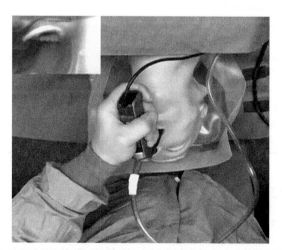

Fig. 2. Suction in upper esophagus stabilized to left of laryngoscope (SALAD approach). (*Courtesy of* Ruben Strayer, MD.)

more than 4600 intubations and demonstrated that, although airway contamination was associated with a decreased first-attempt success rate, this was irrespective of the choice of GlideScope or DL as the first-attempt device used. The use of DL or Macintosh VL, in which a direct approach can be used if the camera is obscured with the aid of a bougie, may be preferred approaches.

Although not studied in a clinical setting, the Ducanto suction-assisted laryngoscopy airway decontamination (SALAD) approach has gained acceptance as a method to manage the soiled airway.[57,58] In the uncommon circumstance in which blood or vomit is overwhelming these management strategies, intubation is not possible and the patient is critically desaturating, rescue oxygenation with a BVM (bag-valve-mask) or SGA (supraglottic airway) is unlikely to work and an FONA approach is indicated.

Ducanto suction-assisted laryngoscopy airway decontamination approach to managing massive airway contamination

- Use rigid large-bore suction to initially decontaminate
- Perform laryngoscopy keeping blade superior against tongue away from fluid
- Advance suction tip into upper esophagus then wedge in place to left of the laryngoscope
- Use second suction as needed
- Rotate laryngoscope blade 30 degrees to the left to open blade channel
- Place endotracheal tube (ETT), inflate the cuff

Management pearls for the patient with the contaminated airway

- Have at least 2 large-bore rigid suction catheters.
- Consider alternative options for hemorrhage control (sutures, packing, epistaxis kit).
- Minimize positive-pressure ventilation (PPV) and use a monometer for provider feedback when mask ventilation is indicated.
- Look for epiglottis as an important landmark for glottis and have a bougie prepared for use with DL.
- If a VL is considered the best option, Macintosh VL may be the preferred device, as it may be used directly if contamination obstructs camera.
- Consider esophageal ETT diversion connected to suction.
- Suction-assisted laryngoscopy airway decontamination (SALAD) approach.
- If intubation fails and patient is desaturating, front of neck airway (FONA) rescue oxygenation approach is indicated.

The Uncooperative or Agitated Patient

Uncooperative, violent, or agitated patients can encumber adequate assessment, leading to missed injuries and inadequate resuscitation. Agitation can be multifactorial and may be the result of head injury, hypoperfusion, hypoxemia, or intoxication. It may not be clear why a patient is agitated and providers must determine if the patient is agitated *AND* injured or agitated *BECAUSE* the patient is injured.

The EAST guidelines recommend that aggressive behavior refractory to initial pharmacologic intervention is a discretionary indication for intubation; specifically that if a patient's level of agitation prevents assessment and resuscitation, intubation and sedation should follow.[15] Sise and colleagues[59] reviewed 1078 trauma patients intubated for discretionary indications (eg, agitation, alcohol intoxication) and found that 62% of patients, once investigated, had a significant head injury. Importantly, there was no significant difference in complications associated with acute airway management in patients intubated for discretionary indications, as compared with those intubated for higher acuity reasons.[59]

In severely agitated patients, RSI is at times undertaken before optimal hemodynamic resuscitation and preoxygenation has been achieved. Patients rendered apneic as part of an RSI without adequate preoxygenation are at high risk of desaturation. The use of ketamine to facilitate cooperation and allow interventions including preoxygenation has been described as "delayed-sequence intubation" by Weingart and colleagues.[60] If given slowly, a dissociative intravenous dose of 1 to 1.5 mg/kg poses little risk of respiratory depression. However, the use of any sedative, particularly in the presence of other intoxicating ingestions, may inhibit airway reflexes. Concerns that ketamine may raise intracranial pressure and worsen outcomes in TBI is not supported by evidence.[61,62]

Management pearls in the agitated trauma patient

- Agitation may be a symptom of traumatic pathology.
- Agitated patients may require facilitated cooperation to ensure adequate preoxygenation.
- Ketamine is an appropriate agent to facilitate cooperation in agitated patients in preparation for airway management.
- Always be prepared to provide definitive airway intervention before administering sedation.

Maxillofacial Injuries

Maxillofacial fractures may present dramatically and affect airway management in one of several ways.[63] Posterior displacement from fractured maxillofacial segments may cause soft tissue collapse and occlude the airway, which may be worsened by the presence of c-spine collar.[64,65] Bleeding may be significant and cause airway management challenges, as previously discussed. In the supine position, the pooling of blood in the oropharynx may stimulate a gag response or vomiting, which in turn may worsen bleeding. Although patients with mandibular fractures in 2 or more locations may be easier to intubate due to increased mobility of the mandible and attached soft tissues, associated condylar fractures may cause a mechanical obstruction limiting mouth opening, making laryngoscopy and intubation difficult.[64,66] Maxillofacial fractures may also cause trismus that may resolve with the neuromuscular blockade; however, differentiating this from a mechanical obstruction before intubation is required and is often difficult.

Airway management begins with careful consideration to patient positioning. Awake, neurologically intact patients without neck pain should be allowed to position themselves however they are most comfortable to control tissue obstruction and allow drainage of blood and secretions. They may be given a rigid suction catheter to use themselves, which is more often tolerated, effective, and less likely to stimulate a gag and resultant vomiting. Adherence to protocols requiring rigid spinal immobilization and supine positioning may result in catastrophe.

The provider should presume that preoxygenation in patients with facial trauma may be difficult, and that reoxygenation with mask ventilation during RSI if the first attempt is unsuccessful may be difficult or impossible. Distortion of facial structures may make obtaining a seal with a BVM device difficult and patients may poorly tolerate PPV, as disruption of tissues may result in worsening bleeding and in cases of associated lower airway trauma, significant subcutaneous emphysema. Practitioners must proceed with the assumption that structural collapse of the airway may occur during an RSI.

The choice of approach is based on the patient's ability to maintain a patent airway and their oxygenation status. For a "have no time" scenario (obstructing and hypoxemic), the primary approach may require a FONA, facilitated by a dissociative ketamine dosing. Alternatively, a "double set-up" may be used: RSI with a single attempt at oral intubation followed immediately by FONA rescue if needed (**Fig. 3**).

If the patient is maintaining adequate oxygenation, the clinician should proceed with a focused physical examination to assess the specific pattern of facial injury and plan accordingly. For example, swelling and tenderness at the temporomandibular joints suggests the presence of condylar factures and the possibility of mechanical trismus. Because anticipated difficulty in patients with facial trauma may involve challenges with intubation, mask ventilation, and possibly supraglottic airway rescue, preservation of spontaneous respiration during attempts to secure the airway should be considered. These patients may be best served when feasible by an "awake" approach with a laryngoscope or flexible intubating endoscope (FIE) or in selected cases a primary FONA.

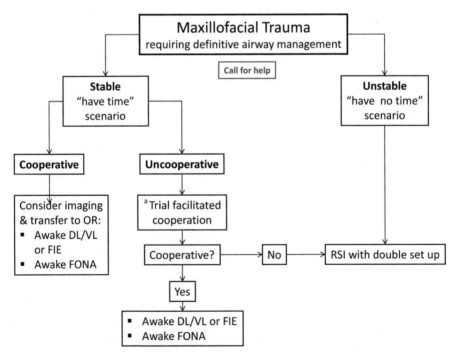

Fig. 3. Approach to maxillofacial trauma. OR, operating room. [a] Facilitated cooperation using ketamine. (*Adapted from* Mercer SJ, Jones CP, Bridge M, et al. Systematic review of the anaesthetic management of non-iatrogenic acute adult airway trauma. Br J Anaesth 2016;117(Suppl 1):i55; with permission.)

Management pearls for the patient with facial injuries
• These patients require careful assessment of damaged anatomy recognizing the unique airway complications associated with facial fractures.
• Both laryngoscopy and mask ventilation may be challenging and a double set-up should be prepared for when rapid sequence intubation (RSI) is the chosen approach.
• An awake approach, although not always practical, should be considered.
• Management of aggressive bleeding should be anticipated.
• Allow patients to assume a position of comfort when safe to do so.

The Traumatized Airway

Airway management for the patient with a primary injury to the larynx or trachea is a high-stakes scenario, in which the loss of a stable airway can happen rapidly and with little warning. Suspicion of a traumatized airway should initiate a call for help to an experienced colleague.

Primary airway trauma is relatively uncommon in the civilian urban setting, with a reported incidence of less than 1% (0.4% for blunt and 4.5% for penetrating injuries).[67] Accordingly, practitioners have infrequent or limited experience in managing these patients and existing management guidelines for care of these patients are mostly based on expert opinion.[68]

Clinical findings suggestive of significant laryngotracheal airway injury include dysphagia, hoarseness, stridor, bleeding in the upper airway, subcutaneous emphysema, expanding hematoma, or in open penetrating injuries, obvious disruption of the larynx or trachea. If airway injury is suspected, aggressive PPV should be avoided. PPV in the setting of airway disruption can create or worsen pneumothorax, pneumomediastinum, or subcutaneous emphysema. Massive subcutaneous emphysema can distort airway anatomy, further complicating management. A potentially catastrophic complication is the conversion of a partial tracheal transection into a complete transection with the force of blindly passing an ETT or a bougie, particularly if relying on distal "hold-up" to confirm placement.[68,69]

For patients with known or suspected airway injury, the safest way to facilitate ETI is placement of the ETT under direct visualization, ideally from the oropharynx to the carina using an FIE.[68,70] Mercer and colleagues[68] described an approach to managing patients with suspected laryngotracheal injury (**Fig. 4**). In the "have time" scenario in the patient who is oxygenating with minimal assistance, awake, and cooperative, the airway can be approached either from above after adequate topicalization, using a FIE, or infraglottically with a FONA approach (most commonly an awake tracheostomy) depending on the location of the injury.

Careful titration of ketamine is often desirable to improve comfort and cooperation while maintaining airway reflexes. Use of an FIE allows both a diagnostic and therapeutic advantage: visualizing the specific pattern of injury, and facilitating careful ETT placement, while avoiding conversion to a complete transection. If an area of partial injury is identified, the FIE can be advanced distally and used as a guide to ensure safe advancement of the ETT beyond the site of injury.

In a "have no time" situation with a deteriorating patient in whom an RSI is considered the only viable option, a double set-up is mandatory, recognizing that the level of airway breach will influence whether FONA can occur through the cricothyroid membrane or if a tracheostomy is required. One option to improve visual navigation past the airway injury is to use a VL-assisted flexible endoscopic intubation.[71] In this

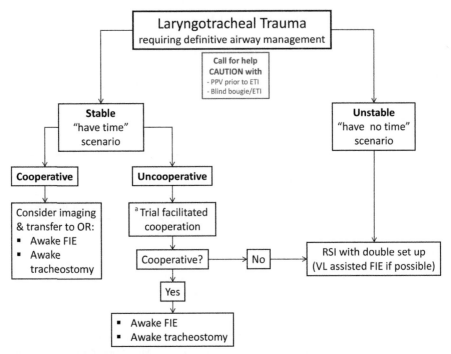

Fig. 4. Approach to laryngotracheal trauma. [a] Facilitated cooperation using ketamine. (*Adapted from* Mercer SJ, Jones CP, Bridge M, et al. Systematic review of the anaesthetic management of non-iatrogenic acute adult airway trauma. Br J Anaesth 2016;117(Suppl 1):i56; with permission.)

scenario, an RSI is initiated in the usual fashion and a VL is used to control soft tissues and obtain a view of the glottic inlet. A flexible intubating endoscope is then advanced through the vocal cords with the visual aid of VL distally to the carina facilitating inspection of the airway, and the ETT is advanced over the FIE into position.

Management pearls for the patient with a primary airway injury

- Decompensation in the patient with a traumatized airway may be rapid and catastrophic.

- PPV should be avoided if possible.

- An awake approach with appropriate topicalization is the preferred approach.

- If an RSI is chosen, a double set-up with a FONA plan for accessing the trachea based on the level of the airway breach.

- ETT placement should ideally be performed with visualization of the airway using a flexible intubating endoscope (FIE).

- Advanced techniques using FIE either primarily in an awake patient or assisted by VL when an RSI is chosen are recommended when resources and skill are available.

THE AWAKE INTUBATION

A successful awake intubation is dependent on careful patient selection, and, in particular, identifying anatomic, pathologic, or physiologic features that would make RSI problematic. There are several specific patient populations, including the burn patient and the patient with penetrating neck injuries, in whom an awake intubation may be the approach of choice, as a strategy to mitigate both predicted difficulty and anticipated dynamic changes in airway anatomy and physiology.

The awake intubation is a "have time" approach, involving placement of an ETT following adequate topicalization in a patient who is able to maintain spontaneous respirations. It is not device-specific and can be performed using DL, VL, or an FIE. Success with awake intubation is dependent on meticulous airway topicalization, and in general requires an awake and cooperative patient.[72,73] The use of sedation is not routine, and has been associated with increased awake intubation failures.[74] Specifically, sedation should never be used in place of adequate airway topicalization. A difficult airway paradox exists here: patients identified as difficult are selected to undergo a technically more challenging awake approach, a procedure that is performed infrequently by most emergency physicians. There is no simple answer to this resource, skill availability dilemma. It is our opinion that physicians who are responsible for acute airway management should acquire and maintain the skills required for awake intubation, as it can be a lifesaving approach in a specific subset of dynamic airway situations.

RAPID SEQUENCE INTUBATION

RSI involves the rapid administration of an induction agent and a neuromuscular blocking agent in quick succession to facilitate ETT placement in a patient who is presumed to have a full stomach. RSI is the most common approach for airway management in trauma.[75,76] Oxygenation with or without ventilation during the procedure (referred to by some as a "modified" RSI) is considered standard by most acute care practitioners.[77–79] Historically, the application of cricoid pressure (CP) to prevent passive aspiration has been considered an essential component of an RSI. However, its routine use remains controversial, with some evidence suggesting it may make various aspects of airway management more challenging. If cricoid pressure is being applied and the practitioner experiences difficulty with laryngoscopy, intubation, or ventilation, CP should be immediately discontinued.[80,81]

Hemodynamic instability and hypoxemia must be aggressively managed before attempting RSI.[22,23] The "rapid" part of an RSI refers to the delivery of the induction drug and neuromuscular blocking agent, and is not meant to imply a hurried or rushed process. RSI in underresuscitated patients may result in unintended poor outcomes, including critical hypoxemia and circulatory collapse.[82,83] The term "resuscitative sequence intubation" has been suggested as a more representative term used to describe the preparation and optimization of the patient's physiologic status before definitive airway management.[84]

Preparation

Numerous preparatory airway acronyms and checklists have been proposed to reduce errors and adverse events associated with RSI.[85,86] Although evidence of outcome benefit may be lacking, based on an increased understanding of the role of human factors in contributing to adverse airway outcomes, it seems a reasonable recommendation that an airway checklist be used in the preparation phase of trauma airway management.[87–91] In general, checklists should be simple, use terminology that is clearly understood by the entire team, and can be performed rapidly (**Fig. 5**).

Optimizing Hemodynamics

Hemodynamic instability in trauma is most commonly caused by hypovolemia due to hemorrhage. Intravascular depletion shifts the gradient between right atrial pressure

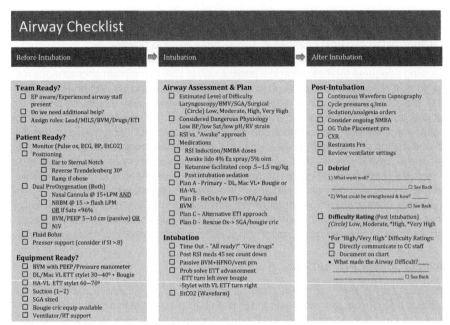

Airway Checklist

Before Intubation ⇒	Intubation ⇒	After Intubation

Team Ready?
- ☐ EP aware/Experienced airway staff present
- ☐ Do we need additional help?
- ☐ Assign roles: Lead/MILS/BVM/Drugs/ETI

Patient Ready?
- ☐ Monitor (Pulse ox, ECG, BP, EtCO2)
- ☐ Positioning
  - ☐ Ear to Sternal Notch
  - ☐ Reverse Trendelenberg 30°
  - ☐ Ramp if obese
- ☐ Dual PreOxygenation (Both)
  - ☐ Nasal Cannula @ 15+LPM AND
  - ☐ NRBM @ 15 -> flush LPM
    OR If Sats <96%
  - ☐ BVM/PEEP 5–10 cm (passive) OR
  - ☐ NIV
- ☐ Fluid Bolus
- ☐ Pressor support (consider if SI >.8)

Equipment Ready?
- ☐ BVM with PEEP/Pressure manometer
- ☐ DL/Mac VL ETT stylet 30–40° + Bougie
- ☐ HA-VL ETT stylet 60–70°
- ☐ Suction (1–2)
- ☐ SGA sized
- ☐ Bougie cric equip available
- ☐ Ventilator/RT support

Airway Assessment & Plan
- ☐ Estimated Level of Difficulty
  Laryngoscopy/BMV/SGA/Surgical
  (Circle) Low, Moderate, High, Very High
- ☐ Considered Dangerous Physiology
  Low BP/low Sat/low pH/RV strain
- ☐ RSI vs. "Awake" approach
- ☐ Medications
  - ☐ RSI Induction/NMBA doses
  - ☐ Awake lido 4% Ez spray/5% oint
  - ☐ Ketamine facilitated coop .5–1.5 mg/kg
  - ☐ Post intubation sedation
- ☐ Plan A - Primary - DL, Mac VL+ Bougie or HA-VL
- ☐ Plan B - ReOx b/w ETI-> OPA/2-hand BVM
- ☐ Plan C - Alternative ETI approach
- ☐ Plan D - Rescue Ox-> SGA/bougie cric

Intubation
- ☐ Time Out – "All ready?" "Give drugs"
- ☐ Post RSI meds 45 sec count down
- ☐ Passive BVM+HFNO/vent prn
- ☐ Prob solve ETT advancement
  -ETT turn left over bougie
  -Stylet with VL ETT turn right
- ☐ EtCO2 (Waveform)

Post-Intubation
- ☐ Continuous Waveform Capnography
- ☐ Cycle pressures q3min
- ☐ Sedation/analgesia orders
- ☐ Consider ongoing NMBA
- ☐ OG Tube Placement prn
- ☐ CXR
- ☐ Restraints Prn
- ☐ Review ventilator settings

- ☐ **Debrief**
  1) What went well? _____
  _____ ☐ See Back
  *2) What could be strengthened & how? _____
  _____ ☐ See Back
- ☐ **Difficulty Rating** (Post Intubation)
  (Circle) Low, Moderate, *High, *Very High

  *For "High/Very High" Difficulty Ratings:
  - ☐ Directly communicate to CC staff
  - ☐ Document on chart
  - What made the Airway Difficult?____
  _____ ☐ See Back

Fig. 5. Intubation checklist example. BP, blood pressure; BVM: bag-valve mask; CXR, chest radiograph; DL: direct laryngoscope; ETI: endotracheal intubation; ETT: endotracheal tube; HFNO: high flow nasal oxygen; LPM: leters per minute; MILS: manual in-line stabilization; NIV: non-invasive ventilation; NMBA: neuromuscular blocking agent; NRBM: non-rebreather mask; OG: orogastric; pulse ox, pulse oximetry. ReOx: reoxygenation; SGA: supraglottic airway; SI: shock index (SBP/HR); VL: video laryngoscope. (*From* SaferAirway. org Toolkit (Emergency Medicine Associates, Germantown, Maryland); with permission.)

and mean systemic pressure, reducing preload and subsequently mean arterial pressure. The transition to PPV, either through a closed system BVM with an attached with positive end-expiratory pressure (PEEP) valve or with mechanical ventilation once intubated, abruptly increases the intrathoracic pressure, further shifting this gradient.

Postintubation hypotension is defined as a systolic blood pressure (SBP) <90 mm Hg or a mean arterial pressure <65 mm Hg within 30 minutes of intubation.[92] Inadequate resuscitation of hemorrhagic shock, transition to PPV, loss of sympathetic drive associated with general anesthesia, and the hemodynamic effect of many induction drugs are all contributing factors. The incidence of post intubation hypotension is high in patients requiring emergency airway management (23%–46%), which is important because even transient drops in blood pressure are associated with adverse outcomes in trauma patients.[23,92–94] Patients with a shock index (defined as heart rate divided by SBP) of greater than 0.8 are at particular risk of developing significant hypotension in the postintubation period.[82,95,96] The combination of hypoxemia and hypotension is additive, with an adjusted odds of death double that of the increased mortality associated with either event alone.[23,97,98]

Early use of blood products is recommended when the etiology of shock in trauma is believed to be from hemorrhage. Vasopressors have traditionally been avoided in trauma based on concerns that they may worsen bleeding. During the peri-intubation phase, early aggressive use of blood products and hemorrhage control measures (splinting, pelvic binding) should remain the mainstay of resuscitation efforts. Careful use of vasopressors should be strongly considered in at-risk head-injured patients to prevent or manage postintubation hypotension. Sustained vasopressor use by infusion beyond the immediate peri-intubation period may be required to mitigate the effects of PPV, postparalysis sedation, and ongoing losses unresponsive to fluid and blood product replacement.

All commonly used induction agents will cause hypotension, particularly when a full dose is administered to a volume-constricted patient. Dosage recommendations for RSI induction agents are largely based on patients without hemodynamic instability. As such, in trauma patients with hypotension or a shock index greater than 0.8, it seems prudent that the dose of the induction agent be reduced by at least 50%.[83,91,95,99] In North America, etomidate has been the most commonly used induction agent used for RSI. Owing to the association between using etomidate and adrenal suppression, many institutions have moved to alternative induction agents.[1,100] With a favorable hemodynamic profile and strong analgesic effect, ketamine is quickly becoming the preferred induction agent for trauma patients.[100] A study comparing standard full-dose ketamine with etomidate in trauma patients showed no survival benefit of one agent over the other.[100] In light of this, it is probably true to suggest that *the dose of the drug is more important than the choice of drug.*

Paralysis should have no direct effect on the patient's hemodynamic status, and in hypoperfused states their dose should be increased. There is some debate regarding which neuromuscular blocking agent is superior for an RSI: both succinylcholine and rocuronium may be safely used and can provide good intubating conditions.[101] It should be emphasized, however, that administering too small a dose (<1.0 mg/kg) of rocuronium, particularly in low-flow states, will result in inadequate intubating conditions and a larger dose is recommended (1.2–1.6 mg/kg).[101,102] Although clinicians may be weary of the prolonged effect of high-dose rocuronium in potentially difficult airway cases, extended, deep paralysis is in fact desirable in this circumstance, as it helps to create optimal conditions for laryngoscopy, BVM and SGA ventilation, and FONA. Having the sick trauma patient wake up to a state that he or she will be able rescue his or her own airway is simply not realistic, and will make efforts to secure the airway even more difficult.

Management of peri-intubation hemodynamic instability

- Resuscitation using blood products (packed red blood cells/massive transfusion) should be done early in the preintubation phase of trauma management.
- In selected scenarios consider the use of vasopressors during the peri-intubation phase.
- Reduce the dose of all induction agents by at least 50% and increase the dose of the paralytic.

Avoiding Hypoxemia

Hypoxemia during emergency department (ED) RSI is common, occurring in more than one-third of cases.[24] Proceeding with an RSI in a patient who is already hypoxemic can result in catastrophic complications. Patients with preintubation oxygen saturations of less than 95% are at risk of abrupt desaturation within 90 seconds of the onset of apnea.[103] Although recent literature has focused on extending safe apnea time with passive high-flow nasal oxygenation (HFNO) with or without noninvasive ventilation, the most important determinant of time to desaturation remains preoxygenation status.[104]

Although high oxygen saturation is reassuring, it is not a true measurement of oxygen reserve. Furthermore, oxygen saturation alone provides little information about the true safe apnea time, which is defined by the relationship between oxygen reserve and the rate of oxygen consumption. Effective management of the preoxygenation phase requires both increasing the patient's oxygen reserve while simultaneously decreasing the rate of oxygen consumption through aggressive resuscitation. Increasing the oxygen reserve has 3 components: denitrogenation of the lungs, recruitment of alveoli with PEEP, and apneic oxygenation.

Denitrogenation is the primary physiologic mechanism of preoxygenation and is dependent on delivery of a high concentration of oxygen, resulting in a 10-fold increase available oxygen. Increased functional residual capacity (FRC) provides an ongoing reservoir to keep hemoglobin saturated. Delivery of close to 100% oxygen for approximately 4 minutes is required to denitrogenate normal lungs and may be most easily accomplished with high-flow, "flush-rate" (40 LPM) oxygen using a conventional non-rebreather mask.[105] In patients with a high minute ventilation or shunt physiology, a closed system BVM with a PEEP valve and a tight-fitting mask is the preferred preoxygenation technique. If respiratory effort support is required, this is best achieved using a mechanical (NIV) as opposed to manual ventilator (BVM).

With atelectasis, pulmonary contusion, and other lung pathologies, the FRC is diminished and the resultant shunt physiology renders preoxygenation with a high Fio_2 less effective in preventing desaturation.[106–108] Alveolar recruitment using an oxygen delivery device with PEEP is necessary to help mitigate the negative effects of shunt physiology. A PEEP valve should be considered standard when using a BVM for preoxygenation, as it will prevent entrainment in BVMs without a dedicated expiratory valve. A PEEP valve attached to a BVM and applied over conventional nasal prongs at high flow ($\geq$15 LPM) in a spontaneously breathing patient will produce continuous positive airway pressure–like conditions. Assisted ventilations are best delivered using a dedicated noninvasive ventilator; however, can be performed with the same BVM/PEEP, nasal cannula combination. It is advisable to use a pressure manometer attached to the BVM when using this combination to minimize high pressures that may result in gastric distention and aspiration.

Alveolar oxygen delivery that continues without respiratory effort is referred to as apneic oxygenation (AO). AO is facilitated by the pressure gradient between the oropharynx and the alveoli created by the differential uptake of oxygen and delivery of CO2 to and from the alveoli, resulting in the passive transfer of oxygen.[104,107] By continuously replenishing the FRC oxygen stores, apneic oxygenation using conventional or specialized nasal prongs to administer high-flow oxygen (10–70 LPM) may extend the safe apnea time after an RSI.[103,104] Numerous studies have evaluated to effectiveness of HFNO as an adjunct to preoxygenation for RSI, and the balance of evidence suggest the procedure as both safe and effective.[104]

Of note, the ability to extend the safe apnea time must not allow providers to become cavalier and should not encourage prolonged intubation attempts.[106,109] By the time peripheral oxygen saturation begins to fall, cerebral hypoxemia has already occurred, a phenomenon known as "pulse-ox lag."[103] Effective situation awareness is required, even (and perhaps especially) when supporting gas exchange by way of passive oxygenation, to stay within the "safe apnea" zone.

Preoxygenation: "the rule of 2s"

- Elevate the head (ear to sternum) and the bed greater than 20° (reverse Trendelenburg).
- Two sources of oxygen for all critically ill patients: high-flow nasal prongs $\geq$15 L/min and NRB/bag-mask ventilation $\geq$15 L/min.
- Two approaches for obstruction: OPA with a jaw thrust for soft tissue obstruction.

- Two attachments for your BVM: positive end-expiratory pressure valve and pressure manometer.
- Two hands on all face masks: to ensure closed system oxygenation and ventilation and perform an aggressive jaw thrust.
- Two providers: the most experienced obtaining a tight mask seal and aggressive jaw thrust giving feedback to the provider squeezing the bag to avoid overventilation and hyperventilation.

Abbreviations: BVM, bag-valve-mask; NRB, non-rebreather mask; OPA, oropharyngeal airway.

FRONT OF NECK AIRWAY TO SECURE THE AIRWAY

Numerous methods are used to access the trachea infraglottically, and the terminology describing the procedure is as variable as the techniques available to do so. Perhaps most accurate is the new term "front of neck airway" (FONA), which eliminates ambiguous verbiage like "surgical airway" or "airway rescue."[110] Although rare (0.05%–1.7% of ED-based intubations), the decision to perform FONA must begin during the initial assessment of the patient's airway, long before the "cannot intubate cannot oxygenate" (CICO) scenario is encountered.[111] This begins with a pre-procedure briefing with team members to define clear triggers for moving ahead with the procedure. Palpation of the anterior neck, and perhaps even marking the anticipated location of the cricothyroid membrane should be done routinely for all emergency airway cases and equipment should be both familiar to team members and immediately available.

Cognitive and team-based preparation is vital, as the decision to proceed with a FONA is often delayed until critical hypoxemia has occurred.[111] It is widely speculated that the most significant delay is often the result of hesitant decision-making and a reluctance to perform a rarely encountered procedure.[112] Open discussion of the emergency surgical airway as a potential outcome familiarizes the team and normalizes the procedure, shifting from the negative connotation of the "failed airway" to the recognition of the ultimately inevitable surgical airway.[113] By normalizing the procedure, at least cognitively, we aim to reduce the psychological distress associated with it.

No specific oxygen saturation level should be used as a trigger to perform FONA, recognizing that a failed oxygenation situation is dynamic and characterized by a rapidly falling oxygen saturation despite maximal efforts to reoxygenate the patient.[111] Failed intubation followed by difficult mask ventilation with falling saturations represents an impending FONA that should be initiated after a single rescue attempt with supraglottic airway device. In rare situations, FONA may be the first and only invasive airway technique attempted, even in the setting of normal oxygen saturation; for example, massive facial trauma disrupting all recognizable airway landmarks. This "surgically inevitable" airway needs to be identified and declared early, such that time is not wasted on fruitless efforts to intubate "from above."

There are several options for the emergency FONA and there remains some controversy regarding the preferred approach. Historically, methods such as transtracheal jet ventilation and percutaneous cricothyroidotomy with a Seldinger technique, have been advocated. However, recent reviews have shown that complications associated with jet ventilation are unacceptably high and wire-guided approaches are not as easy or successful as once believed.[114–117]

There has been a recent push to adopt a modified open technique using a scalpel, finger, and bougie (the "scalpel-bougie" technique). The 2015 Difficult Airway Society guidelines recommend that all clinicians responsible for airway management be able to perform a FONA, and that the scalpel-bougie technique is the technique of choice.[89] The scalpel-bougie technique has several advantages for the emergency clinician: it relies on gross motor skills (which are more likely to be preserved during periods of acute stress), uses familiar equipment (scalpel, bougie, and a #6 ETT), and has a minimal number of steps.

The body of evidence for this rarely needed procedure is (and will likely remain) limited, yet all clinicians need to be mentally and technically prepared to rapidly perform front of neck access to secure the airway. Success for high-acuity, low-opportunity events like this requires frequent, deliberate practice using simulation.[118] FONA trainers need not be expensive or complicated; motor habit can be developed using simple models with Venturi oxygen tubing or an empty roll of bathroom tissue.

SUMMARY

Effective trauma care requires a team approach, with resuscitation priorities clearly communicated and interventions guided by the physiologic priorities that ensure adequate oxygen delivery. Although ensuring oxygenation and ventilation are priorities, airway management as the technical imperative of putting the "tube in the hole" must not overshadow other resuscitative elements.

Providing advanced airway management is part of the A *and* B *and* C parallel resuscitative priorities of trauma care. Safely managing both the anticipated and unanticipated difficult airway requires technical expertise; however, decisions of when and how to intervene are equally important determinants of outcome. Airway management in trauma begins as soon as patient contact is made and rarely starts with placement of an ETT. Gaining intravenous access, beginning fluid resuscitation, and applying oxygen may be lifesaving and/or bridging interventions that allow for the safe execution of downstream more definitive procedures. Whether the team is a doctor, nurse, and transporting paramedics or a group of 10, success is dependent on a shared understanding of the importance of resuscitation before intubation and clear communication of what and when various airway interventions will be performed. Then, securing the airway will have the best chance of making a positive difference in trauma patient outcomes.

REFERENCES

1. Brown CA, Bair AE, Pallin DJ, et al. NEAR III Investigators. Techniques, success, and adverse events of emergency department adult intubations. Ann Emerg Med 2015;65(4):363–70.e1.
2. Kerslake D, Oglesby AJ, Di Rollo N, et al. Tracheal intubation in an urban emergency department in Scotland: a prospective, observational study of 3738 intubations. Resuscitation 2015;89:20–4.
3. Pieters BMA, Wilbers NER, Huijzer M, et al. Comparison of seven videolaryngoscopes with the Macintosh laryngoscope in manikins by experienced and novice personnel. Anaesthesia 2016;71(5):556–64.
4. Cowley RA. A total emergency medical system for the State of Maryland. Md State Med J 1975;24(7):37–45.
5. Rogers FB, Rittenhouse KJ, Gross BW. The golden hour in trauma: Dogma or medical folklore? Injury 2015;46(4):525–7.
6. Border JR, Lewis FR, Aprahamian C, et al. Panel: prehospital trauma care–stabilize or scoop and run. J Trauma 1983;23(8):708–11.

7. Gold CR. Prehospital advanced life support vs "scoop and run" in trauma management. Ann Emerg Med 1987;16(7):797–801.
8. Eckstein M, Chan L, Schneir A, et al. Effect of prehospital advanced life support on outcomes of major trauma patients. J Trauma 2000;48(4):643–8.
9. Meizoso JP, Valle EJ, Allen CJ, et al. Decreased mortality after prehospital interventions in severely injured trauma patients. J Trauma Acute Care Surg 2015; 79(2):227–31.
10. Lockey DJ, Healey B, Crewdson K, et al. Advanced airway management is necessary in prehospital trauma patients. Br J Anaesth 2014;1–6. https://doi.org/10.1093/bja/aeu412.
11. Miraflor E, Chuang K, Miranda MA, et al. Timing is everything: delayed intubation is associated with increased mortality in initially stable trauma patients. J Surg Res 2011;170(2):286–90.
12. Stockinger ZT, McSwain NE Jr. Prehospital endotracheal intubation for trauma does not improve survival over bag-valve-mask ventilation. J Trauma 2004; 56(3):531–6.
13. Stiell IG, Nesbitt LP, Pickett W, et al. The OPALS Major Trauma Study: impact of advanced life-support on survival and morbidity. CMAJ 2008;178(9):1141–52.
14. Lecky F, Bryden D, Little R, et al. Emergency intubation for acutely ill and injured patients. Cochrane Database Syst Rev 2008;(2):CD001429.
15. Mayglothling J, Duane TM, Gibbs M, et al. Emergency tracheal intubation immediately following traumatic injury: an Eastern Association for the Surgery of Trauma practice management guideline. J Trauma Acute Care Surg 2012; 73(5):S333–40.
16. Murphy M, Hung O, Launcelott G, et al. Predicting the difficult laryngoscopic intubation: are we on the right track? Can J Anaesth 2005;52(3):231–5.
17. Law JA, Broemling N, Cooper RM, et al. The difficult airway with recommendations for management–part 2–the anticipated difficult airway. Can J Anaesth 2013;60(11):1119–38.
18. Yentis SM. Predicting difficult intubation–worthwhile exercise or pointless ritual? Anaesthesia 2002;57(2):105–9.
19. Nørskov AK, Wetterslev J, Rosenstock CV, et al. Effects of using the simplified airway risk index vs usual airway assessment on unanticipated difficult tracheal intubation—a cluster randomized trial with 64,273 participants. Br J Anaesth 2016;116(5):680–9.
20. Teoh WH, Kristensen MS. Prediction in airway management: what is worthwhile, what is a waste of time and what about the future? Br J Anaesth 2016;117(1): 1–3.
21. Vannucci A, Cavallone LF. Bedside predictors of difficult intubation: a systematic review. Minerva Anestesiol 2016;82(1):69–83.
22. Mosier JM, Joshi R, Hypes C, et al. The physiologically difficult airway. West J Emerg Med 2015;16(7):1109–17.
23. Spaite DW, Hu C, Bobrow BJ, et al. The effect of combined out-of-hospital hypotension and hypoxia on mortality in major traumatic brain injury. Ann Emerg Med 2017. https://doi.org/10.1016/j.annemergmed.2016.08.007.
24. Bodily JB, Webb HR, Weiss SJ, et al. Incidence and duration of continuously measured oxygen desaturation during emergency department intubation. Ann Emerg Med 2015;1–7. https://doi.org/10.1016/j.annemergmed.2015.06.006.
25. Gebremedhn EG, Mesele D, Aemero D, et al. The incidence of oxygen desaturation during rapid sequence induction and intubation. World J Emerg Med 2014;5(4):279–85.

26. Heffner AC, Swords DS, Nussbaum ML, et al. Predictors of the complication of postintubation hypotension during emergency airway management. J Crit Care 2012;27(6):587–93.

27. Wilson MH, Hinds J, Grier G, et al. Impact brain apnoea–a forgotten cause of cardiovascular collapse in trauma. Resuscitation 2016;105:52–8.

28. Kwan I, Bunn F, Roberts I. Spinal immobilisation for trauma patients. Cochrane Database Syst Rev 2001;(2):CD002803.

29. Oteir AO, Jennings PA, Smith K, et al. Should suspected cervical spinal cord injuries be immobilised? A systematic review protocol. Inj Prev 2014;20(3):e5.

30. Mulligan RP, Friedman JA, Mahabir RC. A nationwide review of the associations among cervical spine injuries, head injuries, and facial fractures. J Trauma 2010; 68(3):587–92.

31. Dupanovic M, Fox H, Kovac A. Management of the airway in multitrauma. Curr Opin Anaesthesiol 2010. https://doi.org/10.1097/ACO.0b013e3283360b4f.

32. Thompson WL, Stiell IG, Clement CM, et al. Association of injury mechanism with the risk of cervical spine fractures. CJEM 2009;11(1):14–22.

33. Manoach S, Paladino L. Manual in-line stabilization for acute airway management of suspected cervical spine injury: historical review and current questions. Ann Emerg Med 2007;50(3):236–45.

34. Kill C, Risse J, Wallot P, et al. Videolaryngoscopy with glidescope reduces cervical spine movement in patients with unsecured cervical spine. J Emerg Med 2013;44(4):750–6.

35. Hindman BJ, Fontes RB, From RP, et al. Intubation biomechanics: laryngoscope force and cervical spine motion during intubation in cadavers—effect of severe distractive-flexion injury on C3–4 motion. J Neurosurg Spine 2016;1–11. https://doi.org/10.3171/2016.3.SPINE1640.

36. Hindman BJ, From RP, Fontes RB, et al. Intubation biomechanics: laryngoscope force and cervical spine motion during intubation in cadavers—cadavers versus patients, the effect of repeated intubations, and the effect of type II odontoid fracture on C1-C2 motion. Anesthesiology 2015;123(5):1042–58.

37. Durga P, Sahu BP. Neurological deterioration during intubation in cervical spine disorders. Indian J Anaesth 2014;58(6):684–92.

38. Crosby ET. Airway management in adults after cervical spine trauma. Anesthesiology 2006;104(6):1293–318.

39. Farmer J, Vaccaro A, Albert TJ, et al. Neurologic deterioration after cervical spinal cord injury. J Spinal Disord 1998;11(3):192–6.

40. Thiboutot F, Nicole PC, Trépanier CA, et al. Effect of manual in-line stabilization of the cervical spine in adults on the rate of difficult orotracheal intubation by direct laryngoscopy: a randomized controlled trial. Can J Anaesth 2009;56(6):412–8.

41. LeGrand SA, Hindman BJ, Dexter F, et al. Craniocervical motion during direct laryngoscopy and orotracheal intubation with the Macintosh and Miller blades: an in vivo cinefluoroscopic study. Anesthesiology 2007;107(6):884–91.

42. Kovacs G, Law JA. Lights camera action: redirecting videolaryngoscopy. EMCrit. 2016. Available at: https://emcrit.org/blogpost/redirecting-videolaryngoscopy/. Accessed February 25, 2017.

43. Bathory I, Frascarolo P, Kern C, et al. Evaluation of the GlideScope for tracheal intubation in patients with cervical spine immobilisation by a semi-rigid collar. Anaesthesia 2009;64(12):1337–41.

44. Michailidou M, O'Keeffe T, Mosier JM, et al. A comparison of video laryngoscopy to direct laryngoscopy for the emergency intubation of trauma patients. World J Surg 2015;39(3):782–8.

45. Suppan L, Tramèr MR, Niquille M, et al. Alternative intubation techniques vs Macintosh laryngoscopy in patients with cervical spine immobilization: systematic review and meta-analysis of randomized controlled trials. Br J Anaesth 2016;116(1):27–36.

46. Gu Y, Robert J, Kovacs G, et al. A deliberately restricted laryngeal view with the GlideScope® video laryngoscope is associated with faster and easier tracheal intubation when compared with a full glottic view: a randomized clinical trial. Can J Anaesth 2016;63(8). https://doi.org/10.1007/s12630-016-0654-6.

47. Levitan R. Tips for using a hyperangulated video laryngoscope. ACEP Now 2015. Available at: http://www.acepnow.com/article/tips-for-using-a-hyperangulated-video-laryngoscope/. Accessed February 25, 2017.

48. Kleine-Brueggeney M, Greif R, Schoettker P, et al. Evaluation of six videolaryngoscopes in 720 patients with a simulated difficult airway: a multicentre randomized controlled trial. Br J Anaesth 2016;116(5):670–9.

49. Norris A, Heidegger T. Limitations of videolaryngoscopy. Br J Anaesth 2016. https://doi.org/10.1093/bja/aew122.

50. Vu M, Vu E, Tallon J, et al. Airway management in trauma and the traumatized airway. In: Kovacs G, Law J, editors. Airway management in emergencies. 2nd edition. Shelton (CT): People's Medical Publishing House-USA; 2011. p. 299–316.

51. Crosby ET. Considerations for airway management for cervical spine surgery in adults. Anesthesiol Clin 2007;25(3):511–33, ix.

52. Duggan LV, Griesdale DEG. Secondary cervical spine injury during airway management: beyond a "one-size-fits-all" approach. Anaesthesia 2015;70(7):769–73.

53. Aprahamian C, Thompson BM, Finger WA, et al. Experimental cervical spine injury model: evaluation of airway management and splinting techniques. Ann Emerg Med 1984;13(8):584–7.

54. Sakles JC, Corn GJ, Hollinger P, et al. The impact of a soiled airway on intubation success in the Emergency Department when using the GlideScope or the direct laryngoscope. Acad Emerg Med 2017;30(1):42–9.

55. Ohchi F, Komasawa N, Mihara R, et al. Evaluation of gum-elastic bougie combined with direct and indirect laryngoscopes in vomitus setting: a randomized simulation trial. Am J Emerg Med 2016. https://doi.org/10.1016/j.ajem.2016.12.032.

56. Mihara R, Komasawa N, Matsunami S, et al. Comparison of direct and indirect laryngoscopes in vomitus and hematemesis settings: a randomized simulation trial. Biomed Res Int 2015;806243. https://doi.org/10.1155/2015/806243.

57. DuCanto J, Serrano K, Thompson R. Novel airway training tool that simulates vomiting: suction-assisted laryngoscopy assisted decontamination (SALAD) system. West J Emerg Med 2017;18(1):117–20.

58. Brainard C, Gerecht R. The art of SUCTIONING. JEMS 2015;40(8):26–30, 32.

59. Sise MJ, Shackford SR, Sise CB, et al. Early intubation in the management of trauma patients: indications and outcomes in 1,000 consecutive patients. J Trauma Inj Infect Crit Care 2009;66(1):32–40.

60. Weingart SD, Trueger NS, Wong N, et al. Delayed sequence intubation: a prospective observational study. Ann Emerg Med 2015;65(4):349–55.

61. Cohen L, Athaide V, Wickham ME, et al. The effect of ketamine on intracranial and cerebral perfusion pressure and health outcomes: a systematic review. Ann Emerg Med 2015;65(1):43–51.e2.

62. Zeiler FA, Teitelbaum J, West M, et al. The ketamine effect on ICP in traumatic brain injury. Neurocrit Care 2014;21(1):163–73.
63. Hutchison I, Lawlor M, Skinner D. ABC of major trauma. Major maxillofacial injuries. BMJ 1990;301:595–9.
64. Bowman-Howard M. Management of the traumatized airway. In: Hagberg C, editor. Handbook of difficult airway management. Philadelphia: Churchill Livingstone; 2000. p. 199–206.
65. Jose A, Nagori S, Agarwal B, et al. Management of maxillofacial trauma in emergency: an update of challenges and controversies. J Emerg Trauma Shock 2016;9(2):73.
66. Krausz AA, El-Naaj IA, Barak M. Maxillofacial trauma patient: coping with the difficult airway. World J Emerg Surg 2009;4:21.
67. Kummer C, Netto FS, Rizoli S, et al. A review of traumatic airway injuries: potential implications for airway assessment and management. Injury 2007;38(1):27–33.
68. Mercer SJ, Jones CP, Bridge M, et al. Systematic review of the anaesthetic management of non-iatrogenic acute adult airway trauma. Br J Anaesth 2016; 117(suppl 1):i49–59.
69. Jain U, McCunn M, Smith CE, et al. Management of the traumatized airway. Anesthesiology 2016;124(1):199–206.
70. Horton CL, Iii CAB, Raja AS, et al. Trauma reports. J Emerg Med 2014;46(6): 814–20.
71. Sowers N, Kovacs G. Use of a flexible intubating scope in combination with a channeled video laryngoscope for managing a difficult airway in the emergency department. J Emerg Med 2016;50(2). https://doi.org/10.1016/j.jemermed.2015. 10.010.
72. Higgs A, Cook TM, McGrath BA. Airway management in the critically ill: the same, but different. Br J Anaesth 2016. https://doi.org/10.1093/bja/aew055.
73. Lapinsky SE. Endotracheal intubation in the ICU. Crit Care 2015;19:258.
74. Cook TM, Woodall N, Harper J, et al. Major complications of airway management in the UK: results of the Fourth National Audit Project of the Royal College of Anaesthetists and the Difficult Airway Society. Part 2: intensive care and emergency departments. Br J Anaesth 2011;106(5):632–42.
75. Dronen S. Rapid-sequence intubation: a safe but ill-defined procedure. Acad Emerg Med 1999;6(1):1–2.
76. Mace SE. Challenges and advances in intubation: rapid sequence intubation. Emerg Med Clin North Am 2008;26(4):1043–68.
77. Salem MR, Clark-Wronski J, Khorasani A, et al. Which is the original and which is the modified rapid sequence induction and intubation? Let history be the judge! Anesth Analg 2013;116(1):264–5.
78. Tobias JD. Rapid sequence intubation: what does it mean? Does it really matter? Saudi J Anaesth 2014;8(2):153–4.
79. Ehrenfeld JM, Cassedy EA, Forbes VE, et al. Modified rapid sequence induction and intubation: a survey of United States current practice. Anesth Analg 2012; 115(1):95–101.
80. Salem MR, Khorasani A, Zeidan A, et al. Cricoid pressure controversies: narrative review. Anesthesiology 2017;9(6):378–91.
81. Algie CM, Mahar RK, Tan HB, et al. Effectiveness and risks of cricoid pressure during rapid sequence induction for endotracheal intubation. Cochrane Database Syst Rev 2015;(4):CD011656.

82. Heffner AC, Swords DS, Neale MN, et al. Incidence and factors associated with cardiac arrest complicating emergency airway management. Resuscitation 2013;84(11):1500–4.

83. Perbet S, De Jong A, Delmas J, et al. Incidence of and risk factors for severe cardiovascular collapse after endotracheal intubation in the ICU: a multicenter observational study. Crit Care 2015;19(1):257.

84. Levitan R. Timing resuscitation sequence intubation for critically ill patients. ACEP Now 2015. Available at: http://www.acepnow.com/article/timing-resuscitation-sequence-intubation-for-critically-ill-patients/.

85. Hardy G, Horner D. BET 2: should real resuscitationists use airway checklists? Emerg Med J 2016;33(6):439–41.

86. Brindley PG, Beed M, Law JA, et al. Airway management outside the operating room: how to better prepare. Can J Anaesth 2017. https://doi.org/10.1007/s12630-017-0834-z.

87. Conroy MJ, Weingart GS, Carlson JN. Impact of checklists on peri-intubation care in ED trauma patients. Am J Emerg Med 2014;32(6):541–4.

88. Smith KA, High K, Collins SP, et al. A preprocedural checklist improves the safety of emergency department intubation of trauma patients. Acad Emerg Med 2015;22(8):989–92. Reardon R, ed.

89. Frerk C, Mitchell VS, Mcnarry AF, et al. Difficult Airway Society 2015 guidelines for management of unanticipated difficult intubation in adults. Br J Anaesth 2015;115:827–48.

90. Woodall N, Frerk C, Cook TM. Can we make airway management (even) safer? Lessons from national audit. Anaesthesia 2011;66(suppl. 2):27–33.

91. Leeuwenburg T. Airway management of the critically ill patient: modifications of traditional rapid sequence induction and intubation. Crit Care Horizons 2015;1:1–10.

92. Green RS, Edwards J, Sabri E, et al. Evaluation of the incidence, risk factors, and impact on patient outcomes of postintubation hemodynamic instability. CJEM 2012;14(2):74–82.

93. Green RS, Turgeon AF, McIntyre LA, et al. Postintubation hypotension in intensive care unit patients: a multicenter cohort study. J Crit Care 2015. https://doi.org/10.1016/j.jcrc.2015.06.007.

94. Heffner AC, Swords D, Kline JA, et al. The frequency and significance of postintubation hypotension during emergency airway management. J Crit Care 2012;27(4):417.e9-13.

95. Trivedi S, Demirci O, Arteaga G, et al. Evaluation of preintubation shock index and modified shock index as predictors of postintubation hypotension and other short-term outcomes. J Crit Care 2015;30(4):861.e1-7.

96. Lai W-H, Wu S-C, Rau C-S, et al. Systolic blood pressure lower than heart rate upon arrival at and departure from the Emergency Department indicates a poor outcome for adult trauma patients. Int J Environ Res Public Health 2016;13(6):528.

97. Wang HE, Brown SP, MacDonald RD, et al. Association of out-of-hospital advanced airway management with outcomes after traumatic brain injury and hemorrhagic shock in the ROC hypertonic saline trial. Emerg Med J 2014;31(3):186–91.

98. Chou D, Harada MY, Barmparas G, et al. Field intubation in civilian patients with hemorrhagic shock is associated with higher mortality. J Trauma Acute Care Surg 2015;1. https://doi.org/10.1097/TA.0000000000000901.

99. Miller M, Kruit N, Heldreich C, et al. Hemodynamic response after rapid sequence induction with ketamine in out-of-hospital patients at risk of shock as defined by the shock index. Ann Emerg Med 2016;68(2):181–8.e2.

100. Upchurch CP, Grijalva CG, Russ S, et al. Comparison of etomidate and ketamine for induction during rapid sequence intubation of adult trauma patients. Ann Emerg Med 2017;69(1):24–33.e2.

101. Tran DTT, Newton EK, Mount VAH, et al. Rocuronium versus succinylcholine for rapid sequence induction intubation. Cochrane Database Syst Rev 2015;(10):CD002788.

102. Welch JL, Seupaul RA. Update: does rocuronium create better intubating conditions than succinylcholine for rapid sequence intubation? Ann Emerg Med 2016. https://doi.org/10.1016/j.annemergmed.2016.09.001.

103. Weingart SD, Levitan RM. Preoxygenation and prevention of desaturation during emergency airway management. Ann Emerg Med 2012;59(3):165–75.

104. Wong DT, Yee AJ, May Leong S, et al. The effectiveness of apneic oxygenation during tracheal intubation in various clinical settings: a narrative review. Can J Anaesth 2017. https://doi.org/10.1007/s12630-016-0802-z.

105. Driver BE, Prekker ME, Kornas RL, et al. Flush rate oxygen for emergency airway preoxygenation. Ann Emerg Med 2017;69(1):1–6.

106. Mosier JM, Hypes CD, Sakles JC. Understanding preoxygenation and apneic oxygenation during intubation in the critically ill. Intensive Care Med 2017;43(2):226–8.

107. Nimmagadda U, Salem MR, Crystal GJ. Preoxygenation: physiologic basis, benefits, and potential risks. Anesth Analg 2017;124(2):507–17.

108. Sirian R, Wills J. Physiology of apnoea and the benefits of preoxygenation. Cont Educ Anaesth Crit Care Pain 2009;9(4):105–8.

109. Sakles JC, Mosier J, Patanwala AE, et al. First pass success without hypoxemia is increased with the use of apneic oxygenation during RSI in the Emergency Department. Acad Emerg Med 2016. https://doi.org/10.1111/acem.12931.

110. Pracy JP, Brennan L, Cook TM, et al. Surgical intervention during a can't intubate can't oxygenate (CICO) event: emergency front-of-neck airway (FONA)?. Br J Anaesth 2016;117(4):426–8

111. Law JA, Broemling N, Cooper RM, et al. The difficult airway with recommendations for management—Part 1-Intubation encountered in an unconscious/induced patient. Can J Anaesth 2013;60(11):1089–118.

112. Hamaekers AE, Henderson JJ. Equipment and strategies for emergency tracheal access in the adult patient. Anaesthesia 2011;66(suppl. 2):65–80.

113. Levitan R, Chow Y. Levitan, the laryngeal handshake and the cartilaginous cage. PHARM Prehospital Retr Med 2013. Available at: http://prehospitalmed.com/2013/11/17/levitan-the-laryngeal-handshake-and-the-cartilaginous-cage/.

114. Duggan LV, Ballantyne Scott B, Law JA, et al. Transtracheal jet ventilation in the "can't intubate can't oxygenate" emergency: a systematic review. Br J Anaesth 2016;117(suppl 1):i28–38.

115. Marshall SD. Evidence is important: safety considerations for emergency catheter cricothyroidotomy. Acad Emerg Med 2016;23(9):1074–6.

116. Cook TM, Woodall N, Frerk C. Major complications of airway management in the UK: results of the Fourth National Audit Project of the Royal College of Anaesthetists and the Difficult Airway Society. Part 1: anaesthesia. Br J Anaesth 2011;106(5):617–31.

117. Langvad S, Hyldmo PK, Nakstad AR, et al. Emergency cricothyrotomy—a systematic review. Scand J Trauma Resusc Emerg Med 2013;21(1):43.

118. Petrosoniak A, Hicks CM. Beyond crisis resource management. Curr Opin Anaesthesiol 2013;26(6):699–706.

The Evolving Science of Trauma Resuscitation

Tim Harris, BM BS, BMed Sci, Dip O&G, DipIMC, FFAEM[a], Ross Davenport, PhD[b],
Matthew Mak, BSc, MSc, MBBS, FRCEM, FHEA[c], Karim Brohi, FRCS, FRCA[d,e,*]

KEYWORDS

- Trauma resuscitation • Hypovolemia • Trauma-induced coagulopathy
- Viscoelastic hemostatic assays • Endothelial damage • Hemostasis

KEY POINTS

- Future research should inform clinicians on the role of permissive hypovolemia, for how long this should be maintained, and how/if this should be applied to patients with traumatic brain injury.
- Our understanding of trauma-induced coagulopathy (TIC) is evolving and may see targeted blood component therapy incorporated early in trauma shock resuscitation.
- The role of viscoelastic hemostatic assays in assessing TIC and directing blood component resuscitation requires further study.
- There is increasing understanding of endothelial damage as a driver of TIC, raising the possibility of targeting repair to improve hemostasis and reduce organ failure.
- More work is required to identify the most appropriate goals for posthemostasis resuscitation balancing the risks of fluid overload and underresuscitation.

INTRODUCTION

The 2 leading causes of death after trauma are blood loss and neurologic injury, which account for more than three-quarters of injury related mortality.[1] Fifty percent of early deaths (<24 hours from injury) are due to hemorrhage, with hemorrhagic shock an important driver for postresuscitation organ failure and late mortality.[1–3] There has been a considerable improvement in our understanding of trauma resuscitation over the past 30 years, particularly in hemorrhage control and trauma resuscitation, seeing outcomes steadily improve. However, blood loss remains a leading cause of preventable death in the initial 24 hours of hospital admission.[4]

[a] Emergency Medicine, Barts Health NHS Trust, Queen Mary University of London, London, UK;
[b] Trauma Sciences, Blizard Institute, Queen Mary University of London, London, UK;
[c] Emergency Medicine, Barts Health NHS Trust, London, UK; [d] Trauma and Neuroscience, Blizard Institute, Queen Mary University of London, London E1 2AT, UK; [e] London's Air Ambulance, Barts Health NHS Trust, London, UK
* Corresponding author. Trauma and Neuroscience, Blizard Institute, Queen Mary University of London, London E1 2AT, UK.
E-mail address: k.brohi@qmul.ac.uk

Emerg Med Clin N Am 36 (2018) 85–106
https://doi.org/10.1016/j.emc.2017.08.009
0733-8627/18/© 2017 Elsevier Inc. All rights reserved.

emed.theclinics.com

This review summarizes the evolution of trauma resuscitation, offering clinicians the knowledge base to enable the highest standards of clinical care. Trauma resuscitation has evolved from a one-size-fits-all approach to one tailored to patient physiology. The most dramatic change is in the management of patients who are actively bleeding, with a balanced blood product–based resuscitation approach (avoiding crystalloids) and surgery focused on hemorrhage control, not definitive care. The key components of this "damage control resuscitation (DCR)" approach are (1) hemorrhage control, (2) permissive hypotension/hypovolemia, and (3) the prevention and correction of trauma-induced coagulopathy (TIC). When hemostasis has been achieved, definitive resuscitation to restore organ perfusion is initiated. This DCR strategy prioritizes TIC, temporarily sacrificing perfusion for haemostasis.[5] This approach is associated with a decrease in mortality, reduced duration of stay in intensive care and hospital, improved coagulation profile, and reduced crystalloid/vasopressor use. There are many areas of trauma resuscitation that remain controversial and subject to ongoing research, such as patients with concomitant traumatic brain injury (TBI), environments with limited access to blood products, and the optimal diagnostic and therapeutic approaches to treating coagulopathy. In this article, we focus on the tools and methods used for trauma resuscitation in the acute phase of trauma care (**Box 1**).

HEMORRHAGE CONTROL

The most effective resuscitation fluid is our patients' own blood; thus, preserving circulating volume and minimizing blood loss is a key component of trauma resuscitation. Strategies include minimal handing, direct pressure on wounds, early and accurate fracture splinting, and rapid surgical or radiologic hemorrhage control.[16]

The management of bleeding patients has 2 aims—to arrest bleeding and to restore blood volume—and is recognized as the single most important step in the management of the severely injured patient.[17] Hemorrhage can be compressed by applying direct pressure to the site or using tourniquets, but there are certain anatomic regions (groin, axilla, neck) that prove difficult for standard tourniquet use. Junctional tourniquets (for injuries in the inguinal and axillary regions) and hemostatic dressings have been developed to control proximal bleeding, but there are few data on their effectiveness, with studies mainly from combat-related case series.[18] A number of different devices and interventions have been developed in an attempt to reduce the morbidity and mortality associated with noncompressible torso hemorrhage, with military campaigns driving forward innovation in this field. Devices such as tourniquets and splints are used alongside interventions, such as resuscitative endovascular balloon occlusion of the aorta to preserve circulating volume until definitive surgical treatment can be undertaken.

THE RECOGNITION OF SHOCK AND ACTIVE BLEEDING

All patients need to be resuscitated from shock and have normal organ perfusion restored. However, in trauma patients who are actively bleeding, attempts to restore

---

Box 1
Damage control resuscitation strategy

Permissive hypotension[6,7]

Early empiric use of red blood cells and clotting products[4,8–14]

Limited fluids that may dilute coagulation proteins[15]

perfusion before achieving hemostasis are counterproductive. Patients who are shocked may have stopped bleeding, whereas patients who are bleeding may not yet be clinically shocked. Because it is the presence or absence of active bleeding that changes the resuscitation strategy, the recognition of ongoing hemorrhage is the key step in the management of trauma patients. Understanding the depth of shock guides ongoing resuscitation.

Recognizing the Actively Bleeding Patient

Homeostasis with peripheral vasoconstriction acts to preserve blood pressure as circulating volume is progressively lost, potentially leading to inadequate cardiac output for organ perfusion even though blood pressure remains within the normal range.[19] Thus, in trauma patients, adequate cardiac output cannot be inferred from blood pressure, and only when blood loss is critical, or rapid, is there a relationship between the two.[19] Patients with overt hypovolemic shock characterized by hypotension, tachycardia, and overt blood loss are readily identified, but trauma patients may be shocked despite normal blood pressure and pulse, termed cryptic shock; this is associated with increased mortality.[20]

The Advanced Trauma Life Support manual and courses have popularized the role of physiologic parameters to estimate and grade the severity of blood loss.[21] However, physiologic data from a large UK database suggests that this approach is not borne out in practice.[22] Data from UK and US databases demonstrate that mortality increases progressively below a systolic blood pressure of 110 mm Hg.[23–27] A 2011 databank analysis of 902,852 records identified that the optimal systolic blood pressure cutoff for hypotension as a predictor of mortality differed with age: namely, 85 mm Hg for those 18 to 35 years, 96 mm Hg for those 36 to 64 years, and 117 mm Hg for those over 65 years of age.[27]

In the absence of obvious external exsanguination, the identification of patients who are actively bleeding can be very challenging. Only dynamic methods such as fluid responsiveness are of practical utility in this patient group. Classically, patients are categorized according to their response to a fluid bolus into responders, nonresponders, or the intermediate 'transient responder' group. Both transient responders and nonresponders are actively bleeding.

The use of an initial fluid bolus to determine responsiveness is itself now controversial. In a patient who has lost 40% of their circulating volume, a bolus of 500 or 1000 mL of crystalloid will lead to a 15% to 30% dilution and worsen existing coagulopathy. Giving 1 to 2 units of red blood cells and fresh frozen plasma as initial bolus will have a similar effect but will potentially use blood products for a large proportion of patients who are not bleeding.

Focus has shifted, therefore, to looking at whether bleeding can be predicted from a patient's physiology and injury characteristics. Various scoring systems have been developed that aim to predict major hemorrhage or massive transfusion (variably defined). The Assessment of Blood Consumption score is widely used and is derived from penetrating disease, systolic blood pressure in the emergency department, and positive Focused Assessment with Sonography in Trauma[28,29]; the Trauma Associated Severe Hemorrhage score is more complex and is based on systolic blood pressure, hemoglobin, intraabdominal fluid on ultrasound/computed tomography scanning, Abbreviated Injury Scale, heart rate, and male gender.[30,31] These and other tools report sensitivities in the region of 70% to 80% for the prediction of massive transfusion requirements, may induce delays in recognition, and clinician gestalt has been shown to perform marginally below this, with sensitivities of around 65%.[29] Trauma Associated Severe Hemorrhage and Assessment of Blood Consumption scores are excellent at defining which patients will not require massive transfusion.[29] The 2016 UK National Institute for Health and Care Excellence (NICE) guidelines for major trauma reviewed these scoring systems and concluded that there was insufficient evidence of clinical usefulness to support the use of any of these tools to predict massive transfusion.[32] A practical approach to identifying these bleeding patients is therefore to use a combination of the severity of the patient's physiology and injuries, and response to initial bolus volume resuscitation (ideally given as red blood cells [RBCs]).

Assessing Shock Severity

There are 2 key shock thresholds that determine outcome from hemorrhagic shock. The lower threshold is that coronary artery perfusion must be maintained to preserve cardiac function. The upper threshold is the endpoint of resuscitation from shock, as indicated by normalization of global perfusion parameters.

Coronary artery perfusion is blood pressure dependent and, therefore, this represents the lowest acceptable blood pressure threshold during a trauma resuscitation. Cerebral perfusion is essentially a proxy for maintaining the coronary circulation in this group of patients. Coronary perfusion occurs principally during diastole, and so maintenance of diastolic pressure (25–35 mm Hg) is the key value to observe and maintain.[33] It is difficult to equate this to a specific systolic or mean arterial blood pressure, or a specific palpable pulse. With the narrowed pulse pressure of hemorrhagic shock, it is reasonable to target systolic blood pressures of 60 to 70 mm Hg. Resuscitative endovascular balloon occlusion of the aorta may increase diastolic pressure, so improving coronary artery perfusion for a given circulating volume. NICE guidance recommends maintenance of a palpable central pulse (carotid or femoral) at minimum throughout resuscitation.[32]

At the other end of shock resuscitation is normalization of systemic parameters of organ perfusion, such as measurements of base deficit and lactate. These parameters give an estimation of the severity of shock state and tend to be used to the response to resuscitation (although again the goal before hemorrhage control is not necessarily to normalize these figures). Although there is disagreement as to which is the best acid–base parameter to use, generally in trauma patients without preexisting comorbidities, there is strong correlation between all the standard parameters of lactic acidosis (base deficit or lactate, arterial or venous),[34,35] and these measures are strong predictors of outcome.[36–41]

Because these parameters depend on blood draws, they do not provide a continuous assessment of the severity of shock and systemic perfusion. Many technologies have been investigated as a means to continuously monitor the depth of shock. These include near infrared spectrometry,[42–44] sublingual videomicroscopy,[45,46] and noninvasive cardiac output monitoring.[47,48] All have their proponents, benefits, and drawbacks, and all require further study. The most important and routinely available continuous measure of the depth of shock is end-tidal capnography. Studies have shown good correlation between cardiac output and end-tidal capnography in models of hemorrhage and reperfusion.[49] Hemodynamic instability is associated with low end-tidal capnography and low cardiac output in ventilated trauma patients.[50] Decreased delivery of CO_2 and increase in alveolar dead space result in a high ventilation/perfusion ratio, which is reflected in decreased CO_2 output from the lungs in a shocked state. End-tidal capnography should be used in all trauma hemorrhage resuscitations where the patient is intubated and ventilated.

PERMISSIVE HYPOTENSION AND THE ELIMINATION OF CRYSTALLOID INFUSIONS

Permissive hypotension is conceptually the most difficult part of the DCR paradigm to understand and to implement. DCR temporarily prioritizes hemostasis over perfusion, and permissive hypotension is the means to this end. Resuscitation during active bleeding aims to maintain blood pressure above, but possibly close to, the coronary perfusion threshold as described.

Restoration of a normal blood pressure is not a goal at any point during trauma resuscitation. Although many registry studies have shown that patients with low blood pressures (with increasing mortality below a systolic blood pressure of 110 mm Hg) have worse outcomes,[23,24,26] this is principally a reflection of the nature of their injuries. It does not follow that normalization of blood pressure will improve outcomes. In bleeding animals[51] and patients,[52–54] increasing or attempting to increase blood pressure with fluid amounts greater than that required to maintain basal coronary–cerebral circulation is undesirable, because it increases bleeding from sites of hemorrhage and because the methods we have available to increase blood pressure are ultimately harmful in this group of patients. Giving fluid infusions (as crystalloid or colloid) causes dilutional coagulopathy, anemia, endothelial damage, and tissue edema, all of which are associated with poor outcomes.[8,52,55–57] Even volume administered with RBCs or balanced blood product resuscitation will induce some degree of dilutional coagulopathy. High-volume fluid resuscitation may increase trauma-related bleeding, organ failure, and mortality.[15,51,54,57,58]

The experimental evidence for permissive hypotension is compelling, but the majority of studies were conducted before balanced blood product–based resuscitation was available. There are no animal or human studies of uncontrolled hemorrhage that show high-volume resuscitation regimens lead to improved outcomes.[52,53,55,59–61] A 2014 metaanalysis of liberal versus restricted fluid resuscitation for victims of trauma shock included prehospital and in-hospital studies, blunt and penetrating disease, and studies targeting specific volume of fluid and/or specific blood pressures.[54] The authors included 4 randomized, controlled trials, reporting no overall mortality difference between liberal and restrictive fluid strategies (relative risk, 1.18; 95% confidence interval [CI], 0.98–1.42). However, when the Turner study was excluded because it involved a very high level of protocol violations then patients treated with liberal fluid resuscitation strategies had a higher mortality (relative risk, 1.25; 95% CI, 1.01–1.55; *I*, 0%). The proportion of patients with penetrating trauma was higher than is observed in most clinicians' practice and patients with TBI were predominantly excluded. A recent pilot randomized, controlled trial has explored prehospital and emergency department resuscitation using crystalloid targeting either a systolic pressure of greater than 70 or 110 mm Hg.[6] There was a decrease in mortality at 24 hours in the lower pressure group for blunt trauma with significant differences in the infused crystalloid volume (1 vs 2 L), but the numbers of deaths were small and a larger trial is warranted.

Clinical studies of permissive hypotension are difficult, and reflect the challenges of identifying and managing these patients in daily practice. All human trials are remarkably consistent in findings that, (1) in practice it is impossible to achieve a set blood pressure target in bleeding patients, and (2) attempts to reach and maintain these targets only leads to increased fluid resuscitation without any improvement in mortality outcomes. However, the 2011 US recommendations for military resuscitation and the UK 2016 NICE guideline on major trauma recommend fluid administration be titrated to a palpable carotid or femoral pulse or systolic pressures of 80 to 85 mm Hg.[8,32] In practice, such targets are rarely achievable.

Vasopressors in Early Trauma Shock Resuscitation

The sympathetic response to trauma and blood loss shifts the blood from the unstressed to stressed circulation (mainly from the splanchnic circulation) enabling preservation of blood pressure in the face of significant blood losses.[62,63] However, vasoplegia occurs rapidly in shock as a result of cytokine release, nitric oxide production; tissue, cellular, and mitochondrial damage; hypoxia; and reperfusion injury.[64–67] This finding offers a potential theoretic framework to administer vasopressors during trauma resuscitation and has been hypothesized to reduce blood loss and provide early hemodynamic stability, thus buying time to definitive surgical haemostasis.[68] However, inopressors have a wide range of potential adverse effects, including arrhythmia, increased cardiac work, increased afterload, reduced tissue perfusion, and increasing blood loss as a result of induced increases in blood pressure, with evidence for harm when applied in the initial phase; indeed, adrenergic stress is associated with numerous adverse effects in critical illness.[69]

Animal work suggests a potential role for vasopressin, alone or in combination with noradrenaline,[70–74] with some work suggesting improved tissue oxygenation combined with a DCR approach and early blood products.[72] Norepinephrine alone has shown mixed results.[70,75,76]

Given the common use of vasopressors in trauma care and their support in the European guidelines for hemorrhagic shock, there are few human data.[77] Vasopressors are commonly used to improve cerebral perfusion. Arginine vasopressin release occurs early in major blood loss and assists in centralizing the remaining circulating volume to the brain, heart, and lungs.[78] However, stores are depleted rapidly.[73] Limited data, including 1 small randomized, controlled trial, suggest that vasopressin may improve outcomes if combined with rapid hemorrhage control and improve blood pressure while not worsening blood loss.[68,72,73,79,80]

However, 3 large observational studies show an association between vasopressin (55% vs 41%; $P = .02$)[81] and vasopressor (noradrenaline/norepinephrine, vasopressin, dopamine, phenylephrine) to be associated independently with higher mortality.[82,83] A systematic review of vasopressor use in early trauma resuscitation including 6 studies identified an increase in mortality associated with vasopressor use in all five included observational studies (all with high risk of bias) and an underpowered randomized, controlled trial.[84] It remains unclear if vasopressor use is causative of poor outcomes or a marker of severity of illness. The role for vasopressin is currently being evaluated in the VITRIS.at trial (Vasopressin in Traumatic Hemorrhagic Shock Study; NCT00379522; EudraCT number 2006-004252-20).

Currently, there is insufficient evidence to define the place of vasopressors in early trauma resuscitation. In our practice, vasopressors have no role in the initial resuscitation phase, because we find we can maintain blood pressures above coronary artery perfusion pressure with blood products and early surgical intervention, where required.

Resuscitation in Patients with Traumatic Brain Injury

The permissive hypotension approach is most conflicted in patients who are bleeding and have a major TBI. Data from patients with isolated TBI shows that those who experience episodes of hypotension have worse outcomes and guidelines advocate maintaining a systolic blood pressure of greater than 100/110 mm Hg to preserve cerebral perfusion.[85–88] Bleeding trauma patients who have TBI do worse than those without TBI. However, neither of these facts directly support an approach that sets higher blood pressure targets in bleeding patients with TBI. Experimental evidence suggests that, in the setting of combined hemorrhage and brain injury, high-dose crystalloid resuscitation to target higher blood pressures is associated with increased cerebral edema, increased intracranial pressure, decreased cerebral perfusion pressure, and reduced cerebral oxygen delivery with the cerebral circulation protected in trauma shock.[89] Human data in this area are almost completely absent, in part because this represents a small group of patients with generally very poor outcomes, and studies on permissive hypotension have excluded patients with TBI. The UK NICE major trauma guideline suggests that the clinician should focus resuscitation on the predominant injury complex, so a restrictive fluid administration is advocated where bleeding is the dominant pathology being treated.[32]

High-volume crystalloid resuscitation is associated with endothelial damage, tissue edema, organ failure, dilutional coagulopathy, impaired clot formation, dilutional anemia, and increased bleeding, all of which are associated with poor outcomes.[8,51,52,55–57,60,90] Over the past decade, as the DCR approach has become more prevalent, multiple retrospective studies of bleeding patients have shown a decrease in crystalloid use associated with decreased, organ failure, decreased abdominal compartment syndrome, and decreased mortality.[51,52,90–92] The presence of acute lung injury and abdominal compartment syndrome in particular are strongly associated with worse TBI outcomes.[91] The presence or absence of TBI is unknown for most patients in the prehospital and early in-hospital phase of care. The concomitant TBI population has not been examined specifically in retrospective studies, but to date there is no compelling evidence that patients with possible TBI should be treated according to a different management paradigm than those who do not. In trauma patients, where hemorrhagic shock seems to be the dominant pathophysiology, a DCR approach with permissive hypotension should be used.[32] Where brain injury seems to be the dominant pathology, then blood pressure targets should be targeted toward the maintenance of cerebral perfusion pressure.

Conclusions: Permissive Hypotension

Several questions remain around the application of permissive hypotension in contemporary trauma care. All experimental and the majority of clinical studies have been conducted in the context of crystalloid-first resuscitation, and whether the plasma or balanced transfusion regimens reduce the requirement for permissive hypotension is yet to be determined. Methods for continuous monitoring and ensuring coronary and cerebral perfusion would allow a personalized approach and remove many of the unknowns from the permissive approach to blood pressure management.

Permissive hypotension has become a central component of the DCR approach. It must be understood as a passive process that is temporarily tolerated until hemorrhage control is achieved. Basal coronary–cerebral circulation is maintained by avoiding crystalloids and the judicious use of balanced blood product transfusions. At all times, hemorrhage control is the goal, not normalization of blood pressure.

PREVENTION AND CORRECTION OF TRAUMA-INDUCED COAGULOPATHY

DCR aims to preserve hemostatic function, reduce blood loss, and directly address TIC, and is associated with improved outcomes.[15] The mechanisms by which this is achieved and detailed pathophysiology of TIC are yet to be fully elucidated but are the focus of investigation for multiple international trauma research consortia (Targeted Action for the Cure of Trauma-Induced Coagulopathy [Euro TACTIC, http://www.tacticgroup.dk/], Trans-Agency Consortium for Trauma-Induced Coagulopathy

[US TACTIC, http://www.tacticproject.org/] and Research Outcomes Consortium [ROC] [https://roc.uwctc.org/tiki/tiki-index.php?page=roc-public-home]).

Pathophysiology of Trauma-Induced Coagulopathy

TIC is a multifactorial failure of the coagulation system to sustain adequate hemostasis after major trauma hemorrhage.[93] The 2 principle processes are an endogenous coagulopathy induced by the injury and shock state, and a dilutional coagulopathy caused by volume resuscitation. The endogenous coagulopathy (acute traumatic coagulopathy [ATC]) is present almost immediately in severely shocked and injured trauma patients and can be detected in the prehospital phase before large volume resuscitation.[94–99] Resuscitation-induced coagulopathy augments this process and may dominate later in the clinical course.[93,100–102] At physiologic extremes, hypothermia and acidemia will also exacerbate the coagulopathy. Around 25% of critically injured trauma patients are coagulopathic on arrival, increasing to close to 100% after receiving a massive transfusion.[94,103] Once TIC is established, it is a poor prognostic indicator, with greater transfusion requirements, higher levels of organ dysfunction, and a 4-fold increase in mortality.[97,98]

Although there seem to be different patterns of the endogenous ATC, it is characterized by the delayed formation of weak clots, increased clot breakdown, and with only minor prolongation of clotting times.[104] Loss or consumption of procoagulant factors (such as factors VII or X) is not the prime driver of ATC.[104] Rather, there is loss or breakdown of fibrinogen and a systemic hyperfibrinolysis owing to increased plasmin activity. ATC also seems to cause platelet dysfunction, with reduced aggregation in response to all standard activators, although platelet count is typically maintained after trauma.[105–107] The changes seem to be driven by the combination of injury and shock, and may be mediated through endothelial dysfunction and glycocalyx degradation.[108–110]

Resuscitation coagulopathy complicates ATC by adding in a progressive reduction in procoagulant factors. Crystalloid and colloid infusions will rapidly dilute circulating coagulation factors, especially when circulating blood volume is already low. RBC alone will also cause this dilutional effect. Even the recommended "balanced" transfusion of 1:1:1 units of red cell, plasma, and platelets only approaches the normal clotting factor concentrations of whole blood.[111] These transfusion products also have reduced functionality owing to processing and storage.[9,112] This reduction in circulating clotting factors is compounded by further endothelial injury caused by crystalloid transfusions, which likely further exacerbates TIC.

Patients, therefore, present with an established endogenous coagulopathy, which is exacerbated by resuscitation in the face of ongoing bleeding. DCR focuses on maintaining the hemostatic potential of blood, by minimizing any resuscitation-induced coagulopathy and correcting any existing coagulopathy.

TREATMENT OF TRAUMA-INDUCED COAGULOPATHY
Treatment of Endogenous Acute Traumatic Coagulopathy: Tranexamic Acid

At present, the only specific recommended treatment for ATC is the administration of the antifibrinolytic tranexamic acid (TXA). Military and civilian studies, including the large CRASH-2 trial (Clinical Randomisation of an Antifibrinolytic in Significant Haemorrhage), have shown that administration of TXA to bleeding trauma patients reduces overall mortality.[113–116] Treatment with TXA is usually recommended empirically because there are questions about the sensitivity of diagnostic tests to identify hyperfibrinolysis in trauma patients.[77]

There are multiple unanswered questions regarding the use of TXA in trauma. It is unknown which patient groups benefit from TXA. CRASH-2 was conducted in all patients suspected of active bleeding, and therefore included a large number of patients who were not bleeding. A subgroup analysis in CRASH-2 found the greatest survival benefit to be in those patients with shock, and was confirmed in a retrospective civilian study.[116] In combat casualties, empiric use of TXA showed the greatest benefit observed in patients who subsequently required a massive transfusion.[114] Given that ATC is driven by the presence of shock, it would seem biologically consistent to administer TXA to those patients who are in shock or who are bleeding and likely to develop shock.

Other questions include the optimal dose and timing of TXA, as well as its mechanism of effect. TXA seems to reduced bleeding-related deaths without affecting transfusion requirements. It also may worsen outcomes if given more than 3 hours after an injury, which may reflect a dynamic change in coagulation profiles of trauma patients. Further mechanistic studies and clinical trials of TXA are ongoing.

Prevention of Resuscitation Coagulopathy

The development of a resuscitation coagulopathy is prevented or reduced by using a balanced transfusion regimen that approaches that of whole blood. In practice, this means providing an equal ratio of RBCs, plasma, and platelet transfusions (note that some of these products may be pooled in some countries).

There have been many retrospective studies showing the potential benefit of this approach over RBC transfusions alone, catchup strategies, or the use of plasma ratios.[10,11,117–120] The PROPPR randomized, controlled trial (Pragmatic, Randomized Optimal Platelet and Plasma Ratios) examined the effectiveness and safety of a 1:1:1 transfusion ratio (fresh frozen plasma:platelets:RBCs) compared with a 1:1:2 ratio in patients with trauma who were predicted to receive a massive transfusion.[121] Overall, there was no significant difference between groups in either 24-hour or 28-day mortality, but deaths from exsanguination were reduced in the 1:1:1 group, with greater numbers achieving anatomic hemostasis and a consistent trend toward improved overall survival. Although there are many further questions raised by these results, this is likely to remain the best quality evidence in this area. Most recent guidelines suggest that a 1:1:1 strategy is started immediately and used throughout DCR.[32,77,122]

Major Hemorrhage Protocols

Massive hemorrhage protocols (MHPs) are central to DCR and designed to specifically target ATC. Protocolized transfusion avoids dilutional coagulopathy through empiric provision of RBCs with simultaneous, high-dose clotting products (plasma, cryoprecipitate or fibrinogen concentrate, and platelets). To enable rapid delivery of a 1:1:1 strategy, MHPs are activated solely based on physiology and suspected active hemorrhage rather a formal diagnosis of coagulopathy by laboratory or point-of-care assays. Volume resuscitation with RBCs and clotting products from the outset avoids the need for crystalloids and colloids, with blood banks providing a continuous supply of "transfusion packs" until hemorrhage control is achieved (through abbreviated surgery or interventional radiology).

Preventing dilutional coagulopathy and avoiding crystalloids from the start has implications for the prehospital care of these patients. Following experience gained in recent military conflicts with prehospital use of RBC and fresh frozen plasma, a number of civilian services are beginning to use blood products at the scene of the injury. However, data supporting the prehospital use of RBC and fresh frozen plasma are all retrospective and the results are conflicted.[10,123,124] Several randomized, controlled trials are underway evaluating the use of blood products as first-line resuscitation in the prehospital phase of care. The REPHILL trial (Resuscitation with Pre-HospltaL bLood products; https://www.clinicaltrialsregister.eu/ctr-search/trial/2015-001401-13/GB) compares RBC and lyophilized plasma (LyoPlas N-w) against standard of care (crystalloid) and the COMBAT trial (Control of Major Bleeding After Trauma Study; https://clinicaltrials.gov/ct2/show/NCT01838863) explores the role of initial resuscitation using plasma as compared with normal saline.

Correction of Trauma-Induced Coagulopathy

Despite early administration of TXA and volume resuscitation with balanced transfusion, patients will still become coagulopathic as they continue to bleed. Different patterns of coagulopathy will develop depending on the nature of the injuries, severity and duration of shock, and the nature and timing of fluids and blood products patients have received. Although most coagulation therapy is empiric, it is important to monitor coagulation status throughout bleeding to ensure that hemostatic competence is maintained. Point-of-care coagulation monitoring may allow for a more precision approach to the management of TIC during DCR.

Laboratory and Point-of-Care Diagnostics

Traditional monitoring of coagulopathy during hemorrhage has relied on standard laboratory tests of coagulation such as prothrombin time, partial thromboplastin time, platelet count, and fibrinogen levels. These are of limited value in trauma hemorrhage owing to the time delays in laboratory processing and the lack of sensitivity of prothrombin time, partial thromboplastin time, and platelet count for the underlying pathophysiology of TIC.[125,126] Of the laboratory tests, the fibrinogen level is the most valuable. Fibrinogen is affected by both ATC and resuscitation, and levels can rapidly become dangerously low.[104,127–129] Although some MHPs routinely supplement fibrinogen with cryoprecipitate or fibrinogen concentrate, the doses used are rarely sufficient to maintain levels or replace losses. Fibrinogen levels should be taken regularly during DCR and sample processing prioritized by the laboratory.

Point-of-care prothrombin time assays have been appraised in trauma but have been found to have limited accuracy.[125] The viscoelastic hemostatic assays (VHAs), namely, thromboelastography (Haemoscope Corp, Niles, IL) and rotational thromboelastometry (Pentapharm GmbH, Munich, Germany) provide more specific information related to the clot strength and lysis aspects of TIC, but have yet to be fully evaluated in trauma patients. VHAs are capable of rapidly diagnosing ATC[130–132] and, importantly, are able to rapidly assess the need for fibrinogen supplementation. The lack of data-driven, trauma-specific algorithms has hampered inclusion of VHAs into standard practice and guidelines[32,133,134]; however, their use is supported by European guidelines for major hemorrhage management.[77] Many European trauma centers and an increasing number of high-volume centers in the UK and the United States are using rotational thromboelastometry/thromboelastography to diagnose and initiate coagulation therapy. An international randomized controlled trial (ITACTIC [Implementing Treatment Algorithms for the Correction of Trauma Induced Coagulopathy], NCT02593877) is currently ongoing to compare empiric MHPs with MHP plus VHAs in trauma resuscitation.

Fibrinogen Replacement

During major hemorrhage, fibrinogen is depleted and not restored to normal levels despite MHPs providing balanced 1:1:1 transfusions therapy.[129] Because fibrin is a critical component of clot, maintaining adequate fibrinogen levels is a central goal of coagulation management. Fibrinogen levels should be maintained at greater than 2 g/L during DCR.[77] There are 2 main sources of fibrinogen replacement: cryoprecipitate and fibrinogen concentrate. Two observational civilian cohort trauma studies[117,135] have reported a decrease in mortality in patients receiving higher fibrinogen content during major transfusion therapy, data that are mirrored by military cohort studies.[114,128] If fibrinogen replacement is incorporated into MHPs it is usually relatively late in the transfusion sequence and at a relatively low dose.[136] A small pilot study of early high-dose cryoprecipitate supplementation (CRYOSTAT [Early Cryoprecipitate in Major Trauma Haemorrhage]) showed it was possible to rapidly restore fibrinogen levels with a trend toward improved survival.[127] The phase III CRYOSTAT-2 trial of 1544 patients is due to commence enrolling in mid-2017. Fibrinogen concentrate may offer an alternative to cryoprecipitate, but it is expensive and evidence to support its efficacy is lacking. Feasibility studies have shown that fibrinogen concentrate can be administered rapidly to bleeding trauma patients in both in-hospital and prehospital environments with improvements in functional fibrinogen (rotational thromboelastometry) and plasma fibrinogen levels with further studies (eg, FEISTY and EFIT-1, NCT02745041) ongoing. Fibrinogen loss is central to the pathophysiology of TIC, fibrinogen levels must be assayed regularly during DCR, and hypofibrinogenemia must be corrected rapidly.

TIC is a multifactorial, described by varying degrees of dysfibrinogenemia, hyperfibrinolysis, endothelial dysfunction, and impaired platelet activity. Early endogenous processes that drive the aberrant response in the coagulation system depend on the magnitude of trauma, and the severity of hemorrhagic shock. DCR and the use of MHPs are associated with improved outcomes, although the mechanisms of how it corrects TIC have yet to be characterized fully. Optimizing TIC treatment to improve outcomes requires further research to understand the dynamic changes in the equilibrium between procoagulant and anticoagulant factors, fibrinogen use, downstream effectors (eg, fibrinolysis), and the individual response to transfusion therapy.

Temperature and Electrolytes

Calcium is a vital cofactor for procoagulant clotting proteases and levels decrease rapidly during massive bleeding,[137–139] in part owing to chelation after transfusion of citrate-containing blood products during DCR. Low ionized calcium is associated with increased mortality and greater transfusion requirements.[137,138] Levels should be checked regularly during resuscitation and replaced to maintain levels within the normal range.[77]

Numerous studies report an independent association between hypothermia and death, with effects significant at a body temperature of less than 35°C.[140–143] The early use of warming blankets and aggressive rewarming on arrival at the hospital may reduce morbidity and mortality.[144] A 2016 European multicenter retrospective study focusing on 564 severely injured patients reported that mild hypothermia did not alter transfusion rates,[130] but a German study involving 15,895 patients found that hypothermia increased the relative risk for transfusion by 2, and increased the duration of stay as well as mortality.[131] Thus, maintaining normocalcemia and normothermia in early resuscitation are key aspects of trauma resuscitations.

WHICH FLUIDS, IF ANY, SHOULD WE USE FOR TRAUMA PATIENTS WHO DO NOT REQUIRE DAMAGE CONTROL RESUSCITATION?

The majority of research into trauma resuscitation focuses on critically unwell patients with trauma shock who require a DCR approach, but this applies to the minority of trauma patients cared for in the emergency department.[29] Whether patients without trauma shock should receive blood products, crystalloids, or indeed any fluid resuscitation is open to debate.

Hypertonic saline has been widely advocated for use in trauma patients. A 2014 metaanalysis of 6 randomized trials involving patients with hemorrhagic shock reported no benefit (95% CI, 0.82–1.14).[132] Two randomized, controlled trials compared hypertonic saline with normal saline, one recruiting patients with severe TBI and hemorrhagic shock, arguably the group most likely to benefit, and the other patients with TBI not in hypovolemic shock; both trials showed no difference in neurologic function at 6 months or mortality.[145,146] Thus, hypertonic saline has no role in trauma resuscitation other than the control of increased intracranial pressure.[147]

A subgroup analysis of the SAFE trial (Comparing Albumin in 0.9% Saline to 0.9% Saline as a Resuscitation Fluid in Intensive Care Units) identified improved outcomes in trauma shock patients resuscitated in with 0.9% saline (relative risk, 1.63; 95% CI, 1.17–2.26; $P = .003$).[148] This effect was more marked in those with more severe injury and may be due to the hypotonicity of the latter solution. In patients with sepsis, starch-based colloids cause an increase in renal failure and mortality.[149–151] Starches have been associated impaired coagulation.[152,153] A metaanalysis of 59 randomized, controlled trials (including 16,889 trauma and surgical patients) found no difference in mortality among patients receiving colloid as compared with crystalloids (32 trials including 16,647 patients; odds ratio, 0.99; 95% CI, 0.92–1.06), but did show an increase in patients who required renal replacement therapy in the colloid group (9 trials including 11,648 patients; odds ratio, 1.35; 95% CI, 1.17–1.57). A 2015 cohort study of 1,051,441 patients undergoing joint arthroplasty also reported an association between the use of either albumin (odds ratio, 1.56; 95% CI, 1.36–1.78) or hydroxyethyl starch (odds ratio, 1.23; 95% CI, 1.13–1.34) and acute renal failure.[150] A 2011 Cochrane review of critically ill patients (trauma, burns, postoperative) reported no benefit for colloids as compared with crystalloids for resuscitation.[154] Given the potential risk of renal impairment, worsening coagulopathy, and the increase in costs, there is no case for the use of colloids in early trauma resuscitation.

Because 0.9% saline is hypertonic and contains supraphysiologic chloride levels, it has been linked to higher levels of acidosis and reduced renal flow.[155] A randomized, controlled trial including 4 intensive care units in New Zealand and 2278 medical and surgical patients compared Plasma-Lyte with 0.9% saline as a resuscitation and maintenance fluid reported no difference in mortality of renal replacement.[156]

Thus, current data do not support the use of hypertonic saline, synthetic colloids, or albumin as resuscitation fluids in trauma. There are no powered human trauma studies to advise clinicians on crystalloid selection.[157] Our practice is not to use any fluid therapy in this group of patients, unless there is evidence of organ impairment that may benefit from increased cardiac output.

SUMMARY

Once considered a public health problem for the young, the age demographics of major trauma are rapidly changing with some predictions that patients over the age of 75 will soon comprise the larger cohort.[158] Managing polypharmacy and medical comorbidities in patients with reduced physiologic reserve represents a significant challenge for the science of trauma resuscitation.

Fluid replacement in trauma patients in need of resuscitation has seen a paradigm shift over the past 30 years. Current best practice embodies a DCR approach with permissive hypotension/hypovolemia, balanced resuscitation with a high ratio of blood clotting products (fresh frozen plasma, cryoprecipitate and platelets:packed red blood cells—1:1:1), avoidance of crystalloid and vasopressors, and early damage control surgery. In clinical practice, specific blood pressure targets are hard to achieve. Preserving the patient's circulating volume and maintaining normothermia are also key components of trauma resuscitation. These approaches are best applied as a continuum from prehospital through the emergency department to operating room care.

Future research should be directed to inform clinicians on the role of permissive hypovolemia in blunt trauma, for how long this should be maintained, and how/if this should be applied to patients with TBI. Our understanding of TIC is evolving rapidly and may see targeted blood component therapy become incorporated early in trauma shock resuscitation and the subject of current research. The role of VHAs in assessing TIC and directing blood component resuscitation requires further study. There is increasing understanding of the role of endothelial damage as a driver for TIC, raising the possibility of targeting repair to improve hemostasis and reduce organ failure. Finally, more work is required to identify the most appropriate goals for posthemostasis resuscitation balancing the risks of fluid overload and underresuscitation.

REFERENCES

1. Kauvar DS, Lefering R, Wade CE. Impact of hemorrhage on trauma outcome: an overview of epidemiology, clinical presentations, and therapeutic considerations. J Trauma Acute Care Surg 2006;60(6):S3–11.
2. Roberts I, Shakur H, Edwards P, et al. Trauma care research and the war on uncertainty: improving trauma care demands large trials: and large trials need funding and collaboration. BMJ 2005;331:1094–6.
3. Shackford SR, Mackersie RC, Holbrook TL, et al. The epidemiology of traumatic death: a population-based analysis. Arch Surg 1993;128(5):571–5.
4. Holcomb JB, Wade CE. Defining present blood component transfusion practices in trauma patients: papers from the trauma outcomes group. J Trauma Acute Care Surg 2011;71(2):S315 7.
5. Duke MD, Guidry C, Guice J, et al. Restrictive fluid resuscitation in combination with damage control resuscitation: time for adaptation. J Trauma Acute Care Surg 2012;73(3):674–8.
6. Schreiber MA, Meier EN, Tisherman SA, et al. A controlled resuscitation strategy is feasible and safe in hypotensive trauma patients: results of a prospective randomized pilot trial. J Trauma Acute Care Surg 2015;78(4):687–95 [discussion: 695–7].
7. Dutton RP, Mackenzie CF, Scalea TM. Hypotensive resuscitation during active hemorrhage: impact on in-hospital mortality. J Trauma 2002;52(6):1141–6.
8. McSwain NE, Champion HR, Fabian TC, et al. State of the art of fluid resuscitation 2010: prehospital and immediate transition to the hospital. J Trauma Acute Care Surg 2011;70(5):S2–10.
9. Weinberg JA, McGwin G Jr, Griffin RL, et al. Age of transfused blood: an independent predictor of mortality despite universal leukoreduction. J Trauma 2008;65(2):279–82 [discussion: 282–4].
10. Holcomb JB, Wade CE, Michalek JE, et al. Increased plasma and platelet to red blood cell ratios improves outcome in 466 massively transfused civilian trauma patients. Ann Surg 2008;248(3):447–58.

11. Holcomb JB, Zarzabal LA, Michalek JE, et al. Increased platelet:RBC ratios are associated with improved survival after massive transfusion. J Trauma 2011; 71(2 Suppl 3):S318–28.

12. Borgman MA, Spinella PC, Holcomb JB, et al. The effect of FFP: RBC ratio on morbidity and mortality in trauma patients based on transfusion prediction score. Vox Sang 2011;101(1):44–54.

13. Rowell SE, Barbosa RR, Allison CE, et al. Gender-based differences in mortality in response to high product ratio massive transfusion. J Trauma 2011; 71(2 Suppl 3):S375–9.

14. Wade CE, del Junco DJ, Holcomb JB, et al. Variations between level I trauma centers in 24-hour mortality in severely injured patients requiring a massive transfusion. J Trauma 2011;71(2 Suppl 3):S389–93.

15. Cotton BA, Reddy N, Hatch QM, et al. Damage control resuscitation is associated with a reduction in resuscitation volumes and improvement in survival in 390 damage control laparotomy patients. Ann Surg 2011;254(4):598–605.

16. Guerado E, Bertrand ML, Valdes L, et al. Suppl 1: M3: resuscitation of polytrauma patients: the management of massive skeletal bleeding. Open Orthop J 2015;9:283.

17. National confidential enquiry into patient outcomes and death, trauma: who cares? London: National Audit Office; 2007.

18. van Oostendorp SE, Tan EC, Geeraedts LM Jr. Prehospital control of life-threatening truncal and junctional haemorrhage is the ultimate challenge in optimizing trauma care; a review of treatment options and their applicability in the civilian trauma setting. Scand J Trauma Resusc Emerg Med 2016;24(1):110.

19. Wo CC, Shoemaker WC, Appel PL, et al. Unreliability of blood pressure and heart rate to evaluate cardiac output in emergency resuscitation and critical illness. Crit Care Med 1993;21(2):218–23.

20. Meregalli A, Oliveira RP, Friedman G. Occult hypoperfusion is associated with increased mortality in hemodynamically stable, high-risk, surgical patients. Crit Care 2004;8(2):1.

21. American College of Surgeons Committee on Trauma. Advanced trauma life support for doctors: student course manual. Chicago (IL): American College of Surgeons; 2008.

22. Guly H, Bouamra O, Spiers M, et al. Vital signs and estimated blood loss in patients with major trauma: testing the validity of the ATLS classification of hypovolaemic shock. Resuscitation 2011;82(5):556–9.

23. Eastridge BJ, Salinas J, McManus JG, et al. Hypotension begins at 110 mm Hg: redefining "hypotension" with data. J Trauma 2007;63(2):291–9 [discussion: 297–9].

24. Edelman DA, White MT, Tyburski JG, et al. Post-traumatic hypotension: should systolic blood pressure of 90-109 mmHg be included? Shock 2007;27(2):134–8.

25. Hasler RM, Nuesch E, Jüni P, et al. Systolic blood pressure below 110mmHg is associated with increased mortality in blunt major trauma patients: multicentre cohort study. Resuscitation 2011;82(9):1202–7.

26. Bruns B, Gentilello L, Elliott A, et al. Prehospital hypotension redefined. J Trauma Acute Care Surg 2008;65(6):1217–21.

27. Oyetunji TA, Chang DC, Crompton JG, et al. Redefining hypotension in the elderly: normotension is not reassuring. Arch Surg 2011;146(7):865–9.

28. Nunez TC, Voskresensky IV, Dossett LA, et al. Early prediction of massive transfusion in trauma: simple as ABC (assessment of blood consumption)? J Trauma Acute Care Surg 2009;66(2):346–52.

29. Cantle PM, Cotton BA. Prediction of massive transfusion in trauma. Crit Care Clin 2017;33(1):71–84.
30. Schreiber MA, Perkins J, Kiraly L, et al. Early predictors of massive transfusion in combat casualties. J Am Coll Surg 2007;205(4):541–5.
31. Yucel N, Lefering R, Maegele M, et al. Trauma Associated Severe Hemorrhage (TASH)-Score: probability of mass transfusion as surrogate for life threatening hemorrhage after multiple trauma. J Trauma 2006;60(6):1228–36 [discussion: 1236–7].
32. National Institute of Health and Clinical Excellence. Major trauma: assessment and initial management. 2016.
33. Sutton RM, Friess SH, Maltese MR, et al. Hemodynamic-directed cardiopulmonary resuscitation during in-hospital cardiac arrest. Resuscitation 2014;85(8): 983–6.
34. Bloom BM, Grundlingh J, Bestwick JP, et al. The role of venous blood gas in the emergency department: a systematic review and meta-analysis. Eur J Emerg Med 2014;21(2):81–8.
35. Bloom B, Pott J, Freund Y, et al. The agreement between abnormal venous lactate and arterial lactate in the ED: a retrospective chart review. Am J Emerg Med 2014;32(6):596–600.
36. Kaplan LJ, Kellum JA. Initial pH, base deficit, lactate, anion gap, strong ion difference, and strong ion gap predict outcome from major vascular injury. Crit Care Med 2004;32(5):1120–4.
37. Rixen D, Raum M, Bouillon B, et al. Base deficit development and its prognostic significance in posttrauma critical illness: an analysis by the trauma registry of the Deutsche Gesellschaft fur unfallchirurgie. Shock 2001;15(2):83–9.
38. Bilello JF, Davis JW, Lemaster D, et al. Prehospital hypotension in blunt trauma: identifying the "crump factor". J Trauma Acute Care Surg 2011;70(5):1038–42.
39. Coats TJ, Smith JE, Lockey D, et al. Early increases in blood lactate following injury. J R Army Med Corps 2002;148(2):140–3.
40. Claridge JA, Crabtree TD, Pelletier SJ, et al. Persistent occult hypoperfusion is associated with a significant increase in infection rate and mortality in major trauma patients. J Trauma Acute Care Surg 2000;48(1):8.
41. Baxter J, Cranfield KR, Clark G, et al. Do lactate levels in the Emergency Department predict outcome in adult trauma patients? A systematic review. J Trauma Acute Care Surg 2016;81(3):555–66.
42. Crookes BA, Cohn SM, Bloch S, et al. Can near-infrared spectroscopy identify the severity of shock in trauma patients? J Trauma Acute Care Surg 2005; 58(4):806–16.
43. Soller BR, Ryan KL, Rickards CA, et al. Oxygen saturation determined from deep muscle, not thenar tissue, is an early indicator of central hypovolemia in humans. Crit Care Med 2008;36(1):176–82.
44. Cohn SM, Nathens AB, Moore FA, et al. Tissue oxygen saturation predicts the development of organ dysfunction during traumatic shock resuscitation. J Trauma 2007;62(1):44.
45. Naumann DN, Dretzke J, Hutchings S, et al. Protocol for a systematic review of the impact of resuscitation fluids on the microcirculation after haemorrhagic shock in animal models. Syst Rev 2015;4:135.
46. Naumann DN, Mellis C, Smith IM, et al. Safety and feasibility of sublingual microcirculation assessment in the emergency department for civilian and military patients with traumatic haemorrhagic shock: a prospective cohort study. BMJ Open 2016;6(12):e014162.

47. Kuster M, Exadaktylos A, Schnuriger B. Non-invasive hemodynamic monitoring in trauma patients. World J Emerg Surg 2015;10:11.
48. Dunham CM, Chirichella TJ, Gruber BS, et al. Emergency department noninvasive (NICOM) cardiac outputs are associated with trauma activation, patient injury severity and host conditions and mortality. J Trauma Acute Care Surg 2012;73(2):479–85.
49. Kodali BS, Urman RD. Capnography during cardiopulmonary resuscitation: current evidence and future directions. J Emerg Trauma Shock 2014;7(4):332–40.
50. Dunham CM, Chirichella TJ, Gruber BS, et al. In emergently ventilated trauma patients, low end-tidal $CO2$ and low cardiac output are associated and correlate with hemodynamic instability, hemorrhage, abnormal pupils, and death. BMC Anesthesiol 2013;13(1):20.
51. Mapstone J, Roberts I, Evans P. Fluid resuscitation strategies: a systematic review of animal trials. J Trauma 2003;55(3):571–89.
52. Bickell WH, Wall MJ Jr, Pepe PE, et al. Immediate versus delayed fluid resuscitation for hypotensive patients with penetrating torso injuries. N Engl J Med 1994;331(17):1105–9.
53. Hussmann B, Heuer M, Lefering R, et al. Prehospital volume therapy as an independent risk factor after trauma. Biomed Res Int 2015;2015:354367.
54. Wang CH, Hsieh WH, Chou HC, et al. Liberal versus restricted fluid resuscitation strategies in trauma patients: a systematic review and meta-analysis of randomized controlled trials and observational studies*. Crit Care Med 2014;42(4): 954–61.
55. Yaghoubian A, Lewis RJ, Putnam B, et al. Reanalysis of prehospital intravenous fluid administration in patients with penetrating truncal injury and field hypotension. Am Surg 2007;73(10):1027–30.
56. Geeraedts LM Jr, Pothof LA, Caldwell E, et al. Prehospital fluid resuscitation in hypotensive trauma patients: do we need a tailored approach? Injury 2015; 46(1):4–9.
57. Cotton BA, Guy JS, Morris JA Jr, et al. The cellular, metabolic, and systemic consequences of aggressive fluid resuscitation strategies. Shock 2006;26(2): 115–21.
58. Ley EJ, Clond MA, Srour MK, et al. Emergency department crystalloid resuscitation of 1.5 L or more is associated with increased mortality in elderly and non-elderly trauma patients. J Trauma 2011;70(2):398–400.
59. Haut ER, Kalish BT, Cotton BA, et al. Prehospital intravenous fluid administration is associated with higher mortality in trauma patients: a National Trauma Data Bank analysis. Ann Surg 2011;253(2):371–7.
60. Hampton DA, Fabricant LJ, Differding J, et al. Prehospital intravenous fluid is associated with increased survival in trauma patients. J Trauma Acute Care Surg 2013;75(1 Suppl 1):S9–15.
61. Holcomb JB, del Junco DJ, Fox EE, et al. The prospective, observational, multicenter, major trauma transfusion (PROMMTT) study: comparative effectiveness of a time-varying treatment with competing risks. JAMA Surg 2013;148(2): 127–36.
62. Cooke WH, Ryan KL, Convertino VA. Lower body negative pressure as a model to study progression to acute hemorrhagic shock in humans. J Appl Physiol (1985) 2004;96(4):1249–61.
63. Lundvall J, Länne T. Large capacity in man for effective plasma volume control in hypovolaemia via fluid transfer from tissue to blood. Acta Physiol Scand 1989; 137(4):513–20.

64. Cohen MJ, Brohi K, Calfee CS, et al. Early release of high mobility group box nuclear protein 1 after severe trauma in humans: role of injury severity and tissue hypoperfusion. Crit Care 2009;13(6):1.
65. Zhang Q, Raoof M, Chen Y, et al. Circulating mitochondrial DAMPs cause inflammatory responses to injury. Nature 2010;464(7285):104–7.
66. Liu LM, Ward JA, Dubick MA. Hemorrhage-induced vascular hyporeactivity to norepinephrine in select vasculatures of rats and the roles of nitric oxide and endothelin. Shock 2003;19(3):208–14.
67. Thiemermann C, Szabó C, Mitchell JA, et al. Vascular hyporeactivity to vasoconstrictor agents and hemodynamic decompensation in hemorrhagic shock is mediated by nitric oxide. Proc Natl Acad Sci U S A 1993;90(1):267–71.
68. Wenzel V, Raab H, Dünser MW. Arginine vasopressin: a promising rescue drug in the treatment of uncontrolled haemorrhagic shock. Best Pract Res Clin Anaesthesiol 2008;22(2):299–316.
69. Dunser MW, Hasibeder WR. Sympathetic overstimulation during critical illness: adverse effects of adrenergic stress. J Intensive Care Med 2009;24(5):293–316.
70. Voelckel WG, Raedler C, Wenzel V, et al. Arginine vasopressin, but not epinephrine, improves survival in uncontrolled hemorrhagic shock after liver trauma in pigs. Crit Care Med 2003;31(4):1160–5.
71. Raedler C, Voelckel WG, Wenzel V, et al. Treatment of uncontrolled hemorrhagic shock after liver trauma: fatal effects of fluid resuscitation versus improved outcome after vasopressin. Anesth Analg 2004;98(6):1759–66.
72. Li T, Fang Y, Zhu Y, et al. A small dose of arginine vasopressin in combination with norepinephrine is a good early treatment for uncontrolled hemorrhagic shock after hemostasis. J Surg Res 2011;169(1):76–84.
73. Liu L, Tian K, Xue M, et al. Small doses of arginine vasopressin in combination with norepinephrine "buy" time for definitive treatment for uncontrolled hemorrhagic shock in rats. Shock 2013;40(5):398–406.
74. Stadlbauer KH, Wagner-Berger HG, Krismer AC, et al. Vasopressin improves survival in a porcine model of abdominal vascular injury. Crit Care 2007; 11(4):R81.
75. Poloujadoff MP, Borron SW, Amathieu R, et al. Improved survival after resuscitation with norepinephrine in a murine model of uncontrolled hemorrhagic shock. Anesthesiology 2007;107(4):591–6.
76. Lee JH, Kim K, Jo YH, et al. Early norepinephrine infusion delays cardiac arrest after hemorrhagic shock in rats. J Emerg Med 2009;37(4):376–82.
77. Rossaint R, Bouillon B, Cerny V, et al. The European guideline on management of major bleeding and coagulopathy following trauma. Crit Care 2016;20(1):100.
78. Westermann I, Dünser MW, Haas T, et al. Endogenous vasopressin and copeptin response in multiple trauma patients. Shock 2007;28(6):644–9.
79. Bayram B, Hocaoglu N, Atila R, et al. Effects of terlipressin in a rat model of severe uncontrolled hemorrhage via liver injury. Am J Emerg Med 2012;30(7): 1176–82.
80. Cohn SM, McCarthy J, Stewart RM, et al. Impact of low-dose vasopressin on trauma outcome: prospective randomized study. World J Surg 2011;35(2): 430–9.
81. Collier B, Dossett L, Mann M, et al. Vasopressin use is associated with death in acute trauma patients with shock. J Crit Care 2010;25(1):173.e9-14.
82. Sperry JL, Minei JP, Frankel HL, et al. Early use of vasopressors after injury: caution before constriction. J Trauma 2008;64(1):9–14.

83. Plurad DS, Talving P, Lam L, et al. Early vasopressor use in critical injury is associated with mortality independent from volume status. J Trauma Acute Care Surg 2011;71(3):565–72.

84. Hylands M, Beaudoin N, Toma A, et al. 1575: vasopressor use following traumatic injury: a systematic review. Crit Care Med 2016;44(12):469.

85. Chesnut RM, Marshall LF, Klauber MR, et al. The role of secondary brain injury in determining outcome from severe head injury. J Trauma 1993;34(2):216–22.

86. Bratton S, Chestnut RM, Ghajar J, et al. Guidelines for the management of severe traumatic brain injury. I. Blood pressure and oxygenation. J Neurotrauma 2006;24:S7–13.

87. Lapierre F, Dearden M, Teasdale GM, et al. EBIC-guidelines for management of severe head injury in adults. Acta Neurochir (Wien) 1997;139:286–94.

88. Carney N, Totten AM, O'Reilly C, et al. Guidelines for the management of severe traumatic brain injury. Neurosurgery 2016.

89. Wan Z, Sun S, Ristagno G, et al. The cerebral microcirculation is protected during experimental hemorrhagic shock. Crit Care Med 2010;38(3):928–32.

90. Smail N, Wang P, Cioffi WG, et al. Resuscitation after uncontrolled venous hemorrhage: does increased resuscitation volume improve regional perfusion. J Trauma Acute Care Surg 1998;44(4):701–8.

91. Neal MD, Hoffman MK, Cuschieri J, et al. Crystalloid to packed red blood cell transfusion ratio in the massively transfused patient: when a little goes a long way. J Trauma Acute Care Surg 2012;72(4):892–8.

92. Stern SA, Dronen SC, Birrer P, et al. Effect of blood pressure on hemorrhage volume and survival in a near-fatal hemorrhage model incorporating a vascular injury. Ann Emerg Med 1993;22(2):155–63.

93. Davenport RA, Brohi K. Cause of trauma-induced coagulopathy. Curr Opin Anaesthesiol 2016;29(2):212–9.

94. Floccard B, Rugeri L, Faure A, et al. Early coagulopathy in trauma patients: an on-scene and hospital admission study. Injury 2012;43(1):26–32.

95. Wohlauer MV, Moore EE, Droz NM, et al. Hemodilution is not critical in the pathogenesis of the acute coagulopathy of trauma. J Surg Res 2012;173(1):26–30.

96. Wafaisade A, Wutzler S, Lefering R, et al. Drivers of acute coagulopathy after severe trauma: a multivariate analysis of 1987 patients. Emerg Med J 2010; 27(12):934–9.

97. Maegele M, Lefering R, Yucel N, et al. Early coagulopathy in multiple injury: an analysis from the German Trauma Registry on 8724 patients. Injury 2007;38(3): 298–304.

98. Brohi K, Singh J, Heron M, et al. Acute traumatic coagulopathy. J Trauma Acute Care Surg 2003;54(6):1127–30.

99. MacLeod JB, Lynn M, McKenney MG, et al. Early coagulopathy predicts mortality in trauma. J Trauma Acute Care Surg 2003;55(1):39–44.

100. Dobson GP, Letson HL, Sharma R, et al. Mechanisms of early trauma-induced coagulopathy: the clot thickens or not? J Trauma Acute Care Surg 2015;79(2): 301–9.

101. Frith D, Goslings JC, Gaarder C, et al. Definition and drivers of acute traumatic coagulopathy: clinical and experimental investigations. J Thromb Haemost 2010;8(9):1919–25.

102. Cohen MJ, Kutcher M, Redick B, et al. Clinical and mechanistic drivers of acute traumatic coagulopathy. J Trauma Acute Care Surg 2013;75(1 0 1):S40.

103. Brohi K, Cohen MJ, Ganter MT, et al. Acute coagulopathy of trauma: hypoperfusion induces systemic anticoagulation and hyperfibrinolysis. J Trauma Acute Care Surg 2008;64(5):1211–7.
104. Davenport RA, Guerreiro M, Frith D, et al. Activated protein C drives the hyperfibrinolysis of acute traumatic coagulopathy. Anesthesiology 2017;126(1):115–27.
105. Stansbury LG, Hess AS, Thompson K, et al. The clinical significance of platelet counts in the first 24 hours after severe injury. Transfusion 2013;53(4):783–9.
106. Solomon C, Traintinger S, Ziegler B, et al. Platelet function following trauma. Thromb Haemost 2011;106(2):322–30.
107. Kutcher ME, Redick BJ, McCreery RC, et al. Characterization of platelet dysfunction after trauma. J Trauma Acute Care Surg 2012;73(1):13.
108. Hunt BJ, Jurd KM. Endothelial cell activation. BMJ 1998;316(7141):1328–30.
109. Johansson PI, Stensballe J, Rasmussen LS, et al. A high admission syndecan-1 level, a marker of endothelial glycocalyx degradation, is associated with inflammation, protein C depletion, fibrinolysis, and increased mortality in trauma patients. Ann Surg 2011;254(2):194–200.
110. Ostrowski SR, Henriksen HH, Stensballe J, et al. Sympathoadrenal activation and endotheliopathy are drivers of hypocoagulability and hyperfibrinolysis in trauma: a prospective observational study of 404 severely injured patients. J Trauma Acute Care Surg 2017;82(2):293–301.
111. Armand R, Hess JR. Treating coagulopathy in trauma patients. Transfus Med Rev 2003;17(3):223–31.
112. Spinella PC, Perkins JG, Grathwohl KW, et al. Warm fresh whole blood is independently associated with improved survival for patients with combat-related traumatic injuries. J Trauma 2009;66(4 Suppl):S69–76.
113. Roberts I, Shakur H, Coats T, et al. The CRASH-2 trial: a randomised controlled trial and economic evaluation of the effects of tranexamic acid on death, vascular occlusive events and transfusion requirement in bleeding trauma patients. Health Technol Assess 2013;17(10):1–79.
114. Morrison JJ, Dubose JJ, Rasmussen TE, et al. Military application of tranexamic acid in trauma emergency resuscitation (MATTERs) study. Arch Surg 2012;147(2):113–9.
115. Morrison JJ, Dubose JJ, Rasmussen TE, et al. Association of cryoprecipitate and tranexamic acid with improved survival following wartime injury: findings from the MATTERs II Study. JAMA Surg 2013;148(3):218–25.
116. Cole E, Davenport R, Willett K, et al. Tranexamic acid use in severely injured civilian patients and the effects on outcomes: a prospective cohort study. Ann Surg 2015;261(2):390–4.
117. Dente CJ, Shaz BH, Nicholas JM, et al. Improvements in early mortality and coagulopathy are sustained better in patients with blunt trauma after institution of a massive transfusion protocol in a civilian level I trauma center. J Trauma Acute Care Surg 2009;66(6):1616–24.
118. Rowell SE, Barbosa RR, Diggs BS, et al. Effect of high product ratio massive transfusion on mortality in blunt and penetrating trauma patients. J Trauma 2011;71(2 Suppl 3):S353–7.
119. Borgman MA, Spinella PC, Perkins JG, et al. The ratio of blood products transfused affects mortality in patients receiving massive transfusions at a combat support hospital. J Trauma 2007;63(4):805–13.
120. Wafaisade A, Maegele M, Lefering R, et al. High plasma to red blood cell ratios are associated with lower mortality rates in patients receiving multiple

transfusion (4</=red blood cell units<10) during acute trauma resuscitation. J Trauma 2011;70(1):81–8 [discussion: 88–9].

121. Holcomb JB, Tilley BC, Baraniuk S, et al. Transfusion of plasma, platelets, and red blood cells in a 1: 1: 1 vs a 1: 1: 2 ratio and mortality in patients with severe trauma: the PROPPR randomized clinical trial. JAMA 2015;313(5):471–82.

122. Spahn DR, Bouillon B, Cerny V, et al. Management of bleeding and coagulop-athy following major trauma: an updated European guideline. Crit Care 2013; 17(2):R76.

123. Rajasekhar A, Gowing R, Zarychanski R, et al. Survival of trauma patients after massive red blood cell transfusion using a high or low red blood cell to plasma transfusion ratio. Crit Care Med 2011;39(6):1507–13.

124. Holcomb JB, Fox EE, Wade CE, et al. The prospective observational multicenter major trauma transfusion (PROMMTT) study. J Trauma Acute Care Surg 2013; 75:S1–2.

125. Davenport R, Manson J, De'Ath H, et al. Functional definition and characteriza-tion of acute traumatic coagulopathy. Crit Care Med 2011;39(12):2652–8.

126. David JS, Durand M, Levrat A, et al. Correlation between laboratory coagulation testing and thromboelastometry is modified during management of trauma pa-tients. J Trauma Acute Care Surg 2016;81(2):319–27.

127. Curry N, Rourke C, Davenport R, et al. Early cryoprecipitate for major haemor-rhage in trauma: a randomised controlled feasibility trial. Br J Anaesth 2015; 115(1):76–83.

128. Stinger HK, Spinella PC, Perkins JG, et al. The ratio of fibrinogen to red cells transfused affects survival in casualties receiving massive transfusions at an army combat support hospital. J Trauma Acute Care Surg 2008;64(2):S79–85.

129. Rourke C, Curry N, Khan S, et al. Fibrinogen levels during trauma hemorrhage, response to replacement therapy, and association with patient outcomes. J Thromb Haemost 2012;10(7):1342–51.

130. Jensen KO, Held L, Kraus A, et al. The impact of mild induced hypothermia on the rate of transfusion and the mortality in severely injured patients: a retrospec-tive multi-centre study. Eur J Med Res 2016;21(1):37.

131. Klauke N, Gräff I, Fleischer A, et al. Effects of prehospital hypothermia on trans-fusion requirements and outcomes: a retrospective observatory trial. BMJ Open 2016;6(3):e009913.

132. Wang JW, Li JP, Song YL, et al. Hypertonic saline in the traumatic hypovolemic shock: meta-analysis. J Surg Res 2014;191(2):448–54.

133. Wikkelsø A, Wetterslev J, Møller AM, et al. Thromboelastography (TEG) or thromboelastometry (ROTEM) to monitor haemostatic treatment versus usual care in adults or children with bleeding. Cochrane Database Syst Rev 2016;(8):CD007871.

134. Hunt H, Stanworth S, Curry N, et al. Thromboelastography (TEG) and rotational thromboelastometry (ROTEM) for trauma-induced coagulopathy in adult trauma patients with bleeding. Cochrane Database Syst Rev 2015;(2):CD010438.

135. Shaz BH, Dente CJ, Nicholas J, et al. Increased number of coagulation products in relationship to red blood cell products transfused improves mortality in trauma patients. Transfusion 2010;50(2):493–500.

136. Stanworth SJ, Davenport R, Curry N, et al. Mortality from trauma haemorrhage and opportunities for improvement in transfusion practice. Br J Surg 2016; 103(4):357–65.

137. Ho K, Leonard A. Concentration-dependent effect of hypocalcaemia on mortality of patients with critical bleeding requiring massive transfusion: a cohort study. Anaesth Intensive Care 2011;39(1):46.

138. Magnotti LJ, Bradburn EH, Webb DL, et al. Admission ionized calcium levels predict the need for multiple transfusions: a prospective study of 591 critically ill trauma patients. J Trauma Acute Care Surg 2011;70(2):391–7.

139. Sihler KC, Napolitano LM. Complications of massive transfusion. Chest 2010; 137(1):209–20.

140. Jurkovich GJ, Greiser WB, Luterman A, et al. Hypothermia in trauma victims: an ominous predictor of survival. J Trauma Acute Care Surg 1987;27(9):1019–24.

141. Wang HE, Callaway CW, Peitzman AB, et al. Admission hypothermia and outcome after major trauma. Crit Care Med 2005;33(6):1296–301.

142. Martin RS, Kilgo PD, Miller PR, et al. Injury-associated hypothermia: an analysis of the 2004 National Trauma Data Bank. Shock 2005;24(2):114–8.

143. Shafi S, Elliott AC, Gentilello L. Is hypothermia simply a marker of shock and injury severity or an independent risk factor for mortality in trauma patients? Analysis of a large national trauma registry. J Trauma Acute Care Surg 2005; 59(5):1081–5.

144. Perlman R, Callum J, Laflamme C, et al. A recommended early goal-directed management guideline for the prevention of hypothermia-related transfusion, morbidity, and mortality in severely injured trauma patients. Crit Care 2016; 20(1):107.

145. Cooper DJ, Myles PS, McDermott FT, et al. Prehospital hypertonic saline resuscitation of patients with hypotension and severe traumatic brain injury: a randomized controlled trial. JAMA 2004;291(11):1350–7.

146. Bulger EM, May S, Brasel KJ, et al. Out-of-hospital hypertonic resuscitation following severe traumatic brain injury: a randomized controlled trial. JAMA 2010;304(13):1455–64.

147. Kamel H, Navi BB, Nakagawa K, et al. Hypertonic saline versus mannitol for the treatment of elevated intracranial pressure: a meta-analysis of randomized clinical trials. Crit Care Med 2011;39(3):554–9.

148. Myburgh J, Cooper DJ, Finter S, et al. Saline or albumin for fluid resuscitation in patients with traumatic brain injury. N Engl J Med 2007;357(9):874–84.

149. Haase N, Perner A, Hennings LI, et al. Hydroxyethyl starch 130/0.38-0.45 versus crystalloid or albumin in patients with sepsis: systematic review with meta-analysis and trial sequential analysis. BMJ 2013;346:f839.

150. Opperer M, Poeran J, Rasul R, et al. Use of perioperative hydroxyethyl starch 6% and albumin 5% in elective joint arthroplasty and association with adverse outcomes: a retrospective population based analysis. BMJ 2015;350:h1567.

151. Perner A, Haase N, Guttormsen AB, et al. Hydroxyethyl starch 130/0.42 versus Ringer's acetate in severe sepsis. N Engl J Med 2012;367(2):124–34.

152. Harrois A, Hamada SR, Duranteau J. Fluid resuscitation and vasopressors in severe trauma patients. Curr Opin Crit Care 2014;20(6):632–7.

153. Groeneveld AJ, Navickis RJ, Wilkes MM. Update on the comparative safety of colloids: a systematic review of clinical studies. Ann Surg 2011;253(3):470–83.

154. Perel P, Roberts I, Ker K. Colloids versus crystalloids for fluid resuscitation in critically ill patients. Cochrane Database Syst Rev 2011;(3):CD000567.

155. Waters JH, Gottlieb A, Schoenwald P, et al. Normal saline versus lactated Ringer's solution for intraoperative fluid management in patients undergoing abdominal aortic aneurysm repair: an outcome study. Anesth Analg 2001; 93(4):817–22.

156. Young P, Bailey M, Beasley R, et al. Effect of a buffered crystalloid solution vs saline on acute kidney injury among patients in the intensive care unit: the SPLIT randomized clinical trial. JAMA 2015;314(16):1701–10.
157. Annane D, Siami S, Jaber S, et al. Effects of fluid resuscitation with colloids vs crystalloids on mortality in critically ill patients presenting with hypovolemic shock: the CRISTAL randomized trial. JAMA 2013;310(17):1809–17.
158. Kehoe A, Smith JE, Edwards A, et al. The changing face of major trauma in the UK. Emerg Med J 2015;32(12):911–5.

Secondary Gains
Advances in Neurotrauma Management

Brit Long, MD[a],*, Alex Koyfman, MD[b]

KEYWORDS

- Neurotrauma • Traumatic brain injury • Spinal cord injury • Intracranial pressure
- Mean arterial pressure • Tier

KEY POINTS

- Neurotrauma is the leading cause of trauma-related death in patients ages 1 to 45 years. It is categorized by mechanism, imaging findings, and anatomic involvement.
- Cerebral blood flow requires adequate cerebral perfusion pressure, defined by mean arterial pressure minus intracranial pressure.
- Initial management requires assessing neurologic status, maintaining adequate mean arterial pressure, treating elevated intracranial pressure (ICP), avoiding secondary injury, and obtaining emergent neuroimaging.
- Airway considerations such as preoxygenation, head of bed elevation, first pass success, and postintubation analgesia and sedation are essential in avoiding further worsening of traumatic insults including hypotension and hypoxemia.
- Neurosurgical consultation is required for optimal management, and the use of neurocritical care teams can improve patient outcome.

INTRODUCTION

Neurotrauma is associated with significant morbidity and mortality, with traumatic brain injury (TBI) the leading cause of death in North America between the ages of 1 and 45 years of age.[1–5] Approximately 78% of patients are initially assessed and managed in the emergency department (ED), with males and young adults the 2 primary populations affected.[1,2] Spinal cord injury is rare, and more than 80% are male.[6–9] Central nervous system (CNS) injuries can be categorized by mechanism, radiologic appearance, and anatomic involvement.[1–3] Traumatic neurologic injury not only causes an initial primary injury, but it is associated with several secondary insults.[1–5] Emergency physicians, by providing-high quality, evidence-based

---

Disclosure Statement: This review does not reflect the views or opinions of the U.S. government, Department of Defense, SAUSHEC EM Program, or U.S. Air Force.
[a] Department of Emergency Medicine, San Antonio Military Medical Center, 3841 Roger Brooke Drive, Fort Sam Houston, TX 78234, USA; [b] Department of Emergency Medicine, The University of Texas Southwestern Medical Center, 5323 Harry Hines Boulevard, Dallas, TX 75390, USA
* Corresponding author.
E-mail address: Brit.long@yahoo.com

neuroresuscitation, can help to prevent these secondary injuries; this article discusses the current evidence available to guide this process and optimize management.

NEUROLOGIC INJURIES

Intracranial pressure (ICP) is a measure of several components of the CNS: brain parenchyma, blood, and cerebrospinal fluid (CSF).[2,10,11] Any increase in one value mandates a decrease in another.[10–17] Once compensatory methods are exhausted, further volume leads to drastic increases in ICP. Cerebral perfusion pressure (CPP) is related to ICP, and an increase in ICP may decrease cerebral perfusion. The goal of resuscitation and management in neurotrauma is to ensure an adequate MAP for cerebral perfusion. Clinically, an increase in ICP and decrease in cerebral perfusion can be difficult, if not impossible, to measure directly in the ED. Herniation may result from increase in ICP (**Table 1**). Examples of herniation are demonstrated in **Fig. 1**.

Head injury classification is most commonly based on the Glasgow Coma Scale (GCS). The majority of TBI is mild (GCS 14–15). Moderate TBI is defined by a GCS of 9 to 13.[2,11] Approximately 40% of patients with moderate TBI have an abnormality on neuroimaging. For patients with minor and moderate head injury, mortality is less than 20%, but long-term disability is often worse in this subset. Severe TBI is defined by a GCS of 3 to 8, with mortality approaching 40%.[1–5,10,11,18,19] Other scoring systems are available and are discussed elsewhere in this article.

Blunt Injury

Blunt impact to the head causes acceleration and deceleration of the brain within the cranium, and these forces cause compression, distortion, and shearing of tissues.

Table 1
Herniation syndromes

Herniation	Pathophysiology	Presentation
Uncal subtype: Kernohan's notch	• Parasympathetic fibers of cranial nerve III compression • Pyramidal tract compression • Compression of cerebral peduncle in uncal herniation • Secondary condition caused by primary injury on opposite hemisphere	• Ipsilateral fixed and dilated pupil • Contralateral motor paralysis • Ipsilateral hemiplegia/hemiparesis, called Kernohan's sign • False localizing sign
Central transtentorial	• Midline lesion with compression of midbrain	• Bilateral nonresponsive midpoint pupils, bilateral Babinski, increased muscular tone
Cerebellotonsillar	• Cerebellar tonsil herniation through foramen magnum	• Pinpoint pupils, flaccid paralysis, sudden death
Upward posterior fossa/transtentorial	• Cerebellar and midbrain movement upwards through tentorial opening	• Pinpoint pupils, downward conjugate gaze, irregular respirations • Death

Data from Refs.[10–17]

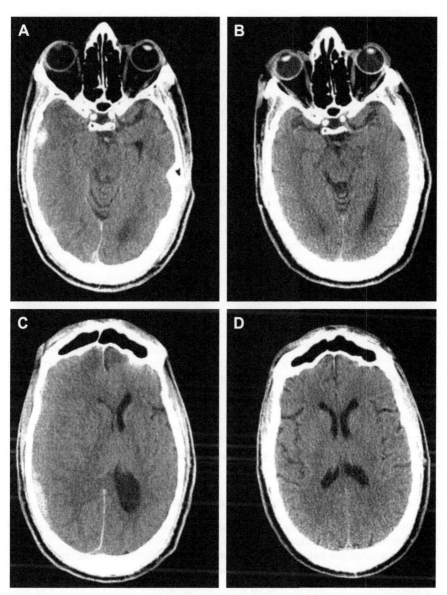

Fig. 1. Head computed tomography (CT) scan illustrating subfalcine and uncal herniation associated with an acute-on-chronic subdural hematoma (SDH). (*A*) Uncal herniation. Right sided holohemispheric mixed density SDH. There is right uncal herniation with flattening of the suprasellar cistern and midbrain compression. (*B*) Comparison: normal brain CT at the level of the midbrain. (*C*) Subfalcine herniation. A more superior slice in the same patient that shows compression of the right lateral ventricle and subfalcine herniation. (*D*) Comparison: normal brain CT at the level of the basal ganglia or lateral ventricles. (*From* Miyakoshi A, Cohen WA. Monitoring in neurocritical care. Philadelphia: Elsevier; 2013. p. 258–70.e4.)

This movement results in contusions, hematomas, and axonal injuries. Common injuries are shown in **Table 2**.

Penetrating Injury

Although much less common, penetrating head injury is associated with high morbidity and mortality.[2,11,20] Most penetrating TBI is due to firearm projectiles, which are associated with a wavelike pattern of tissue compression and expansion. Kinetic energy from the projectile determines the amount of injury, so higher velocity projectiles result in more extensive damage.[20]

Blast Injury

This injury pattern is comparatively rare in civilian trauma, but has specific diagnostic and management considerations. Any explosion can cause energy transmission through the cranium and central vasculature.[20,21] This insult may result in malignant cerebral edema that occurs rapidly (within 1 hour of injury). Vasospasm occurs in 50% of patients, which may result in further neurologic decline owing to ischemia.[2,20,21]

SPINAL CORD INJURY

Blunt spinal injury is due to cord compression, spinal distraction, or shearing with vertebral and disk damage.[2,6–9] Owing to trauma, the spinal canal may be compromised, leading to spinal artery blood flow obstruction, resulting in further ischemia.[2,7–9] Penetrating injury involves spinal cord laceration or transection, which is rare. The cervical and thoracic regions are affected most commonly if penetrating injury does occur.[6–9]

Vascular Injury

An incidence of 1.2% of coexistent vascular injury is present with neurotrauma, primarily involving extracranial and vertebral artery injury. These injuries are more common in patients with cervical spine trauma.[2,22]

WHAT ARE SECONDARY INJURIES, AND ARE THEY DANGEROUS?

Neurotrauma begins a cascade of inflammatory cytokines that worsens ischemia and edema, resulting in secondary injury and poor patient outcomes.[10,11,23,24] The following elements are believed to be linked to the development of secondary injury and provide rational targets for neuroresuscitation in the ED:

- Hypotension: Present in 30% of patients, resulting in higher likelihood of poor outcome (odds ratio, 2.67).[25–29]
- Hypoxia: Present in 50% of patients, resulting in a higher likelihood of poor outcome (odds ratio, 2.14).[2,11,25–29]
- Hyperoxia: Pao_2 levels of greater than 300 to 470 mm Hg are associated with worse outcomes.[2,11,25–29]
- Hyperpyrexia: Elevated core body temperature worsens morbidity by secondary brain injury aggravation.[2,11]
- Coagulopathy: Coagulopathy is often associated with the traumatic event and may cause worsening of the neurologic injury, hemorrhage enlargement, and death. Acute TBI may cause coagulopathy itself through tissue factor and phospholipid release.[27,30]

Table 2
Direct injury categories

Injury	Pathophysiology	Common Locations	Characteristics
Contusion	• Coup and contrecoup injury from trauma	• Orbitofrontal region • Anterior temporal region	• Up to one-third may expand
Epidural hematoma	• Middle meningeal artery and vein injury	• Close to site of skull fracture	• Convex shape • Does not cross suture lines
Subdural hematoma	• Bridging vein injury	• Cerebral convexities • Tentorium and falx	• Concave shape • Crosses suture lines • More common in those with brain atrophy
Subarachnoid hemorrhage	• Pial vessel injury or laceration	• Cerebral convexities • Interpeduncular cisterns • Ventricles	• May be present in a few sulci or fissures, more diffuse if severe • Most common CT finding in moderate TBI
Diffuse axonal injury	• Shearing mechanism results in white matter damage • Diffuse axonal swelling	• Gray-white matter junction in hemispheres • Severe injuries may affect corpus callosum and midbrain	• May present in profound coma without elevated ICP • Associated with significant morbidity and mortality
Depressed skull fracture	• Fracture through cranial vault	• Any site of cranial trauma	• Often associated with underlying damage to central vasculature or parenchyma

Abbreviations: CT, computed tomography; ICP, intracranial pressure; TBI, traumatic brain injury.
Data from Refs.[1–5,11,13,18]

- Glucose dysregulation: Hyperglycemia and hypoglycemia are predictors of poor neurologic status and GCS 5 days after the initial event.[2,25,27]

PHYSIOLOGIC GOALS

Hypotension is associated with increased morbidity and mortality in TBI. A CPP goal of 50 to 70 mm Hg should be used, although without direct monitoring of cerebral tissue this is difficult in the ED. Per the Brain Trauma Foundation, a systolic blood pressure of at least 100 mm Hg (ages 50–69) and 110 mm Hg for those 15 to 49 years or older than 70 years is a better target than CPP. Otherwise, a MAP of 70 mm Hg is advised.[11,27–29] However, other authors recommend a MAP of 80 mm Hg as target. Hypertension is rare and suggests herniation is imminent or occurring acutely. Avoiding cerebral hypotension is recommended, although aggressive CPP targeting is not associated with improved outcomes.[25–29] Hypoxia also results in a significant increase in mortality. Key targets of resuscitation are shown in **Box 1**.

EVALUATION AND MANAGEMENT

Initial management should focus on airway, breathing, circulation, disability, and exposure in the primary survey, while maintaining spinal precautions.[27,28,31] Considerations for ED care are discussed in **Box 2**. Markers of increased mortality and morbidity include hypoxia, hypotension, advanced age, poor admission GCS motor score, pupillary function, and intracranial hypertension.[2,11,23,25–28] A GCS of less than 8 may require intubation for airway protection. Other indications include failure to oxygenate or ventilate, or neurologic decline with rapid drop in GCS. These indications are discussed elsewhere in this article.[31] Pupillary response and motor examination are vital components of assessment.[27–29] A decrease in mental status, new focal neurologic finding, penetrating injury, or concern for herniation (such as a unilateral dilated pupil) warrants neuroimaging after initial resuscitation measures, because patients commonly experience worsening neurologic injury in the early stages of neurotrauma.[32–36] The emergency physician should manage these patients with neurosurgical consultation for definitive care, although this expertise may not be available in initial stages of resuscitation.[11]

Neuroimaging with a computed tomography (CT) scan is preferred in the acute management phase, although stabilization is required for other injuries first.[11,27,28] CT scans can detect fractures, hematomas, and signs of cerebral edema. Any sign of clinical deterioration warrants an immediate follow-up CT scan after treatment. The evolution of intracranial pathology is common, especially with parenchymal lesions such as intracerebral hemorrhage.[2,32–34,37,38] Routine follow-up imaging is often institution dependent.

TIERS OF MANAGEMENT OF INTRACRANIAL PRESSURE

ICP and neurologic resuscitation are aimed at restoring and maintaining cerebral metabolism through sufficient oxygen and glucose delivery.[10,11,16,17,23,26–28,35,36,39] A tiered approach may be used for ICP management. Close evaluation of clinical herniation is warranted. These signs include unilateral pupillary dilation, acute unilateral weakness, decreased mental status, posturing, and Cushing's triad (hypertension, bradycardia, and changes in respiratory pattern). The following tier system is recommended by the Brain Trauma Foundation.[27] Once suspected ICP elevation is controlled and the patient is stabilized, neuroimaging should be completed. Airway

---

Box 1
Goal physiologic parameters

- Pulse oximetry $\geq$90%
- Pao_2 $\geq$100 mm Hg
- $Paco_2$ 35 to 45 mm Hg
- Mean arterial pressure $\geq$70–80 mm Hg
- pH 7.35 to 7.45
- Intracranial pressure $\leq$20 mm Hg
- Brain tissue oxygen pressure $\geq$15 mm Hg
- Glucose 80 to 180 mg/dL
- Cerebral perfusion pressure $\geq$60 mm Hg
- Serum Na 135 to 145; hypertonic saline goal is 145 to 155
- International Normalized Ratio $\leq$1.4
- Platelets $\geq$75 $\times$ $10^3/mm^3$
- Hemoglobin >8 mg/dL

Data from Swadron SP, LeRoux P, Smith WS, et al. Emergency neurological life support: traumatic brain injury. Neurocrit Care 2012;17:S112–21.

---

protection via intubation may be required in the appropriate setting, discussed elsewhere in this article.

Tier 0

Initial management in tier 0 includes head of bed elevation, maintaining a neck neutral position, and avoiding neck constriction.[27,28,40,41] Hyperthermia may be present and can contribute to secondary injury. A goal temperature between 36°C and 38°C is

---

Box 2
Emergency department considerations

- Maintain spinal precautions.
- Conduct primary and secondary surveys, while addressing life-threatening injuries.
- Advanced airway management may be needed for airway protection, hypoxia, and control of ventilation.
- Obtain rapid intravenous access.
- Optimize oxygenation, blood pressure, and ventilation.
- Target oxygen saturation 94%–98%, with a systolic blood pressure of >100 mm Hg.
- Assess Glasgow Coma Scale, motor function, and pupillary function.
- Obtain a noncontrast head computed tomography scan.
- Any sign of worsening neurologic status, including decreased mental status, posturing, and vital sign abnormality, warrants hyperosmolar therapy.
- Obtain neurosurgical consultation for decreased Glasgow Coma Scale, penetrating injury, or abnormal computed tomography scan.

recommended. Adequate analgesia and avoidance of agitation are important to reduce ICP.[10,11,23,42] Laryngeal stimulation should be minimized.[11,31] Per the Brain Trauma foundation, systolic blood pressure should remain at greater than 100 mm Hg (>110 mm Hg in those >70 years of age), or the MAP at greater than 70 mm Hg.[43–45] However, other authors recommend 80 mm Hg. If these measures are not effective, the physician should move to tier 1 management. Owing to concern for hypotension, invasive blood pressure monitoring using an arterial line may be warranted if placement does not delay further study and intervention. There is little evidence present discussing invasive arterial blood pressure monitoring.

Tier 1

Hyperosmotic agents should be used with signs of increased ICP or altered mental status. Of note, mannitol is often the first agent recommended per the Brain Trauma Foundation, although studies suggest that mannitol and hypertonic saline (HTS) are equivalent, except in the situation involving hypotension (HTS is then recommended).[27,28,40,41] Literature evaluating mannitol and HTS is discussed elsewhere in this article, although the authors prefer HTS. Mannitol can be provided as a 0.25 to 1.0 g/kg intravenous (IV) bolus; however, in the hypotensive patient, mannitol should be avoided owing to its diuretic effects. HTS at 3% concentration can also be used at 150- to 250-mL IV boluses, with a serum sodium target greater than 145 mEq/L (maximum 155–160 mEq/L). CSF drainage via external ventricular drainage is required if acute obstructive hydrocephalus is discovered, although this procedure requires neuroimaging.[46,47] If ICP is not controlled with these measures, tier 2 measures are needed.

Tier 2

Per the Brain Trauma Foundation, tier 2 measures include first HTS bolus, which can be administered in concentrations ranging from 3.0% to 23.4%. We prefer a bolus of 250 mL of 3% HTS. Concentrations of greater than 3% should be provided through central access. Goal serum sodium is greater than 145 mEq/L. If HTS was provided in tier 1, a second bolus may be provided. If ICP remains elevated, propofol 1 to 3 mg/kg IV bolus is needed to reduce ICP, with infusion of 200 μg/kg/min.[11,27,28,40,41] IV fluids and vasopressors may be needed to maintain blood pressure.

Tier 3

Tier 3 measures are the most aggressive, with the greatest potential for adverse events. Pentobarbital coma may be needed, with a bolus 10 mg/kg IV over 30 minutes, followed by 5 mg/kg/h IV for 3 hours and maintenance of 1 to 4 mg/kg/h. This infusion is continued for 24 to 96 hours. Although this approach is recommended, propofol may be used, which is readily available in the ED. Moderate hypothermia with target core temperature 32°C to 34°C with external cooling devices or cooled IV fluids may decrease ICP. Hyperventilation targeting $Paco_2$ 30 to 35 mm Hg may be considered, although cerebral oxygenation should be monitored to reduce ischemia. Surgical decompression is another potential therapy in consultation with neurosurgery.[11,27,28,40,41]

These treatments are explored further, with more in-depth explanations of the literature and intricacies of these therapies.

HOW SHOULD THE AIRWAY BE MANAGED?

Airway protection and blood pressure support for severe neurotrauma are priorities. Rapid sequence intubation with in-line stabilization of the cervical spine may be necessary. First pass success is vital to avoid the adverse effects of hypoxia and avoid repeated laryngeal stimulation.[11,31] Considerations of intubation are discussed in **Box 3**. Adequate preoxygenation with apneic oxygenation and head of bed elevation are important in preventing hypoxia.[48,49]

Patients may experience hypertensive response to laryngoscopy or suctioning attempts.[31,50,51] Lidocaine was originally thought to help prevent sympathomimetic responses to endotracheal tube placement; however, lidocaine has not demonstrated an ability to reduce ICP or improve neurologic outcome.[31,52,53] Fentanyl at doses of 2 to 5 μg/kg IV before intubation can reduce the hyperdynamic response to intubation.[31,54,55] Several studies have evaluated esmolol (1.5 mg/kg IV) before intubation to blunt the hemodynamic response to intubation, although this medication should be avoided in patients with hypotension, hemorrhagic shock, or signs of multiple trauma.[11,31,56,57] Its role in premedication remains to be defined. Authors recommend fentanyl if concerned for hypertensive response to laryngoscopy, which also provides analgesia.

Induction medications are a vital component of intubation. Traditionally, ketamine was contraindicated for induction in intubation for head injury,[58–60] but the literature suggests it is useful in this setting owing to its hemodynamic neutrality.[31,61,62] It has demonstrated safety in patients with CNS trauma and TBI, with evidence suggesting increase in cerebral perfusion and no change on ICP.[31,61,62] Propofol is a phenol derivative with high lipid solubility and rapid onset of action.[27,31,63,64] Studies demonstrate a neuroprotective effect through a reduction in ICP and oxidative stress.[27,31,63,64] However, this effect must be balanced with the potential hypotension caused by propofol.[31,65] Etomidate causes less hypotension and cardiovascular depression when compared with propofol or benzodiazepines.[31] It has a rapid onset and lasts 5 minutes, while reducing ICP and maintaining or increasing CPP.[66–68] However, it may lower the seizure threshold and may increase nausea/vomiting and

---

Box 3
Intubation considerations

- Preparation: proper positioning, preoxygenate, and use apneic oxygenation with nasal cannula, facemask, or noninvasive positive pressure ventilation if needed.

- Head of bed elevation to improve cerebral perfusion pressure and decrease aspiration.

- Among neurotrauma patients, 80% experience catecholamine surge after intubation, which is often worsened with extensive airway manipulation and suctioning.

- Premedication regimens are controversial. Fentanyl at 2–5 μg/kg intravenously may decrease catecholamine surge. Lidocaine and defasciculating doses of neuromuscular blockers have shown no benefit.

- Esmolol at 1.5 mg/kg intravenously before intubation in hemodynamically stable patients may help control the hemodynamic response to intubation.

- Induction agent may include ketamine (does not adversely affect patients with neurotrauma) and etomidate, as these medications possess hemodynamic-sparing properties.

- Propofol has neuroprotective effects, but hypotension may occur.

- Postintubation analgesia and sedation are essential.

Data from Bucher J, Koyfman A. Intubation of the neurologically injured patient. J Emerg Med 2015;49(6):920–7; and Seder DB, Riker RR, Jagoda A, et al. Emergency neurological life support: airway, ventilation, and sedation. Neurocrit Care 2010;17:S4–20.

myoclonic movements (resulting in increased ICP).[66–68] These authors recommend ketamine or etomidate for induction.

Paralysis should be used to assist first pass success while intubating; however, a neurologic examination should be conducted before paralysis if possible.[68–71] Subsequent paralysis complicates the picture, and the neurologic examination when combined with neuroimaging can impact clinical decision making. Defasciculating doses of paralytics such as succinylcholine or pancuronium to reduce fasciculations or reduce the chance of ICP elevation are not beneficial.[69–71] Succinylcholine is a depolarizing neuromuscular blocker with a duration of 2 to 10 minutes, whereas rocuronium is a nondepolarizing neuromuscular agent with a duration of close to 40 minutes to 1 hour.[31,68] Any paralytic agent requires analgesia and sedation with intubation. Succinylcholine may allow a faster time to recovery and an ability to assess neurologic function, as compared with rocuronium.[31,68] The choice of paralytic rests on the provider, because either agent is safe and efficacious when used appropriately.

One vital aspect to consider is the need for postintubation sedation and analgesia. An intubated patient with inadequate analgesia and sedation may display a sympathomimetic response.[27,28,31,68] Physicians should order postintubation medications at similar times as the induction and paralytic agents to avoid this pitfall. Analgesics, including fentanyl and remifentanil, offer fast and predictable pain relief. These agents function as an adjunct to other sedative agents and should be used in these patients with sedatives.[31,68] Morphine and hydromorphone have a longer duration of action and may accumulate with prolonged infusion. Propofol is an optimal sedative agent, because it possesses fast onset and offset, allowing for repeat neurologic assessment.[63,64] However, if used, the blood pressure should be carefully monitored owing to the potential for hypotension. The cardiovascular effects can be minimized by titrating the infusion, rather than providing bolus doses.[27,28,31] Propofol infusion syndrome may occur if infusion of greater than 4 mg/kg/h for more than 48 hours is used.[72] Benzodiazepines can be used for sedation and may reduce cerebral blood flow and ICP, while increasing seizure threshold. However, they can reduce blood pressure and cause respiratory depression.[27,31,68] Tolerance can also develop in prolonged infusions. Patient reassessment is difficult with this infusion, because the accumulation of metabolites results in a prolonged duration of action, and patients also demonstrate increased delirium. Dexmedetomidine is a selective alpha-2 receptor agonist with anxiolytic and sedative effects and an elimination time of 2 hours. Hypotension and bradycardia are the most common side effects.[31,73,74] This medication may reduce ICP and increase cerebral perfusion, although further study is needed.

Once intubation is completed, hypoxia and hyperoxia should be avoided. Oxygenation should not decrease to less than 90% or to less than 60 mm Hg, although hyperoxia with a Pao_2 of greater than 300 to 470 mm Hg is discouraged.[31,35] $Paco_2$ levels of 35 to 45 mm Hg, or an end-tidal CO_2 of 30 to 40 mm Hg, are encouraged. Hyperventilation should be avoided, except in the setting of active herniation. Ventilator settings should target these mentioned Pao_2 and $Paco_2$ levels.[27,31,68]

HOW SHOULD YOU TREAT HYPOTENSION?

A single systolic blood pressure reading of less than 90 mm Hg is a predictor of worse outcome in TBI, whereas MAP greater than 80 mm Hg is preferable in the resuscitation phase.[25,29,36,41,43–45,75,76] The multitrauma patient with head trauma who is hypotensive presents a challenge. Permissive hypotension to reduce the risk of clot disruption in penetrating trauma may be beneficial. However, in the patient with moderate to severe head trauma, permissive hypotension is contraindicated. We recommend a MAP of

70–80 mm Hg. First-line management includes fluid resuscitation. Although some may use HTS for fluid resuscitation, the literature suggests no difference between normal saline and HTS for patients with no evidence of herniation.[27,41,77] If hypotensive, the patient should receive blood products and HTS. Hypoosmotic fluids such as albumin should be avoided.[2,11,27] Albumin is associated with higher mortality, as demonstrated in a subset of TBI patients in the SAFE trial (Saline versus Albumin Fluid Evaluation).[78]

ARE VASOPRESSORS NEEDED?

The patient with shock from a neurogenic source often requires the use of IV fluid and vasopressors.[8,76,79–81] Patients with neurogenic shock with hypotension and bradycardia should receive IV fluids before vasopressors. Loss of sympathetic tone is common within the first week of injury.[8,9,76,79–82] A goal MAP of 85 mm Hg is recommended by the American Association of Neurological Surgeons and Congress of Neurological Surgeons, which is different other conditions in neurotrauma including TBI.[82] The American Association of Neurological Surgeons and Congress of Neurological Surgeons recommend dopamine, norepinephrine, or phenylephrine for blood pressure management. We prefer IV fluid resuscitation first with blood products, followed by norepinephrine targeting MAP 80 mm Hg, because norepinephrine provides an optimal increase in afterload and inotropy, which is needed with the loss of sympathetic tone.[76,79–82]

WHEN SHOULD YOU SPEAK WITH THE NEUROSURGEON?

Neurosurgical consultation is advised for a GCS of 13 or less, seizure, lateralizing findings on examination, abnormal head CT scan, signs of CSF leak, basilar skull fracture, penetrating injury, cerebrovascular injury, or C-spine injury.[2,11,27,28,75,82,83] Rapid neurosurgical team involvement is associated with improved outcomes.[27,28,83]

WHAT HYPEROSMOLAR THERAPIES ARE AVAILABLE, AND WHICH IS THE MOST EFFECTIVE?

Hyperosmolar therapy is a staple of neurotrauma management through reduction in ICP, decreased brain water and edema, and improved cerebral blood flow. This combination ultimately results in improved cerebral perfusion.[2,11,41,77,78,84–87] Any findings suggestive of increased ICP such as pupillary change, decrease in the GCS of 2 or more points, or posturing warrants empiric treatment with 20% mannitol 0.25 to 1.00 g/kg IV as a rapid infusion over 5 minutes or 3% NaCl 150 to 250 mL IV over 10 minutes (although concentrations vary up to 23.4%).[10,11,27,28] HTS is preferred if the systolic blood pressure is approaching 90 mm Hg or below owing to its volume expander effects. These measures also increase perfusion and cerebral blood flow.[27,41,77,78,84–86] However, in terms of ICP reduction, a metaanalysis from 2015 demonstrates no difference in neurologic outcome or mortality between HTS and mannitol.[77] HTS may provide longer term ICP control.[88,89]

Mannitol has been in use for more than 5 decades as a hyperosmolar agent and is administered as a 20% solution.[2,77,90–92] This solution deforms RBCs and decreases blood viscosity, allowing cerebral blood flow in hypoperfused areas.[90–92] If autoregulation is intact, compensatory vasoconstriction will decrease total cerebral blood volume and decrease ICP.[91–94] Rebound increases in ICP are possible, and mannitol can cause diuresis and increase the risk of renal failure.[2,42,77,95–97] IV fluids should be provided with the diuresis that can occur, and placement of a Foley catheter will likely be needed for monitoring of urine output.[41]

HTS can be provided in concentrations ranging from 2.0% to 23.4%, with similar effects as mannitol in improving cerebral blood flow and decreasing parenchymal water content.[2,77,98–101] HTS can function as a volume expander, while improving blood pressure. The risk of rebound ICP is less than that with mannitol. HTS is impermeable to an intact blood–brain barrier, as opposed to mannitol.[2,11,27,41,42] The most common side effect of HTS is hyperchloremic metabolic acidosis.[2,11] The attributes of HTS are beneficial in patients with low blood pressure and neurotrauma.[99–101] Ultimately, both agents are effective in decreasing ICP and improving CPP. We prefer HTS saline 3% concentration in 250 mL IV boluses, which can be repeated.

WHEN IS MONITORING OF INTRACRANIAL PRESSURE REQUIRED?

Placement of an ICP monitor is difficult in an ED, and it requires consultation with a neurosurgeon.[2,11,27,102] However, these monitors may assist in management, because prolonged intracranial hypertension is associated with poor outcome specifically in patients with a GCS of less than 8.[2,26,27,102,103] Indications are discussed further in **Box 4**. Of note, patients with any abnormality on the head CT scan have an increased risk of intracranial hypertension that approaches 63%, compared with those with a normal CT.[103,104] The value in ICP monitoring is that it can be difficult to diagnose elevated ICP clinically in certain patients, such as those with severe neurotrauma.[104] Especially in the sedated patient, examination can be difficult. Pupillary examination and posturing may be the only signs of an increased ICP.[2,102–104]

The most reliable monitors involve invasive placement of a ventricular catheter or intraparenchymal monitor.[2,11,102–104] Ventriculostomy or external ventricular drain also allows drainage of CSF, which can be therapeutic.[11,102–104] Elevated ICP may be controlled in approximately 50% of patients with external ventricular drain insertion after failure of other measures.[11,70–75]

IS THERE A BEDSIDE TECHNIQUE TO EVALUATE FOR INCREASED INTRACRANIAL PRESSURE?

Ocular ultrasound imaging can measure the optic nerve sheath diameter (ONSD), which correlates closely with ICP.[105–108] The normal optic nerve sheath is up to 5 mm in diameter, which increases with elevated ICP. To measure the ONSD, a high-resolution linear array probe should be used, with a large amount of water-soluble transmission gel applied to the patient's closed eyelid. The depth should be adjusted so the eye fills

---

Box 4
Intracranial pressure monitoring indications

- GCS 3–8 with abnormal CT scan.
- GCS 3–8 with normal CT scan and 2 of the following: age >40 years, motor posturing, SBP <90 mm Hg.
- GCS 9–15 with CT scan showing mass lesion (>1-cm contusion, intracranial hemorrhage >3 cm), effaced cisterns, or midline shift of >5 mm.
- After craniectomy.
- Inability to follow neurologic examination (such as with sedation).

Abbreviations: CT, computed tomography; GCS, Glasgow Coma Scale; SBP, systolic blood pressure.
Data from Refs.[26,27,102–104]

the screen. Both eyes should be scanned in sagittal and transverse planes. The ONSD should be measured 3 mm posterior to the globe for both eyes, with an average between 2 separate measurements. If the ONSD is greater than 5 mm, increased ICP should be suspected. Multiple studies have demonstrated sensitivities of greater than 90% for detection of ICP with ultrasound imaging, with specificities also of greater than 90%.[105–108] At this time, ultrasound imaging can be used for the evaluation of ICP and should supplement, rather than replace, clinical examination.

WHEN IS SURGERY REQUIRED?

Surgical management of TBI includes repair of depressed skull fracture and evacuation of intracranial mass.[109–114] Decompressive craniectomy is indicated for refractory intracranial hypertension. Indications for specific injuries are shown in **Table 3**. However, decompressive craniectomy may not improve functional outcome while decreasing ICP.[113] The DECRA trial (DEcompressive CRAniectomy) evaluated bifrontotemporal decompression in randomized patients with severe TBI failing other treatments.[109–111] The group undergoing craniectomy experienced worse outcomes.[109–111]

Unstable thoracic spinal fractures include burst fracture, compression fracture with greater than 50% of vertebral height loss, fracture/dislocation, or Chance fracture.[112] Patients with unstable spinal fractures or subluxation may experience improved neurologic outcomes if decompression is completed within 24 hours of injury, demonstrated in the STASCIS trial (Surgical Timing in Acute Spinal Cord Injury Study).[112]

IS HYPOTHERMIA EFFECTIVE IN NEUROTRAUMA?

Hypothermia may act as a neuroprotectant.[2,11,27,121–123] To date, no benefit is present for hypothermia in patients with neurotrauma in mortality or neurologic outcome in

Table 3 Surgical indications for neurologic injuries	
Lesion	**Surgical Indication**
Epidural hematoma	• GCS <9 with anisocoria • Size >30 cm³
Subdural hematoma	• Thickness >10 mm or midline shift >5 mm regardless of GCS • GCS decline by >2 • Fixed and dilated or asymmetric pupils • ICP >20 mm Hg
Parenchymal lesion	• Lesion ≥50 cm³ • GCS 6–8 with midline shift ≥5 mm, cistern compression, or frontal/temporal contusion ≥20 cm³ • Continued neurologic decline, refractory intracranial hypertension, or mass effect on CT owing to lesion
Posterior fossa lesion	• Mass effect on CT • Neurologic decline owing to lesion
Depressed skull fracture	• Open fracture greater than cranium thickness • Open fracture with dural penetration, significant associated intracranial hematoma, depression >1 cm, frontal sinus involvement, gross deformity, wound infection, pneumocephalus, gross wound contamination

Abbreviations: CT, computed tomography; GCS, Glasgow Coma Scale; ICP, intracranial pressure.
Data from Refs.[109–120]

several metaanalyses.[121–123] However, intracranial hypertension is reduced with hypothermia.[121–123] Targeted management of temperature reduces the cerebral metabolic rate, the release of excitatory neurotransmitters, and blood–brain barrier destruction.[124–126] Hypothermia remains experimental, and further research is required.

SHOULD YOU REVERSE COAGULOPATHY WITH TRAUMATIC INTRACEREBRAL HEMORRHAGE?

Close to one-third of patients who experience severe TBI develop a coagulopathy, associated with poor neurologic outcomes and mortality. This coagulopathy can be due to patient medications, but acute neurotrauma can result in coagulopathy through systemic release of tissue factor, which lead to intravascular coagulation and consumptive coagulopathy.[127,128] Tests such as the prothrombin time, partial thromboplastin time, International Normalized Ratio, and thromboelastography can be used to assess coagulation status.[129] Patients on warfarin can be given IV vitamin K and either prothrombin complex concentrate or fresh frozen plasma. Prothrombin complex concentrate provides significantly less volume with faster time to coagulation reversal.[127,128,130] Prothrombin complex concentrate may also reverse novel oral anticoagulants, although medication-specific antidotes are currently available.[127,128,130] Platelet transfusion in patients with ICH on antiplatelet medications may be harmful in spontaneous ICH, as recently demonstrated in the PATCH trial (Platelet Transfusion versus Standard Care after Acute Stroke Due to Spontaneous Cerebral Haemorrhage Associated with Antiplatelet Therapy).[131] In patients with traumatic hemorrhage and thromboelastography that demonstrates platelet dysfunction, desmopressin and platelet transfusion may be needed.[27,129]

IS THERE ANY ROLE FOR A PHARMACOLOGICALLY INDUCED COMA?

Barbiturates such as phenobarbital may be used to reduce ICP if refractory to other treatment.[11,27,41,132–137] The mechanism of action is thought to be due to suppression of cerebral metabolism, modification of vascular resistance, and decrease of neuronal excitotoxicity.[133,134] This therapy is associated with multiple side effects, including hypotension, gastroparesis, and immunosuppression.[135,136] Close to 1 in 4 patients experiences hypotension, and a 2012 Cochrane Review found no change in outcomes for severe TBI with barbiturate coma.[137] This measure is a last stage effort to decrease elevated ICP with herniation. These authors prefer propofol infusion first, before attempting barbiturates.

CORTICOSTEROIDS USED TO BE RECOMMENDED, BUT WHAT ABOUT NOW?

Corticosteroids were first used in the 1960s for cerebral edema treatment. Researchers hypothesized that steroids reduced CSF production, altered vascular permeability, and decreased free radicals.[138,139] However, the CRASH trial (Corticosteroid Randomisation after Significant Head Injury) suggests worse outcomes for patients with TBI given steroids.[140] This trial of 10,008 patients from 49 countries demonstrated increased mortality in the group given steroids.[140] For spinal injury, the NASCIS study (National Acute Spinal Cord Injury Study) suggests high-dose steroids within 8 hours of injury improves recovery.[141] However, other studies question this benefit.[142–145] The American Association of Neurological Surgeons and Congress of Neurological Surgeons do not recommend steroids in the setting of SCI.[9,27]

SHOULD SEIZURES BE TREATED IN NEUROTRAUMA?

Seizures occur in up to 30% of TBI patients and 50% of patients with penetrating head injury.[2,11,27,41] Early posttraumatic seizures occur within 7 days of injury and late seizures beyond 7 days. Active seizure requires immediate treatment, because prolonged seizures increase secondary brain injury and increase the ICP.[2,11,27,28,41] Benzodiazepines are a first-line treatment for active seizures. Phenytoin may reduce the incidence of early seizure, but not delayed seizure.[146] Levetiracetam is equivalent to phenytoin, and it also is associated with a lesser risk of side effects and adverse events.[147] Risk factors for seizure include a GCS of less than 10, cortical contusion, any intracranial hematoma, depressed skull fracture, penetrating head injury, or seizure within 24 hours of injury.[147,148] If any of these risk factors are present, seizure prophylaxis is recommended.

DOES TRANEXAMIC ACID HAVE A PLACE IN NEUROTRAUMA?

Tranexamic acid (TXA) has demonstrated usefulness and efficacy in oral bleeding, epistaxis, postpartum hemorrhage, and major trauma.[149–152] The CRASH-2 study found improved measures of coagulopathy and survival in patients requiring massive transfusion if given within the first 3 hours after an injury.[149] However, the effects of TXA in neurotrauma is under study. For patients with nontraumatic intracranial hemorrhage (subarachnoid hemorrhage and intracerebral hemorrhage), limited data suggest that, although it reduces bleeding, it may increase size of the cerebral penumbra.[150,151] The CRASH-2 Intracranial Bleeding Study evaluated use of TXA in TBI patients, finding a trend toward reduction in intracranial hemorrhage growth and lower mortality, but the results were not statistically significant.[150] The current CRASH-3 trial is recruiting patients to assess TXA on TBI.[151] A study in 2017 evaluating TXA in TBI found less hemorrhage growth in patients receiving TXA.[152] At this time, further study is needed, but TXA is likely beneficial.

WHEN IS BURR HOLE EVACUATION REQUIRED, AND HOW IS IT COMPLETED?

Ideal treatment for extraaxial hematoma is provided by a neurosurgeon, but in remote locations this is not always possible.[153–156] Performing an emergency burr hole can be successful, and there have been several advances in the safety of this technique. This procedure should only be attempted in cases of raised and deteriorating ICP refractory to medical management when neurosurgical intervention is not readily available.[153–156] Contraindications include a GCS of greater than 8, no imaging obtained, and neurosurgical intervention available. An important advancement is the production of clutch drill bits, which allows the drill to disengage once the inner table of the skull is penetrated. This procedure requires identification of the site of injury based on imaging, with burr hole placement over the center of the hematoma on the correct side. Hair should be shaved 5 cm over the site, with a 3-cm line marked for incision. The area should be sterilized, and an incision made down to bone. Bleeding should be controlled with direct pressure. The periosteum needs to be pushed off the bone with a scalpel or swab, followed by insertion of a self-retaining retractor. A drill should be pushed down firmly perpendicular to the skull. An assistant must keep the patient's head still, and a saline wash can help to clean away material. Once the drill begins, it should be kept going, because stopping the drill disengages the clutch mechanism. Once the drill bit stops spinning, the drill can then be removed. A blunt hook can then remove any remaining bone fragments, allowing extradural blood to be removed. If a subdural hematoma is present, open the dura with a sharp hook to tent the dura and a scalpel to incise the dura. Subdural hematoma can be difficult to remove owing to clotting, and careful suction or forceps may be needed. If no blood is found, ensure that the site is correct.[153–156]

WHAT IS NEUROGENIC SHOCK, AND IS IT DIFFERENT FROM SPINAL SHOCK?

Neurogenic shock is a form of distributive shock found in spinal cord injuries above T6, resulting in loss of sympathetic tone to the systemic vasculature.[75,76,79–82] This leads to hypotension, vasodilatation, and bradycardia with increased vagal tone. Brady-cardia should trigger the consideration for neurogenic shock, although this entity may be complicated by concomitant hemorrhage.[75,76,79–82] Providers should always consider hemorrhagic shock in the patient with hypotension and trauma.

Spinal shock is a different entity, characterized by an incomplete spinal cord syn-drome with the loss of sensation and motor function (flaccid paralysis) below the injury level.[157,158] Reflexes are depressed or absent below the level of injury, which may take weeks for resolution.[157,158]

WHAT ARE THE PITFALLS IN EVALUATION AND MANAGEMENT?

A variety of pitfalls are present in neuroresuscitation. These pitfalls include failure to obtain adequate neurologic examination before sedation and paralysis, inadequate postintubation sedation and analgesia, and failure to achieve the neuroresuscitation targets as described. Various trials have evaluated the use of other medications that target aspects of neurotrauma. Progesterone IV has not demonstrated efficacy in 2 separate trials and should not be used.[159,160]

Hyperventilation was previously used to reduce ICP.[2,11,23,27,41,42] Increasing the respiratory rate or tidal volume produces a decrease in $Paco_2$, which leads to cere-bral vasoconstriction. This measure reduces cerebral blood volume and ICP acutely.[2,11,23,27,42] However, hyperventilation may result in secondary ischemia if used for prolonged periods. Hyperventilation has demonstrated worse clinical outcomes in patients hyperventilated to a $Paco_2$ of less than 30 mm Hg for 5 days.[161–165] This condition has also been observed in patients hyperventilated for more than 6 hours.[163,164] Hyperventilation reduces cerebral blood flow and in-creases the amount of ischemic tissue. A risk of increased cerebral edema is present when hyperventilation is discontinued.[163,164] Most guidelines recommend the avoid-ance of hyperventilation within the first 48 hours.[11,27,68] Mild hyperventilation can be considered for acute neurologic deterioration, but only temporarily, owing to an increased risk of cerebral ischemia. A $Paco_2$ of less than 30 mm Hg should be avoided.[2,11,27]

WHAT AFFECTS PROGNOSIS?

Patient outcome depends on multiple factors, including arrival GCS, CT abnormalities, age, other injuries, hypotension, hypoxemia, pyrexia, elevated ICP, decreased CPP, decreased pupillary function, and coagulopathy. Biomarkers have been evaluated including alpha-synuclein, S-100Beta protein, and neuro-specific enolase of the blood or CSF.[166–168] These markers require further validation before use. A GCS of less than 8 is associated with a 30% mortality, and only 25% are functionally independent in the long term.[169–171] In spinal trauma, the level and degree of deficit affect prognosis. The higher the lesion (such as C5 vs L1), the worse the outcome. Incomplete injuries are associated with improved outcomes and functional ability.[172,173] Complete loss of function below a specific spinal level is a poor prognostic sign.

NEWER DIRECTIONS

Care of patients with neurotrauma is now a well-defined specialty. Specialized neuro-critical care teams reduce duration of stay and in-hospital mortality.[2,83] Specialized imaging include MRI and real-time monitoring of further cerebral physiology such as transcranial Doppler ultrasound imaging may provide benefit, although further studies are needed.[174,175]

A number of assessment scores are available, often dependent on the physician and institution. The GCS is a 15-point score composed of eye, motor, and verbal responses, first described in 1974.[176] It is used universally and can be performed quickly. The FOUR score (Full Outline of Unresponsiveness Score) demonstrates a greater ability to assess the neurologic function of intubated patients and an ability to predict the mortality of critical patients when compared with GCS.[177–179] This score was first described in 2005 and is a 16-point score that assesses eye, motor, brain-stem reflexes, and respirations.[176] Ultimately, either score may be used to evaluate initial neurologic status and with reassessments.

SUMMARY

Neurotrauma is the leading cause of death in North America in those between 1 and 45 years of age. Primary and secondary injuries result in severe morbidity and mortality. Neurotrauma includes head contusion, epidural hematoma, subdural hematoma, subarachnoid hemorrhage, diffuse axonal injury, skull fracture, and traumatic spinal cord injury. CPP requires adequate cerebral blood flow. Evaluation and management in the ED entails initial stabilization and resuscitation while assessing neurologic status. Targeting mean arterial pressure, oxygen levels, and neurologic status are key components. ICP management should follow a tiered approach. Intubation of the patient with neurotrauma should be completed with several considerations. Steroids are not recommended currently. The criteria for the placement of an ICP monitor and surgical decompression require consultation with neurosurgery.

REFERENCES

1. Faul M, Xu L, Wald MM, et al. Traumatic brain injury in the United States: emergency department visits, hospitalizations and deaths 2002–2006. Atlanta (GA): Centers for Disease Control and Prevention, National Center for Injury Prevention and Control; 2010.
2. Wan-Tsu WC, Badjatia N. Neurotrauma. Emerg Med Clin North Am 2014;32: 889–905.
3. Rutland-Brown W, Langlois JA, Thomas KE, et al. Incidence of traumatic brain injury in the United States, 2003. J Head Trauma Rehabil 2006;21:544.
4. Tagliaferri F, Compagnone C, Korsic M, et al. A systematic review of brain injury epidemiology in Europe. Acta Neurochir (Wien) 2006;148:255.
5. Hillier SL, Hiller JE, Metzer J. Epidemiology of traumatic brain injury in South Australia. Brain Inj 1997;11:649.
6. Center NSCIS. Spinal cord injury facts and figures at a glance. Birmingham (AL): 2013. Available at: https://www.nscisc.uab.edu/PublicDocuments/fact_figures_docs/Facts 2013.pdf. Accessed May 16, 2016.
7. Devivo MJ. Epidemiology of traumatic spinal cord injury: trends and future implications. Spinal Cord 2012;50(5):365–72.
8. Stein DM, Roddy V, Mark J, et al. Emergency neurological life support: traumatic spine injury. Neurocrit Care 2012;17:S102–11.

9. Hadley MN, Walters BC, Aarabi B, et al. Guidelines for the management of acute cervical spine and spinal cord injuries. Neurosurgery 2013;72(Suppl 2):1–259.

10. Oddo M, Le Roux PD. What is the etiology, pathogenesis and pathophysiology of elevated intracranial pressure?. In: Neligan P, Deutschman CS, editors. The evidenced based practice of critical care. Philadelphia: Elsevier Science; 2009. p. 399–405.

11. Swadron SP, LeRoux P, Smith WS, et al. Emergency neurological life support: traumatic brain injury. Neurocrit Care 2012;17:S112–21.

12. Barr RM, Gean AD, Le TH. Craniofacial trauma. In: Brant WE, Helms CA, editors. Fundamentals of diagnostic radiology. Philadelphia: Lippincott, Williams & Wilkins; 2007. p. 69. ISBN 0-7817-6135-2.

13. Gruen P. Surgical management of head trauma. Neuroimaging Clin N Am 2002; 12(2):339–43.

14. Smith J, Tiandra JJ, Clupie GJA, et al. Textbook of surgery. Wiley-Blackwell; 2006. p. 446.

15. Orlando Regional Healthcare, Education and Development. 2004. "Overview of adult traumatic brain injuries". Available at http://text.123doc.org/document/1404616-overview-of-adult-traumatic-brain-injuries.htm. Accessed June 16, 2016.

16. Bouma GJ, Muizelaar JP. Cerebral blood flow, cerebral blood volume, and cerebrovascular reactivity after severe head injury. J Neurotrauma 1992;9(Suppl 1):S333.

17. Bouma GJ, Muizelaar JP, Bandoh K, et al. Blood pressure and intracranial pressure-volume dynamics in severe head injury: relationship with cerebral blood flow. J Neurosurg 1992;77:15.

18. Thurman DJ, Alverson C, Dunn KA, et al. Traumatic brain injury in the United States: a public health perspective. J Head Trauma Rehabil 1999;14:602.

19. Zaloshnja E, Miller T, Langlois JA, et al. Prevalence of long-term disability from traumatic brain injury in the civilian population of the United States, 2005. J Head Trauma Rehabil 2008;23:394.

20. Aarabi B, Tofighi B, Kufera JA, et al. Predictors of outcome in civilian gunshot wounds to the head. J Neurosurg 2014;120(5):1138–46.

21. Magnuson J, Leonessa F, Ling GS. Neuropathology of explosive blast traumatic brain injury. Curr Neurol Neurosci Rep 2012;12(5):570–9.

22. Stein DM, Boswell S, Sliker CW, et al. Blunt cerebrovascular injuries: does treatment always matter? J Trauma 2009;66(1):132–43 [discussion: 143–4].

23. Robertson CS, Valadka AB, Hannay HJ, et al. Prevention of secondary ischemic insults after severe head injury. Crit Care Med 1999;27:2086.

24. Howells T, Elf K, Jones PA, et al. Pressure reactivity as a guide in the treatment of cerebral perfusion pressure in patients with brain trauma. J Neurosurg 2005; 102:311.

25. Chestnut RM, Marshall LF, Klauber MR, et al. The role of secondary brain injury in determining outcome from severe head injury. J Trauma 1993;34(2):216–22.

26. Marmarou A, Anderson RL, Ward JD, et al. Impact of ICP instability and hypotension on outcome in patients with severe head trauma. J Neurosurg 1991; 75(Suppl):S59–66.

27. Carney N, Totten AM, O'Reilly C, et al. Guidelines for the management of severe traumatic brain injury, fourth edition. Neurosurgery 2017;80(1):6–15.

28. Stevens RD, Huff JS, Duckworth J, et al. Emergency neurological life support: intracranial hypertension and herniation. Neurocrit Care 2012;17(Suppl 1): S60–5.

29. McHugh GS, Engel DC, Butcher I, et al. Prognostic value of secondary insults in traumatic brain injury: results from the IMPACT study. J Neurotrauma 2007; 24:287.

30. Harhangi BS, Kompanje EJ, Leebeek FW, et al. Coagulation disorders after traumatic brain injury. Acta Neurochir (Wien) 2008;150:165.

31. Bucher J, Koyfman A. Intubation of the neurologically injured patient. J Emerg Med 2015;49(6):920–7.

32. Oertel M, Kelly DF, McArthur D, et al. Progressive hemorrhage after head trauma: predictors and consequences of the evolving injury. J Neurosurg 2002;96:109.

33. Narayan RK, Maas AI, Servadei F, et al. Progression of traumatic intracerebral hemorrhage: a prospective observational study. J Neurotrauma 2008;25:629.

34. Thomas BW, Mejia VA, Maxwell RA, et al. Scheduled repeat CT scanning for traumatic brain injury remains important in assessing head injury progression. J Am Coll Surg 2010;210:824.

35. Muizelaar JP, Marmarou A, Ward JD, et al. Adverse effects of prolonged hyperventilation in patients with severe head injury: a randomized clinical trial. J Neurosurg 1991;75(5):731–9.

36. Pietropaoli J, Rogers F, Shackford S, et al. The deleterious effects of intraoperative hypotension on outcome in patients with severe head injuries. J Trauma 1992;33(3):403–7.

37. Servadei F, Murray GD, Penny K, et al. The value of the "worst" computed tomographic scan in clinical studies of moderate and severe head injury. European Brain Injury Consortium. Neurosurgery 2000;46:70.

38. Chang EF, Meeker M, Holland MC. Acute traumatic intraparenchymal hemorrhage: risk factors for progression in the early post-injury period. Neurosurgery 2006;58:647.

39. Nordstrom C, Reinstrup P, Xu W, et al. Assessment of the lower limit for cerebral perfusion pressure in severe head injuries by bedside monitoring of regional energy metabolism. Anesthesiology 2003;98(4):809–14.

40. Emergency Neurological Life Support: elevated ICP or herniation. 2014. Available at: http://enlsprotocols.org/files/ICP.pdf. Accessed November 16, 2016.

41. Weingart S. EMCrit: Podcast 78 – Increased intra-cranial pressure (ICP) and herniation, aka brain code. Available at: http://emcrit.org/podcasts/high-icp-herniation/. Accessed November 16, 2016.

42. Rosner MJ, Daughton S. Cerebral perfusion pressure management in head injury. J Trauma 1990;30:933.

43. Berry C, Ley EJ, Bukur M, et al. Redefining hypotension in traumatic brain injury. Injury 2012;43(11):1833–7.

44. Brenner M, Stein DM, Hu PF, et al. Traditional systolic blood pressure targets underestimate hypotension-induced secondary brain injury. J Trauma Acute Care Surg 2012;72(5):1135–9.

45. Butcher I, Murray GD, McHugh GS, et al. Multivariable prognostic analysis in traumatic brain injury: results from the IMPACT study. J Neurotrauma 2007; 24(2):329–37.

46. Haddad SH, Arabi YM. Critical care management of severe traumatic brain injury in adults. Scand J Trauma Resusc Emerg Med 2012;20:12.

47. Helmy A, Vizcaychipi M, Gupta AK. Traumatic brain injury: intensive care management. Br J Anaesth 2007;99(1):32–42.

48. Weingart SD, Levitan RM. Preoxygenation and prevention of desaturation during emergency airway management. Ann Emerg Med 2012;59:165–75.e1.

49. Dixon BJ, Dixon JB, Carden JR, et al. Preoxygenation is more effective in the 25 degrees head-up position than in the supine position in severely obese patients: a randomized controlled study. Anesthesiology 2005;102:1110–5 [discussion: 1115A].

50. Perkins ZB, Wittenberg MD, Nevin D, et al. The relationship between head injury severity and hemodynamic response to tracheal intubation. J Trauma Acute Care Surg 2013;74:1074.

51. Hassan HG, el-Sharkawy TY, Renck H, et al. Hemodynamic and catecholamine responses to laryngoscopy with vs. without endotracheal intubation. Acta Anaesthesiol Scand 1991;35:442–7.

52. Lin CC, Yu JH, Lin CC, et al. Postintubation hemodynamic effects of intravenous lidocaine in severe traumatic brain injury. Am J Emerg Med 2012;30:1782–7.

53. Robinson N, Clancy M. In patients with head injury undergoing rapid sequence intubation, does pretreatment with intravenous lignocaine/lidocaine lead to an improved neurological outcome? A review of the literature. Emerg Med J 2001;18(6):453–7.

54. Dahlgren N, Messeter K. Treatment of stress response to laryngoscopy and intubation with fentanyl. Anaesthesia 1981;36:1022–6.

55. Cork RC, Weiss JL, Hameroff SR, et al. Fentanyl preloading for rapid-sequence induction of anesthesia. Anesth Analg 1984;63:60–4.

56. Singh H, Vichitvejpaisal P, Gaines GY, et al. Comparative effects of lidocaine, esmolol, and nitroglycerin in modifying the hemodynamic response to laryngoscopy and intubation. J Clin Anesth 1995;7:5–8.

57. Ugur B, Ogurlu M, Gezer E, et al. Effects of esmolol, lidocaine and fentanyl on haemodynamic responses to endo- tracheal intubation: a comparative study. Clin Drug Invest 2007;27:269–77.

58. Shaprio HM, Wyte SR, Harris AB. Ketamine anaesthesia in patients with intracranial pathology. Br J Anaesth 1972;44:1200–4.

59. Gibbs JM. The effect of intravenous ketamine on cerebrospinal fluid pressure. Br J Anaesth 1972;44:1298–302.

60. Gardner AE, Dannemiller FJ, Dean D. Intracranial cerebrospinal fluid pressure in man during ketamine anesthesia. Anesth Analg 1972;51:741–5.

61. Jabre P, Combes X, Lapostolle F, et al. Etomidate versus ketamine for rapid sequence intubation in acutely ill patients: a multicentre randomised controlled trial. Lancet 2009;374:293–300.

62. Cohen L, Athaide V, Wickham ME, et al. The effect of ketamine on intracranial and cerebral perfusion pressure and health outcomes: a systematic review. Ann Emerg Med 2015;65:43–51.

63. Rossaint J, Rossaint R, Weis J, et al. Propofol: neuroprotection in an in vitro model of traumatic brain injury. Crit Care 2009;13:R61.

64. Kelly DF, Goodale DB, Williams J, et al. Propofol in the treatment of moderate and severe head injury: a randomized, prospective double-blinded pilot trial. J Neurosurg 1999;90:1042.

65. Hug CC Jr, McLeskey CH, Nahrwold ML, et al. Hemodynamic effects of propofol: data from over 25,000 patients. Anesth Analg 1993;77:S21–9.

66. Bergen JM, Smith DC. A review of etomidate for rapid sequence intubation in the emergency department. J Emerg Med 1997;15:221–30.

67. Moss E, Powell D, Gibson RM, et al. Effect of etomidate on intracranial pressure and cerebral perfusion pressure. Br J Anaesth 1979;51:347–52.

68. Seder DB, Riker RR, Jagoda A, et al. Emergency neurological life support: airway, ventilation, and sedation. Neurocrit Care 2010;17:S4–20.

69. Kovarik WD, Mayberg TS, Lam AM, et al. Succinylcholine does not change intracranial pressure, cerebral blood flow velocity, or the electroencephalogram in patients with neurologic injury. Anesth Analg 1994;78:469–73.

70. Brown MM, Parr MJ, Manara AR. The effect of suxamethonium on intracranial pressure and cerebral perfusion pressure in patients with severe head injuries following blunt trauma. Eur J Anaesthesiol 1996;13:474–7.

71. Koenig KL. Rapid-sequence intubation of head trauma patients: prevention of fasciculations with pancuronium versus minidose succinylcholine. Ann Emerg Med 1992;21:929–32.

72. Otterspoor LC, Kalkman CJ, Cremer OL. Update on the propofol infusion syndrome in ICU management of patients with head injury. Curr Opin Anaesthesiol 2008;21:544.

73. Barrientos-Vega R, Mar Sanchez-Soria M, Morales-Garcia C, et al. Prolonged sedation of critically ill patients with midazolam or propofol: impact on weaning and costs. Crit Care Med 1997;25:33–40.

74. Jakob SM, Ruokonen E, Grounds RM, et al. Dexmedetomidine vs. midazolam or propofol for sedation during prolonged mechanical ventilation: two randomized controlled trials. JAMA 2012;307:1151–60.

75. ATLS Subcommittee, American College of Surgeons' Committee on Trauma, International ATLS Working Group. Advanced trauma life support (ATLS®): the ninth edition. J Trauma Acute Care Surg 2013;74(5):1363–6.

76. Jia X, Kowalski RG, Sciubba DM, et al. Critical care of traumatic spinal cord injury. J Intensive Care Med 2013;28:12.

77. Boone MD, Oren-Grinberg A, Robinson TM, et al. Mannitol or hypertonic saline in the setting of traumatic brain injury: what have we learned? Surg Neurol Int 2015;6:177.

78. The SAFE Study Investigators. A comparison of albumin and saline for fluid resuscitation in the intensive care unit. N Engl J Med 2004;350:2247–56.

79. Vale FL, Burns J, Jackson AB, et al. Combined medical and surgical treatment after acute spinal cord injury: results of a prospective pilot study to assess the merits of aggressive medical resuscitation and blood pressure management. J Neurosurg 1997;87:239.

80. Levi L, Wolf A, Belzberg H. Hemodynamic parameters in patients with acute cervical cord trauma: description, intervention, and prediction of outcome. Neurosurgery 1993;33:1007–16 [discussion: 16–7].

81. Blood pressure management after acute spinal cord injury. Neurosurgery 2002; 50:S58.

82. Guidelines for the management of Acute Cervical Spine and Spinal Cord Injuries. 2007. Available at: http://www.aans.org/en/Education%20and%20Meetings/*/media/Files/Education%20and%20Meetingf/Clinical%20Guidelines/TraumaGuidelines.ashx. Accessed May 14, 2016.

83. Suarez JI, Zaidat OO, Suri MF, et al. Length of stay and mortality in neurocritically ill patients: impact of a specialized neurocritical care team. Crit Care Med 2004;32(11):2311–7.

84. Freshman S, Battistella F, Matteucci M, et al. Hypertonic saline (7.5%) versus mannitol: a comparison for treatment of acute head injuries. J Trauma 1993; 35(3):344–8.

85. Thenuwara K, Todd MM, Brian JE. Effect of mannitol and furosemide on plasma osmolality and brain water. Anesthesiology 2002;96(2):416–21.

86. Wang LC, Papangelou A, Lin C, et al. Comparison of equivolume, equiosmolar solutions of mannitol and hypertonic saline with or without furosemide on brain water content in normal rats. Anesthesiology 2013;118(4):903–13.

87. Scalfani M, Dhar R, Zazulia A, et al. Effect of osmotic agents on regional blood flow in traumatic brain injury. J Crit Care 2012;27(5):526.e7-1.

88. Battison C, Andrews PJ, Graham C, et al. Randomized, controlled trial on the effect of a 20% mannitol solution and a 7.5% saline/6% dextran solution on increased intracranial pressure after brain injury. Crit Care Med 2005;33:196.

89. Vialet R, Albanèse J, Thomachot L, et al. Isovolume hypertonic solutes (sodium chloride or mannitol) in the treatment of refractory posttraumatic intracranial hypertension: 2 mL/kg 7.5% saline is more effective than 2 mL/kg 20% mannitol. Crit Care Med 2003;31:1683.

90. Kassell N, Baumann K, Hitchon P, et al. The effects of high dose mannitol on cerebral blood flow in dogs with normal intracranial pressure. Stroke 1982;13(1):59–61.

91. Muizelaar JP, Wei EP, Kontos HA, et al. Mannitol causes compensatory cerebral vasoconstriction and vasodilation in response to blood viscosity changes. J Neurosurg 1983;59(5):822–8.

92. Mendelow AD, Teasdale GM, Russell T, et al. Effect of mannitol on cerebral blood flow and cerebral perfusion pressure in human head injury. J Neurosurg 1985;63(1):43–8.

93. Muizelaar JP, Ward JD, Marmarou A, et al. Cerebral blood flow and metabolism in severely head-injured children. Part 2: autoregulation. J Neurosurg 1989;71:72.

94. Juul N, Morris GF, Marshall SB, et al. Intracranial hypertension and cerebral perfusion pressure: influence on neurological deterioration and outcome in severe head injury. The Executive Committee of the International Selfotel Trial. J Neurosurg 2000;92:1.

95. McManus M, Soriano S. Rebound swelling of astroglial cells exposed to hypertonic mannitol. Anesthesiology 1998;88(6):1586–91.

96. Palma L, Bruni G, Fiaschi A, et al. Passage of mannitol into the brain around gliomas: a potential cause of rebound phenomenon. A study on 21 patients. J Neurosurg Sci 2006;50(3):63–6.

97. Fang L, You H, Chen B, et al. Mannitol is an independent risk factor of acute kidney injury after cerebral trauma: a case-control study. Ren Fail 2010;32(6):673–9.

98. Wade C, Grady J, Kramer G, et al. Individual patient cohort analysis of the efficacy of hypertonic saline/dextran in patients with traumatic brain injury and hypotension. J Trauma 1998;42(Suppl 5):S61–5.

99. Prough DS, Whiteley JM, Taylor CL, et al. Regional CBF following resuscitation from hemorrhagic shock with HTS influence of a subdural mass. Anesthesiology 1991;75(2):319–27.

100. Shackford SR, Zhuang J, Schmoker J. Intravenous fluid tonicity: effect on intracranial pressure, cerebral blood flow, and cerebral oxygen delivery in focal brain injury. J Neurosurg 1992;76(1):91–8.

101. Shackford S, Schmoker J, Zhuang J. The effect of hypertonic resuscitation on pial arteriolar tone after brain injury and shock. J Trauma 1994;37(6):899–908.

102. Brain Trauma Foundation, American Association of Neurological Surgeons, Congress of Neurological Surgeons, et al. Guidelines for the management of severe traumatic brain injury. VI. Indications for intracranial pressure monitoring. J Neurotrauma 2007;24(Suppl 1):S37.

103. Narayan RK, Kishore PR, Becker DP, et al. Intracranial pressure: to monitor or not to monitor? J Neurosurg 1982;56(56):650–9.
104. Servadei F, Antonelli V, Giuliani G, et al. Evolving lesions in traumatic subarachnoid hemorrhage: prospective study of 110 patients with emphasis on the role of ICP monitoring. Acta Neurochir Suppl 2002;81:81–4.
105. Girisgin AS, Kalkan E, Kocak S, et al. The role of optic nerve ultrasonography in the diagnosis of elevated intracranial pressure. Emerg Med J 2007;24(4):251–4.
106. Potgieter DW, Kippin A, Ngu F, et al. Can accurate ultrasonographic measurement of the optic nerve sheath diameter (a non-invasive measure of intracranial pressure) be taught to novice operators in a single training session? Anaesth Intensive Care 2011;39(1):95–100.
107. Sekhon MS, McBeth P, Zou J, et al. Association between optic nerve sheath diameter and mortality in patients with severe traumatic brain injury. Neurocrit Care 2014;21(2):245–52.
108. Hassen GW, Bruck I, Donahue J, et al. Accuracy of optic nerve sheath diameter measurement by emergency physicians using bedside ultrasound. J Emerg Med 2015;48(4):450–7.
109. Cooper DJ, Rosenfeld JV, Murray L, et al. Decompressive craniectomy in diffuse traumatic brain injury. N Engl J Med 2011;364(16):1493–502.
110. Honeybul S, Ho KM, Lind CR. What can be learned from the DECRA study. World Neurosurg 2013;79(1):159–61.
111. Sahuquillo J, Martinez-Ricarte F, Poca MA. Decompressive craniectomy in traumatic brain injury after the DECRA trial. Where do we stand? Curr Opin Crit Care 2013;19(2):101–6.
112. Fehlings MG, Vaccaro A, Wilson JR, et al. Early versus delayed decompression for traumatic cervical spinal cord injury: results of the surgical timing in acute spinal cord injury study (STASCIS). PLoS One 2012;7(2):e32037.
113. Hutchinson PJ, Kolias AG, Timofeev IS, et al. Trial of decompressive craniectomy for traumatic intracranial hypertension. N Engl J Med 2016;375(12):1119–30.
114. Bullock MR, Chestnut R, Ghajar J, et al. Guidelines for the surgical management of traumatic brain injury. Neurosurgery 2006;58(Suppl):S2-S1-3.
115. Bullock MR, Chesnut R, Ghajar J, et al. Surgical management of acute epidural hematomas. Neurosurgery 2006;58:S7.
116. Bullock MR, Chesnut R, Ghajar J, et al. Surgical management of acute subdural hematomas. Neurosurgery 2006;58:S16.
117. Bullock MR, Chesnut R, Ghajar J, et al. Surgical management of posterior fossa mass lesions. Neurosurgery 2006;58:S47.
118. Bullock MR, Chesnut R, Ghajar J, et al. Surgical management of traumatic parenchymal lesions. Neurosurgery 2006;58:S25.
119. Bullock MR, Chesnut R, Ghajar J, et al. Surgical management of depressed cranial fractures. Neurosurgery 2006;58:S56.
120. Compagnone C, Murray GD, Teasdale GM, et al. The management of patients with intradural post-traumatic mass lesions: a multicenter survey of current approaches to surgical management in 729 patients coordinated by the European Brain Injury Consortium. Neurosurgery 2005;57:1183.
121. Sydenham E, Roberts I, Alderson P. Hypothermia for traumatic head injury. Cochrane Database Syst Rev 2009;(2):CD00104.
122. Clifton GL, Valadka A, Zygun D, et al. Very early hypothermia induction in patients with severe brain injury (the National Acute Brain Injury Study: Hypothermia II): a randomised trial. Lancet Neurol 2011;10(2):131–9.

123. Peterson K, Carson S, Carney N. Hypothermia treatment for traumatic brain injury: a systematic review and meta-analysis. J Neurotrauma 2008;25(1):62–71.

124. Bering E. Effect of body temperature change on cerebral oxygen consumption of the intact monkey. Am J Physiol 1961;200(3):417–9.

125. Busto R, Globus MY, Dietrich WD, et al. Effect of mild hypothermia on ischemia-induced release of neurotransmitters and free fatty acids in rat brain. Stroke 1989;20(7):904–10.

126. Smith SL, Hall ED. Mild pre- and posttraumatic hypothermia attenuates blood-brain barrier damage following controlled cortical impact injury in the rat. J Neurotrauma 1996;13(1):1–9.

127. Morgenstern LB, Hemphill JC 3rd, Anderson C, et al. Guidelines for the management of spontaneous intracerebral hemorrhage: a guideline for healthcare professionals from the American Heart Association/American Stroke Association. Stroke 2010;41:2108.

128. Manno EM, Atkinson JL, Fulgham JR, et al. Emerging medical and surgical management strategies in the evaluation and treatment of intracerebral hemorrhage. Mayo Clin Proc 2005;80:420.

129. Eller T, Busse J, Dittrich M, et al. Dabigatran, rivaroxaban, apixaban, argatroban and fondaparinux and their effects on coagulation POC and platelet function tests. Clin Chem Lab Med 2014;52:835.

130. Dickneite G, Hoffman M. Reversing the new oral anticoagulants with prothrombin complex concentrates (PCCs): what is the evidence? Thromb Haemost 2014;111:189.

131. Baharoglu MI, Cordonnier C, Al-Shahi Salman R, et al. Platelet transfusion versus standard care after acute stroke due to spontaneous cerebral haemorrhage associated with antiplatelet therapy (PATCH): a randomised, open-label, phase 3 trial. Lancet 2016;387(10038):2605–13.

132. Eisenberg HM, Frankowski RF, Contant CF, et al. High-dose barbiturate control of elevated intracranial pressure in patients with severe head injury. J Neurosurg 1988;69(1):15–23.

133. Kassell N, Hitchon P, Gerk M, et al. Alterations in cerebral blood flow, oxygen metabolism, and electrical activity produced by high dose sodium thiopental. Neurosurgery 1980;7(6):598–603.

134. Goodman JC, Valadka AB, Gopinath SP, et al. Lactate and excitatory amino acids measured by microdialysis are decreased by pentobarbital coma in head-injured patients. J Neurotrauma 1996;13(10):549–56.

135. Stover JF, Stocker R. Barbiturate coma may promote reversible bone marrow suppression in patients with severe isolated traumatic brain injury. Eur J Clin Pharmacol 1998;54(7):529–34.

136. Bochicchio GV, Bochicchio K, Nehman S, et al. Tolerance and efficacy of enteral nutrition in traumatic brain-injured patients induced into barbiturate coma. JPEN J Parenter Enteral Nutr 2006;30(6):503–6.

137. Roberts I, Sydenham E. Barbiturates for acute traumatic brain injury. Cochrane Database Syst Rev 2012;(12):CD000033.

138. Maxwell RE, Long DM, French LA. The effects of glucosteroids on experimental cold-induced brain edema. Gross morphological alterations and vascular permeability changes. J Neurosurg 1971;34(4):477–87.

139. Hall ED. The neuroprotective pharmacology of methylprednisolone. J Neurosurg 1992;76(1):13–22.

140. Roberts I, Yates D, Sandercock P, et al. Effect of intravenous corticosteroids on death within 14 days in 10008 adults with clinically significant head injury (MRC

CRASH trial): randomised placebo-controlled trial. Lancet 2004;364(9442): 1321–8.

141. Bracken M, Shepard M, Collins W, et al. A randomized, controlled trial of methylprednisolone or naloxone in the treatment of acute spinal-cord injury. Results of the second national acute spinal cord injury study. N Engl J Med 1990; 322(20):1405–11.

142. Bracken MB, Shepard MJ, Holford TR, et al. Administration of methylprednisolone for 24 or 48 hours or tirilazad mesylate for 48 hours in the treatment of acute spinal cord injury. JAMA 1997;277(20):1597–604.

143. Bracken M. Steroids for acute spinal cord injury. Cochrane Database Syst Rev 2012;(1):CD001046.

144. Early Acute Management in Adults with Spinal Cord Injury Clinical Practice Guidelines. 2008. Available at: www.pva.org. Accessed May 20, 2016.

145. Stevens RD, Bhardwaj A, Kirsch JR, et al. Critical care and perioperative management in traumatic spinal cord injury. J Neurosurg Anesthesiol 2003;15: 215–29.

146. Temkin NR, Dikmen SS, Wilensky AJ, et al. Randomized, double-blind study of phenytoin for the prevention of post-traumatic seizures. N Engl J Med 1990; 323(8):497–502.

147. Inaba K, Menaker J, Branco BC, et al. A prospective multicenter comparison of levetiracetam versus phenytoin for early posttraumatic seizure prophylaxis. J Trauma Acute Care Surg 2013;74(3):766–71 [discussion: 771–3].

148. Torbic H, Forni A, Anger KE, et al. Use of antiepileptics for seizure prophylaxis after traumatic brain injury. Am J Health Syst Pharm 2013;70(9):759–66.

149. Roberts I, Shakur H, Coats T, et al. The CRASH-2 trial: a randomised controlled trial and economic evaluation of the effects of tranexamic acid on death, vascular occlusive events and transfusion requirement in bleeding trauma patients. Health Technol Assess 2013;17(10):1–79.

150. Perel P, Al-Shahi Salman R, Kawahara T, et al. CRASH-2 (Clinical Randomisation of an Antifibrinolytic in Significant Haemorrhage) intracranial bleeding study: the effect of tranexamic acid in traumatic brain injury–a nested randomised, placebo-controlled trial. Health Technol Assess 2012;16(13):iii–xii, 1–54.

151. Dewan Y, Komolafe EO, Mejía-Mantilla JH, et al. CRASH-3-tranexamic acid for the treatment of significant traumatic brain injury: study protocol for an international randomized, double-blind, placebo-controlled trial. Trials 2012;13:87.

152. Jokar A, Ahmadi K, Salehi T. The effect of tranexamic acid in traumatic brain injury: a randomized controlled trial. Chin J Traumatol 2017;20(1):49–51.

153. Wilson MH, Wise D, Davies G, et al. Emergency burr holes: "how to do it". Scand J Trauma Resusc Emerg Med 2012;20:24.

154. Bishop CV, Drummond KJ. Rural neurotrauma in Australia: implications for surgical training. ANZ J Surg 2006;76(1–2):53–9.

155. Rinker CF, McMurry FG, Groeneweg VR, et al. Emergency craniotomy in a rural Level III trauma center. J Trauma 1998;44(6):984–9.

156. Wester K. Decompressive surgery for "pure" epidural hematomas: does neurosurgical expertise improve the outcome? Neurosurgery 1999;44(3):495–500.

157. Ditunno JF, Little JW, Tessler A, et al. Spinal shock revisited: a four-phase model. Spinal Cord 2004;42:383.

158. Nanković V, Snur I, Nanković S, et al. Spinal shock. Diagnosis and therapy. Problems and dilemmas. Lijec Vjesn 1995;117(Suppl 2):30 [in Croatian].

159. Wright DW, Yeatts SD, Silbergleit R, et al. Very early administration of progesterone for acute traumatic brain injury. N Engl J Med 2014;371(26):2457–66.

160. Skolnick BE, Maas AI, Narayan RK, et al, SYNAPSE Trial Investigators. A clinical trial of progesterone for severe traumatic brain injury. N Engl J Med 2014; 371(26):2467–76.

161. Stocchetti N, Maas AI, Chieregato A, et al. Hyperventilation in head injury: a review. Chest 2005;127:1812.

162. Imberti R, Bellinzona G, Langer M. Cerebral tissue PO2 and SjvO2 changes during moderate hyperventilation in patients with severe traumatic brain injury. J Neurosurg 2002;96:97.

163. Coles JP, Minhas PS, Fryer TD, et al. Effect of hyperventilation on cerebral blood flow in traumatic head injury: clinical relevance and monitoring correlates. Crit Care Med 2002;30:1950.

164. Coles JP, Fryer TD, Coleman MR, et al. Hyperventilation following head injury: effect on ischemic burden and cerebral oxidative metabolism. Crit Care Med 2007;35:568–78.

165. Marion DW, Puccio A, Wisniewski SR, et al. Effect of hyperventilation on extracellular concentrations of glutamate, lactate, pyruvate, and local cerebral blood flow in patients with severe traumatic brain injury. Crit Care Med 2002;30:2619.

166. Mondello S, Buki A, Italiano D, et al. α-Synuclein in CSF of patients with severe traumatic brain injury. Neurology 2013;80:1662.

167. Mercier E, Boutin A, Lauzier F, et al. Predictive value of S-100β protein for prognosis in patients with moderate and severe traumatic brain injury: systematic review and meta-analysis. BMJ 2013;346:f1757.

168. Chabok SY, Moghadam AD, Saneei Z, et al. Neuron-specific enolase and S100BB as outcome predictors in severe diffuse axonal injury. J Trauma Acute Care Surg 2012;72:1654.

169. Roozenbeek B, Lingsma HF, Lecky FE, et al. Prediction of outcome after moderate and severe traumatic brain injury: external validation of the International Mission on Prognosis and Analysis of Clinical Trials (IMPACT) and Corticoid Randomisation after Significant Head injury (CRASH) prognostic models. Crit Care Med 2012;40:1609.

170. Yuan F, Ding J, Chen H, et al. Predicting outcomes after traumatic brain injury: the development and validation of prognostic models based on admission characteristics. J Trauma Acute Care Surg 2012;73:137.

171. McMillan TM, Teasdale GM, Weir CJ, et al. Death after head injury: the 13 year outcome of a case control study. J Neurol Neurosurg Psychiatry 2011;82:931.

172. Tee JW, Chan PC, Fitzgerald MC, et al. Early predictors of functional disability after spine trauma: a level 1 trauma center study. Spine (Phila Pa 1976) 2013; 38:999.

173. Waters RL, Adkins RH, Yakura JS, et al. Motor and sensory recovery following incomplete tetraplegia. Arch Phys Med Rehabil 1994;75:306.

174. Trabold F, Meyer PG, Blanot S, et al. The prognostic value of transcranial Doppler studies in children with moderate and severe head injury. Intensive Care Med 2004;30(1):108–12.

175. Ract C, Le Moigno S, Bruder N, et al. Transcranial Doppler ultrasound goal-directed therapy for the early management of severe traumatic brain injury. Intensive Care Med 2007;33(4):645–51.

176. Teasdale G, Jennett B. Assessment of coma and impaired consciousness. A practical scale. Lancet 1974;2(7872):81–4.

177. Wijdicks EF, Bamlet WR, Maramattom BV, et al. Validation of a new coma scale: the FOUR score. Ann Neurol 2005;58(4):585–93.

178. Sadaka F, Patel D, Lakshmanan R. The FOUR score predicts outcome in patients after traumatic brain injury. Neurocrit Care 2012;16(1):95–101.
179. Wijdicks EF, Kramer AA, Rohs T Jr, et al. Comparison of the full outline of unresponsiveness score and the Glasgow Coma Scale in predicting mortality in critically ill patients. Crit Care Med 2015;43(2):439–44.

Critical Decisions in the Management of Thoracic Trauma

Morgan Schellenberg, MD, MPH, Kenji Inaba, MD, FRCSC*

KEYWORDS

- Thoracic trauma • Resuscitation • Resuscitative thoracotomy • POCUS • EFAST

KEY POINTS

- Every trauma patient should undergo a rapid clinical examination to screen for traumatic injuries to the thorax.
- There are several imaging modalities that should be considered in the emergency department, which include ultrasound, plain radiographs, and computed tomography scan. It is important to be aware of the indications and pitfalls of each.
- Many thoracic injuries can be managed nonoperatively. Invasive bedside procedures, such as chest tube placement, are critical skills for all emergency medicine physicians who treat trauma patients.
- Resuscitative thoracotomy is a procedure that should be familiar to the emergency medicine physician and is indicated for select patients following penetrating and blunt trauma.

INTRODUCTION

The initial assessment of any injured patient must proceed expeditiously and in a systematic fashion. Injuries to the thorax are common after both blunt and penetrating trauma and, therefore, all patients who present to the emergency department (ED) after trauma should be screened for thoracic injury according to the Advanced Trauma Life Support (ATLS) protocol.[1] Because chest injury can impact each of the ABCs (Airway, Breathing, and Circulation), a rapid evaluation of the chest is performed early in the evaluation of the injured patient to look for any life-threatening injuries. Non–life-threatening injuries to the thorax are detected as part of the detailed secondary survey.

Disclosure Statement: The authors have no conflicts of interest or disclosures of funding to declare.
Division of Trauma and Surgical Critical Care, LAC+USC Medical Center, University of Southern California, 2051 Marengo Street, IPT C5L100, Los Angeles, CA 90033, USA
* Corresponding author.
E-mail address: kenji.inaba@med.usc.edu

HOW DO I MANAGE LIFE-THREATENING THORACIC INJURIES?

In the thorax, immediately life-threatening injuries include tension pneumothorax, massive hemothorax, open pneumothorax from a chest wall defect, and cardiac or great vessel injury. These injuries and their management in the ED are reviewed here.

DECOMPRESSING THE CHEST IN A HYPOTENSIVE PATIENT WITH THORACIC TRAUMA

Although shock in the trauma patient is hemorrhagic until proven otherwise, consideration of a tension pneumothorax should occur with any hypotensive trauma patient. The practical clinical findings associated with tension pneumothoraces include hypotension and tachycardia with poor oxygenation. The classically described absent ipsilateral breath sounds can be difficult to detect in the noisy, chaotic trauma bay, and tracheal deviation may be missed if a cervical collar is in place. Therefore, clinical suspicion should remain high even when breath sounds are equivocal.

If a tension pneumothorax is suspected, the chest should be rapidly decompressed. A chest radiograph (CXR) is unnecessary and potentially harmful if it delays intervention. An ultrasound probe, if readily available in the trauma bay, can be placed on the chest to assess lung sliding, the absence of which is suggestive of pneumothorax. However, tension pneumothorax is a clinical diagnosis, and the clinician should not wait for radiographic confirmation before intervening.

In the classic description of needle decompression, a large-bore angiocatheter is placed into the pleural space at the second intercostal space in the midclavicular line (2IC/MCL). More contemporarily, the fifth intercostal space at the anterior axillary line has been found to yield greater success rates because of decreased chest wall thickness at that site.[2,3] Needle decompression may fail in up to 58% of cases when performed at the 2IC/MCL position.[4] Because of this, needle decompression as a means to treat tension pneumothorax should be limited to settings in which finger thoracostomy or chest tube placement is not feasible.

The first portion of tube thoracostomy, in which decompression of the pleural space is achieved by opening the parietal pleura and confirming entry by inserting a finger into the pleural space (referred to by some as a finger thoracostomy), is a better and more reliable means for decompressing the thorax. A scalpel is used to make a 2-cm to 3-cm skin incision in the fourth or fifth intercostal space in the anterior axillary line and then is used to cut through the subcutaneous fat and intercostal muscle. A small cut is made in the pleura and the physician's finger is then used to widen the opening into the pleural space, thereby decompressing the chest. This should take mere seconds to perform and should be followed up with the insertion of a chest tube through the aperture as soon as time and the patient's condition permit. The clinician will know the pleural space has been entered with the evacuation of a gush of air or blood, and the patient's hemodynamics should normalize accordingly. If they do not, another etiology for the patient's altered physiology must immediately be considered. Entering the pleural space under direct visualization with digital confirmation provides visual and tactile feedback that the pleural space has been decompressed. This is not true for needle decompression, in which the absence of air return may simply be a result of the catheter becoming kinked, blocked, or malpositioned.

Which Patients Require Tube Thoracostomy?

Pneumothoraces and hemothoraces causing respiratory or circulatory compromise require drainage by way of chest tube connected to a closed suction system and underwater seal. A large hemothorax can present with absent breath sounds, poor oxygenation, or hypotension, but is more typically detected on supine CXR by visualizing a layered opacity throughout the hemithorax, with point-of-care ultrasound demonstrating a pleural effusion, or by way of finger thoracostomy during the primary survey.

Not every patient with a pneumothorax or hemothorax needs a chest tube. Most hemothoraces should be drained with tube thoracostomy because of the risk of developing empyema or fibrothorax, although diminutive hemothoraces can be left undrained.[5,6] Patients with an asymptomatic pneumothorax clearly visible on CXR and any symptomatic pneumothoraces, including those with signs of tension pneumothorax, should have a chest tube placed. Patients with an occult pneumothorax, identified on computed tomography (CT) of the chest but not seen on CXR, likely do not require tube thoracostomy if the pneumothorax is stable and asymptomatic.[6–9] The Eastern Association for the Surgery of Trauma (EAST) Practice Management Guidelines support this approach even if the patient undergoes positive pressure ventilation.[6] In other words, occult pneumothoraces seldom progress to tension physiology, even with mechanical ventilation. Indications for delayed chest tube placement in patients with traumatic occult pneumothoraces are poorly defined but could reasonably include pneumothoraces that become visible on follow-up CXR and patients who become symptomatic.[8]

A chest wall defect causing an open pneumothorax also requires rapid chest tube placement. The chest wall defect, usually obvious on clinical examination, can cause tension pathophysiology and circulatory collapse. An occlusive dressing taped on 3 sides should be placed to cover the defect and a tube thoracostomy should quickly follow.

Chest Tube Insertion

Inserting a chest tube requires a scalpel, 2 Kelly clamps, the chest tube itself, a needle driver, suture (usually 0 silk), scissors, and an underwater seal system. Using sterile technique, the fourth or fifth intercostal space is identified as the site for chest tube insertion in the anterior axillary line. The appropriate location can be approximated by the intercostal space in line with the nipple. The chest should be prepped widely to landmark the axilla, sternal border, and costal margin. Especially in the awake patient, generous infiltration of local anesthetic, including to the rib periosteum and parietal pleura, is critical. The skin incision, approximately 2 to 3 cm in length, is typically oriented in a transverse direction and a Kelly clamp is then used to spread the subcutaneous tissue and intercostal muscle. The pleura should be entered just above the superior border of the rib below to avoid the neurovascular bundle traveling along the costal groove inferiorly in the rib above. In young patients, entry into the pleural space can require a significant amount of force; it is important to brace the hand advancing the Kelly clamp with the opposite hand against the chest wall, to halt overzealous entry into the thorax when the pleura is punctured. The opening into the pleura is then widened by spreading the Kelly, and a finger is inserted next to confirm entry into the pleural space and ensure the lung is not adherent to the chest wall at that site. A chest tube is then guided into the pleural space with the physician's finger. Care should be taken to ensure the distal-most drainage hole is within the pleural space, a distance that can be approximated by inserting the chest tube a hand's width farther into the chest than the last drainage hole. The tube is then sutured in place and connected to underwater seal and wall suction at −20 cm H20.

Does Size Matter?

Traditionally, the insertion of large-bore chest tubes ($\geq$36 Fr) was advocated for traumatic hemothoraces and pneumothoraces. More recently, clinicians have moved toward the placement of smaller chest tubes. One study compared the use of 28 to 32-Fr with 36 to 40-Fr chest tubes in trauma and found no difference in the successful evacuation of hemothoraces or pneumothoraces with smaller-bore chest tubes.[10] One article argued that chest tubes as small as 14 Fr can successfully drain hemothoraces among stable trauma patients,[11] but further confirmation of these findings is required before chest tubes this small are adopted into widespread practice. At our institution, 28-Fr chest tubes are used in most trauma patients requiring tube thoracostomy.

CARDIAC TAMPONADE LEADING TO TRAUMATIC ARREST

Traumatic cardiac tamponade occurs almost exclusively after penetrating injuries to the chest. Blunt cardiac injury causing free wall rupture and tamponade is exceedingly rare and usually catastrophic.[12] Patients with cardiac tamponade are deceptively stable at first, but can deteriorate rapidly and are exquisitely sensitive to routine resuscitation interventions, such as volume resuscitation, sedation, and positive pressure ventilation. Because these patients are normotensive until they arrest, clinical suspicion of tamponade must be high after penetrating injuries to the thorax.

Pericardiocentesis is an optional technique taught by ATLS for decompressing cardiac tamponade. Once a staple of diagnosis and management, the diagnostic component of pericardiocentesis has been supplanted by the pericardial view in Focused Assessment with Sonography for Trauma (FAST).[13] The therapeutic capacity of pericardiocentesis is now emphasized as a temporizing measure when cardiac tamponade is present but a surgeon with the capacity to fix a cardiac injury is not. If a surgeon is available and the patient has vital signs, time should not be wasted attempting a pericardiocentesis in the trauma bay; the patient should instead be transported emergently to the operating room (OR) for median sternotomy and cardiac repair. Pericardiocentesis thus has only a very limited role as a temporizing measure when cardiac tamponade is identified on FAST, but the patient requires transfer to a surgical center before definitive repair.[13] If the patient loses vital signs, a resuscitative thoracotomy should be performed.

The Ultimate Emergency Room "Procedure": Resuscitative Thoracotomy

The indications for resuscitative thoracotomy (RT) are controversial. Resuscitation after a traumatic cardiac arrest is a blood product–intensive and resource-intensive undertaking, and if no one is available to surgically halt the bleeding that induced the arrest, opening the chest will be a uniformly fatal procedure. Conversely, not performing an RT when it is indicated carries a 100% mortality. Although RT should not be restricted to trauma centers, patients who present to an ED with a very limited blood bank or lacking surgical or intensive care unit support should not undergo RT, as outcomes are likely to be very poor.

Survival after RT is variable. In the largest systematic review of outcomes (n = 4620), overall survival was 7.4%.[14] In this 25-year review, the 3 key predictors of survival after RT were anatomic location of the injury (highest among cardiac injuries, 19.4% survival), mechanism of injury (highest after penetrating trauma, 8.8% survival), and signs of life on arrival to ED (11.5% survival).[14] In some practice settings, ultrasound also may be used to decide who should undergo this procedure. A prospective study showed that arrested patients without cardiac motion or pericardial fluid on FAST died uniformly (negative predictive value 100%).[15] The positive predictive value of cardiac motion on FAST, defined in the study as organized, nonfibrillating contractions, was 16.7%. If ultrasound is used, the absence of cardiac motion and pericardial fluid can be used to avoid initiating this procedure, as the survival is extremely low.

Both the EAST and the Western Trauma Association (WTA) have published guidelines about the indications for RT. The EAST guidelines are centered around signs of life, defined by the American College of Surgeons Committee on Trauma as any of the following: pupillary response, respiratory effort, palpable carotid pulse, measurable or palpable blood pressure, extremity movement, or cardiac electrical activity.[16,17] EAST strongly endorses RT for patients with penetrating thoracic trauma who arrive pulseless to the ED but show signs of life.[16] For patients with penetrating thoracic trauma who present without signs of life, patients with penetrating extrathoracic trauma with or without signs of life, and patients with blunt trauma and signs of life, EAST conditionally recommends RT. RT is not recommended for patients who present pulseless after blunt injury, without signs of life.[16] WTA, on the other hand, stratifies patients first according to duration of cardiac arrest. For blunt traumatic arrests with less than 10 minutes of cardiopulmonary resuscitation (CPR) and penetrating traumatic arrests with less than 15 minutes of CPR, RT is considered beneficial.[18] WTA also supports RT for longer durations of arrest if signs of life (respiratory or motor effort, electrical activity, or pupillary activity) are present.[18]

In summary, deciding which patients are candidates for RT requires integrating information on the mechanism and anatomic location of injury, duration of cardiac arrest, presence or absence of signs of life, findings on bedside ultrasound, and the available resources and personnel. At our institution, we are liberal with the indications for RT and perform it on all patients with traumatic cardiac arrest after penetrating trauma, as well as most patients who arrest after blunt trauma. We do not use ultrasound routinely to select candidates for the procedure, but use it selectively in arrested patients with blunt trauma if they have had a prolonged down time to identify patients who are unlikely to survive.

How Do I Perform a Resuscitative Thoracotomy?

The goals of an RT are to release pericardial tamponade, control intrathoracic hemorrhage, apply an aortic cross-clamp, and perform internal cardiac massage. Very infrequently, an air embolism may be evacuated from the left ventricle by way of needle aspiration.[19] When resources permit, the patient's airway should be secured, a right-sided chest tube should be placed, and intravenous access should be obtained concurrently with RT.

To perform a left anterolateral thoracotomy, the first step in RT, a skin incision is made boldly in the fifth intercostal space, approximated by the rib space below the nipple in men and in the inframammary fold in women, starting from the midline and curving upward toward the axilla to follow the curvature of the ribs, all the way down to the stretcher. The subcutaneous fat, chest wall musculature, and intercostal muscle are incised sharply with a scalpel. The intercostal muscle and underlying parietal pleura can be divided en masse with scissors, if preferred, which will decrease the chances of iatrogenic lung injury on entering the chest.

After entering the chest, a Finochetto retractor is used to spread the ribs and the lung is retracted superiorly and posteriorly to allow visualization of the pericardium. The pericardium is opened anterior and parallel to the phrenic nerve, and the heart is then delivered and inspected for injury. Any lacerations are repaired using a 2.0 prolene suture. The left hemithorax is inspected for any other signs of bleeding; for example, from the lung, intercostal vessels, or pulmonary hilum. An aortic cross-clamp is applied after first identifying the aorta just above the diaphragm as the structure immediately anterior to the vertebral bodies, and opening the mediastinal pleura bluntly with a finger anteriorly and posteriorly to the aorta to allow secure clamp placement. Internal cardiac massage is then performed using 2 hands with compression initiated at the cardiac apex.

Intracardiac medication delivery, such as 1 mg of epinephrine into the left ventricle, and defibrillation are initiated as warranted. Evacuation of blood from the right chest tube should prompt extension into a clamshell thoracotomy. Additionally, if a cardiac injury is discovered and visualization is poor through the left anterolateral thoracotomy, the physician should not hesitate to extend the incision across the midline and into the right chest as a clamshell thoracotomy to facilitate repair. A complete description of the procedural approach to RT can be found elsewhere.[19,20]

Finding Yourself Face to Face with an Opened Chest: What to Do Once You're In

- Open the pericardium and deliver the heart. Check for and repair any cardiac injuries.
- Stop any major intrathoracic bleeding.
- Cross-clamp the aorta just above the diaphragm.
- Begin open cardiac massage and resuscitation.
- Inject intracardiac epinephrine into the left ventricle.
- Extend into a clamshell thoracotomy if there is blood in the right chest.

The goal of RT is ultimately to facilitate return of spontaneous circulation (ROSC). If ROSC is achieved, the patient should be brought immediately to the OR for definitive management.

The decision to cease resuscitative efforts after RT, much like the decision to initiate RT, is complex and requires rapid integration of a number of considerations, including the mechanism and location of injury, the skill set of the physician, and the resources of the hospital. If ROSC is not achieved after repairing identified injuries in the chest, cross clamping the aorta, injecting intracardiac epinephrine, and administering blood, resuscitation should be stopped. This is a team decision and should be made with input from all providers in the trauma bay.

WHAT KIND OF IMAGING DOES MY PATIENT NEED TO DIAGNOSE OR EXCLUDE THORACIC INJURY?

Once immediately life-threatening thoracic injuries have been excluded or managed, a secondary survey should be performed. The 3 most commonly used investigations to screen for thoracic injury are the portable, often supine, anteroposterior (AP) CXR, point-of-care ultrasound (POCUS), including extended FAST (EFAST), and CT scan with arterial-phase intravenous contrast. As with most decision making in trauma, the selection of imaging investigations in the workup of thoracic trauma hinges on the clinical stability of the patient. It is worth emphasizing that unstable patients do not belong in the CT scanner, as anyone who has had the uncomfortable experience of running a code in the radiology department can attest to.

CHEST RADIOGRAPH: THE UTILITY INVESTIGATION IN THORACIC TRAUMA

The CXR is considered by most to be the standard initial imaging investigation for all trauma patients, whether stable or unstable. The traditional single-view AP CXR is typically obtained as a portable radiograph and therefore has the benefits of being fast and inexpensive with a low radiation burden, and screens the entire thorax for injury without having to remove the patient from the trauma bay. Although an upright CXR is typically advocated for in textbooks, in practice these radiographs are most frequently taken supine. The CXR allows for the assessment not only of the lungs and pleural space but also of the mediastinum, aorta, diaphragm, and bony structures, including ribs, thoracic vertebrae, clavicles, sternum, and scapulae. Indeed, ATLS states that "the chest radiograph [is] a necessary part of any evaluation after traumatic injury"[1] and is one screening factor in the decision to obtain a CT scan.

Although it is somewhat contentious, for these reasons the authors recommend that all patients undergo a CXR in the trauma bay to screen for thoracic injury. Some patients can safely have a CXR omitted, but these are the minority. For example, patients with penetrating trauma remote from the thorax do not require CXR, but the clinician must maintain a high degree of suspicion for unusual bullet trajectories. All blunt multisystem trauma patients should have a supine CXR performed in the trauma bay.

Stable patients with an abnormal CXR should proceed next to CT scan. The appropriate management of patients after a normal CXR is more controversial and is explored further in the section on CT thorax, later in this article.

HAS POINT-OF-CARE ULTRASOUND REPLACED THE STANDARD CHEST RADIOGRAPH?

In trauma, POCUS is referred to as FAST. FAST is a quick and radiation-free imaging modality that is rapidly performed in the trauma bay and therefore is appropriate for stable and unstable patients. There are 4 conventional views in FAST. One of these, the subxyphoid pericardial view, plays an important role in the workup of thoracic trauma, as it assesses the heart for cardiac motion and tamponade. More recently, the EFAST has entered into clinical use with the addition of thoracic views to assess for hemothorax and pneumothorax.[21–25]

The subxyphoid pericardial view has a sensitivity that approaches 100% and specificity of 97% at detecting penetrating cardiac injuries.[26] Although it is rare, physicians must be aware of the possibility of a falsely negative pericardial EFAST. A laceration to the pericardium in the setting of a cardiac injury can allow blood to decompress into the left hemithorax, leading to a falsely normal ultrasound of the pericardial sac.[27] The clinician should have a high degree of suspicion for a false-negative pericardial EFAST in patients with penetrating precordial wounds and left hemothoraces, particularly in the setting of hypotension or ongoing chest tube drainage.

In the assessment for pneumothorax in EFAST, ultrasound views of the chest are obtained by scanning the lung fields in intercostal spaces in the midclavicular line (spaces 2 to 4) and in the midaxillary line (spaces 6 to 8).[24] Pneumothorax is detected if lung sliding (the normal movement of the visceral on parietal pleural during breathing) and "comet tail" artifacts (hyperechoic signals that result from normal pleural apposition) are absent, or a lung point (the junctional interface between normal and partially collapsed lung) is observed.

Several well-designed studies have demonstrated the excellent sensitivity and specificity of EFAST in the evaluation for pneumothorax. When compared with the gold standard of CT scan, EFAST has a sensitivity of 86% to 100% and specificity of 97% to 100% in pneumothorax detection.[23,28,29] This diagnostic yield makes EFAST superior to CXR in the investigation of pneumothorax, because CXR has a sensitivity of 27% to 83% and specificity of 99% to 100%.[23,29] EFAST thus detects pneumothoraces that would be occult on CXR, although these injuries generally do not require chest tube placement unless the patient is symptomatic.

With the superiority of EFAST over CXR at detecting pneumothoraces, one of the questions that follows is whether or not CXR can now be omitted in the evaluation of thoracic trauma. Indeed, some studies have argued that EFAST should replace portable CXR in screening trauma patients for thoracic injury.[21,30] However, although

EFAST is excellent in the assessment for pneumothorax, it does not provide any assessment of the bony elements of the thorax, the mediastinum (apart from the evaluation for pericardial effusion), or the diaphragm, all of which are assessed on CXR. Ultrasound is also a user-dependent test whose validity is constrained by the experience of the clinician, which is true to a much lesser extent with CXR. Therefore, EFAST and CXR should be considered complementary rather than competing diagnostic tests. Given the ease of performing a CXR and the low cost and radiation burden associated with it, the authors propose that instead of omitting a CXR from the diagnostic workup, a better question may be whether or not the CT chest can be forgone in the context of a normal CXR and EFAST. This has not yet been clearly studied.

CROSS-SECTIONAL IMAGING: WHO REALLY NEEDS A COMPUTED TOMOGRAPHY SCAN OF THE THORAX?

CT scan of the chest is the gold standard imaging modality in thoracic trauma for stable patients, with sensitivity of 74% to 82% and specificity of 99% to 100%.[31,32] Despite its excellent diagnostic capability, CT scan has important limitations. It is costly,[33,34] exposes the patient to an effective radiation dose of roughly 9 mSv,[35] and perhaps most importantly, necessitates the transport of the patient out of the trauma bay at a critical time in the clinical course.[36] Therefore, it is important to carefully select patients who will derive benefit from this diagnostic intervention.

Stable patients with an abnormal physical examination, EFAST, or CXR require CT chest for further assessment of their injuries. One study of 141 patients with major blunt trauma found that an abnormal physical examination (chest wall tenderness, decreased air entry, and/or abnormal respiratory effort) increased the diagnostic yield of CT chest by odds ratios of 4.1 to 6.7 depending on the specific physical examination findings.[36] Rodriguez and colleagues[37] developed the NEXUS Chest Rule, in which stable patients with blunt trauma who lack all 7 criteria (age >60, rapid deceleration mechanism, chest pain, intoxication, distracting injury, tenderness to chest wall palpation, and abnormal mental status) do not require either CXR or CT chest.[38–40] If one or more feature is present, the NEXUS Chest Rule recommends CXR as the next investigation, with the subsequent decision about the need for CT chest based on the mechanism of injury, the findings on CXR, and the physical examination.

Patients with a normal primary survey and CXR or EFAST present more of a diagnostic challenge. A large study of 3639 patients with blunt trauma showed that of the patients with a normal CXR who went on to receive a CT chest, only 2.7% had a clinically significant injury.[33] Put differently, if none of the 3383 patients in this study with a normal CXR went on to receive a CT chest, 90 would have had a clinically significant missed injury, including 12 patients with a major missed injury, such as an aortic or other great vessel injury. This rate of missed injuries must be balanced against the cost and radiation exposure necessitated by a CT chest, as well as the risks associated with transporting the patient out of the ED. Limiting a CT chest to patients with a high-risk mechanism or abnormal physical examination, EFAST, or CXR is a reasonable approach. However, there is no clear definition of what specifically constitutes a high-risk mechanism at this time, and clinical judgment must be used.

WHERE TO NEXT? DISPOSITION FROM THE EMERGENCY DEPARTMENT
The Intensive Care Unit

Most thoracic injuries can be managed nonoperatively, including rib fractures, flail chest, and pulmonary contusions. Notably, flail chest, in which at least 2 consecutive ribs are fractured in 2 or more places, can cause significant contusion to the underlying lung parenchyma as the flail segment of ribs moves paradoxically against the remainder of the chest wall on inspiration and expiration. The resultant pulmonary contusion can contribute to respiratory decompensation. Surgical options for flail chest (open reduction and internal fixation with rib plating) are current being explored.[41] For now, the cornerstones of management include aggressive pain control,[42] alveolar recruitment, and judicious use of intravenous fluids, especially in the first few days after injury. Because respiratory failure resulting from inadequate analgesia, poor secretion clearance, evolving pulmonary contusions, and volume overload can occur precipitously, these patients are typically best monitored in the intensive care unit for the period immediately after injury.

Blunt cardiac injury (BCI) is an injury pattern that warrants special consideration. Clinically significant BCI is infrequent and can manifest as either mechanical or electrical cardiac dysfunction. Mechanical BCI, such as injury to the papillary muscles or, at its extreme, septal or cardiac wall rupture, is exceedingly rare among patients who arrive alive to hospital. In a large case series of 811,531 patients with blunt trauma who arrived alive to the ED, the rate of cardiac rupture was 0.045%.[12] On autopsy study, however, blunt cardiac rupture is common (20%).[43] Mechanical BCI is therefore frequently fatal, and most patients who sustain this type of injury die at the scene or en route to hospital.

Electrical BCI, which manifests as arrhythmia, is far more common and is usually self-limited. Most cases occur after high-speed motor vehicle collisions, as a result of rapid deceleration or direct blows to the chest (for example, from the steering wheel).[44] The optimal workup of these patients is unclear. One early study showed that a normal electrocardiogram (ECG) and troponin at admission ruled out clinically significant BCI.[45] The same institution then repeated this prospective study with a larger sample (n = 333) of patients who had sustained significant blunt thoracic trauma, and found that a normal ECG and troponin were required both at admission and 8 hours later to exclude clinically significant BCI.[46] The EAST guidelines recommend that BCI can be safely ruled out if both the ECG and serial troponins are normal.[47] Our approach to BCI screening is to admit patients with significant blunt thoracic trauma for 24 hours of continuous cardiac monitoring, and obtain an ECG and 3 sets of troponins. Echocardiography should be reserved for patients who have hypotension, an abnormal ECG, or up-trending troponin levels.

Endovascular Therapies

The emerging role for endovascular management of thoracic vascular injuries, in which the injured vascular segment is excluded from the circulation,[48] has garnered much attention in recent literature. Endovascular management of blunt thoracic aortic injury, for example, has been shown to result in less blood loss, paraplegia, and mortality, with a similar risk of stroke, as compared with open repair of these injuries. Although most patients with free aortic rupture die on scene, patients with traumatic aortic dissections, intimal flaps, or contained ruptures are typically stable when they present to hospital and are candidates for endovascular repair, the approach now endorsed by major trauma societies, such as EAST.[49] The use of endovascular therapies is increasing, with one study using the National Trauma Data Bank showing a significant increase in the use of endovascular techniques for both penetrating and blunt trauma, as well as a significant decrease in mortality of these patients over the same period.[50]

The Operating Room

It has been previously suggested that initial chest tube output of greater than 1.5 L of blood or greater than 150 to 200 mL/h for 2 to 4 consecutive hours, or total chest tube output greater than 1.5 L in 24 hours, were indications for operative intervention.[1,6,51,52] Most surgeons now rely primarily on the patient's physiology, that is, clinical evidence of shock, to guide intervention.[6] However, many surgeons would still consider operative intervention with evidence of ongoing bleeding or chest tube output greater than 1 L, regardless of the patient's hemodynamic status. Early involvement of the surgical team is most prudent, although with increased acceptance of nonoperative management and a rise in the use of catheter-based interventions, few patients now require urgent or emergent thoracotomy apart from patients suffering traumatic cardiac arrest.

SUMMARY

Thoracic injury is common after both blunt and penetrating trauma, and can range from a relatively benign occult pneumothorax to a cardiac injury causing rapid exsanguination and clinical death. Expedient assessment of the injury burden is critical, and familiarity with the imaging options (CXR, EFAST, and CT chest) for further workup of thoracic trauma is important. The emergency medicine physician must be adept at decompressing tension pneumothoraces, quickly placing chest tubes, and performing RT when indicated. Swift management of life-threatening thoracic injuries and appropriate workup of others will allow the ED physician to successfully manage patients from the moment they arrive in the ED to the time at which they are brought to the OR, interventional radiology suite, intensive care unit, ward, or discharged home.

REFERENCES

1. American College of Surgeons Committee on Trauma. Advanced trauma life support (ATLS), ninth edition. Chicago: Hearthside Publishing Services; 2012.
2. Inaba K, Ives C, McClure K, et al. Radiologic evaluation of alternative sites for needle decompression of tension pneumothorax. Arch Surg 2012;147(9):813–8.
3. Inaba K, Branco BC, Eckstein M, et al. Optimal positioning for emergent needle thoracostomy: a cadaver-based study. J Trauma 2011;71(5):1099–103.
4. Martin M, Shatterly S, Inaba K, et al. Does needle thoracostomy provide adequate and effective decompression of tension pneumothorax? J Trauma 2012;73(6):1412–7.
5. Dubose J, Inaba K, Demetriades D, et al. Management of post-traumatic retained hemothorax: a prospective, observational, multicenter AAST study. J Trauma 2012;72(1):11–22.
6. Mowery NT, Gunter OL, Collier BR, et al. Practice management guidelines for management of hemothorax and occult pneumothorax. J Trauma 2011;70(2):510–8.
7. Kirkpatrick AW, Rizoli S, Ouellet JF, et al. Occult pneumothoraces in critical care: a prospective multicenter randomized controlled trial of pleural drainage for mechanically ventilated trauma patients with occult pneumothoraces. J Trauma 2013;74(3):747–55.
8. Moore FO, Goslar PW, Coimbra R, et al. Blunt traumatic occult pneumothorax: is observation safe? Results of a prospective, AAST multicenter study. J Trauma 2011;70(5):1019–25.
9. Ball CG, Kirkpatrick AW, Feliciano DV. The occult pneumothorax: what have we learned? Can J Surg 2009;52(5):E173–9.
10. Inaba K, Lustenberger T, Recinos G, et al. Does size matter? A prospective analysis of 28-32 versus 36-40 french chest tube size in trauma. J Trauma 2012;72(2):422–7.

11. Kulvatunyou N, Joseph B, Friese RS, et al. 14 french pigtail catheters placed by surgeons to drain blood on trauma patients: is 14-Fr too small? J Trauma 2012; 6(73):1423–7.

12. Teixeira PG, Inaba K, Oncel D, et al. Blunt cardiac rupture: a 5-year NTDB analysis. J Trauma 2009;67:788–91.

13. Lee TH, Ouellet JF, Cook M, et al. Pericardiocentesis in trauma: a systematic review. J Trauma 2013;75(4):543–9.

14. Rhee PM, Acosta J, Bridgeman A, et al. Survival after emergency department thoracotomy: review of published data from the past 25 years. J Am Coll Surg 2000;190:288–98.

15. Inaba K, Chouliaras K, Zakaluzny S, et al. FAST ultrasound examination as a predictor of outcomes after resuscitative thoracotomy: a prospective evaluation. Ann Surg 2015;262:512–8.

16. Seamon MJ, Haut ER, Arendonk KV, et al. An evidence-based approach to patient selection for emergency department thoracotomy: a practice management guideline from the Eastern Association for the Surgery of Trauma. J Trauma 2015;79(1):159–73.

17. American College of Surgeons Committee on Trauma. Practice management guidelines for emergency department thoracotomy. J Am Coll Surg 2001;193: 303–9.

18. Burlew CC, Moore EE, Moore FA, et al. Western Trauma Association critical decisions in trauma: resuscitative thoracotomy. J Trauma 2012;73(6):1359–64.

19. Burlew CC, Moore EE. Emergency department thoracotomy. In: Mattox KL, Moore EE, Feliciano DV, editors. Trauma. 7th edition. New York: The McGraw Hill Companies; 2013. p. 236–50.

20. Demetriades D, Zakaluzny S. Emergency room resuscitative thoracotomy. In: Demetriades D, Inaba K, Velmahos G, editors. Atlas of surgical techniques in trauma. Cambridge: Cambridge University Press; 2015. p. 18–28.

21. Soult MC, Weireter LJ, Britt RC, et al. Can routine trauma bay chest X-ray be bypassed with an extended focused assessment with sonography for trauma examination? Am Surg 2015;81(4):336–40.

22. Matsushima K, Frankel HL. Beyond focused assessment with sonography for trauma: ultrasound creep in the trauma resuscitation area and beyond. Curr Opin Crit Care 2011;17:606–12.

23. Nandipati KC, Allamaneni S, Kakarla R, et al. Extended focused assessment with sonography for trauma (EFAST) in the diagnosis of pneumothorax: experience at a community based level I trauma center. Injury 2011;42:511–4.

24. Brook OR, Beck-Razi N, Abadi S, et al. Sonographic detection of pneumothorax by radiology residents as part of extended focused assessment with sonography for trauma. J Ultrasound Med 2009;28:749–55.

25. Kirkpatrick AW, Sirois M, Laupland KB, et al. Hand-held thoracic sonography for detecting post-traumatic pneumothoraces: the extended focused assessment with sonography for trauma (EFAST). J Trauma 2004;57:288–95.

26. Rozycki GS, Feliciano DV, Ochsner MG, et al. The role of ultrasound in patients with possible penetrating cardiac wounds: a prospective multicenter study. J Trauma 1999;46(4):543–51.

27. Ball CG, Williams BH, Wyrzykowski AD, et al. A caveat to the performance of pericardial ultrasound in patients with penetrating cardiac wounds. J Trauma 2009; 67(5):1123–4.

28. Governatori NJ, Saul T, Siadecki SD, et al. Ultrasound in the evaluation of penetrating thoraco-abdominal trauma: a review of the literature. Med Ultrason 2015; 17(4):528–34.

29. Wilkerson RG, Stone MB. Sensitivity of bedside ultrasound and supine anteroposterior chest radiographs for the identification of pneumothorax after blunt trauma. Acad Emerg Med 2010;17(1):11–7.

30. Wisbach GG, Sise MJ, Sack DI, et al. What is the role of chest x-ray in the initial assessment of stable trauma patients? J Trauma 2007;62:74–9.

31. Strumwasser A, Chong V, Chu E, et al. Thoracic computed tomography is an effective screening modality in patients with penetrating injuries to the chest. Injury 2016;47(9):2000–5.

32. Ahmed N, Kassavin D, Kuo YH, et al. Sensitivity and specificity of CT scan and angiogram for ongoing internal bleeding following torso trauma. Emerg Med J 2013;30(3):e14.

33. Kea B, Gamarallage R, Vairamuthu H, et al. What is the clinical significance of chest CT when the chest x-ray result is normal in patients with blunt trauma? Am J Emerg Med 2013;31:1268–73.

34. Barrios C, Pham J, Malinoski D, et al. Ability of a chest X-ray and an abdominal computed tomography scan to identify traumatic thoracic injury. Am J Surg 2010; 200:741–5.

35. Rodriguez RM, Baumann BM, Raja AS, et al. Diagnostic yields, charges, and radiation dose of chest imaging in blunt trauma evaluations. Acad Emerg Med 2014;21:644–50.

36. Traub M, Stevenson M, McEvoy S, et al. The use of chest computed tomography versus chest X-ray in patients with major blunt trauma. Injury 2007;38:43–7.

37. Rodriguez RM, Hendey GW, Mower WR. Selective chest imaging for blunt trauma patients: the national emergency X-ray utilization studies (NEXUS-chest algorithm). Am J Emerg Med 2017;35:164–70.

38. Rodriguez RM, Anglin D, Langdorf MI, et al. NEXUS chest: validation of a decision instrument for selective chest imaging in blunt trauma. JAMA Surg 2013; 148(10):940–6.

39. Rodriguez RM, Hendey GW, Mower WR, et al. Derivation of a decision instrument for selective chest radiography in blunt trauma. J Trauma 2011;71(3):549–53.

40. Rodriguez RM, Hendey GW, Marek G, et al. A pilot study to derive clinical variables for selective chest radiography in blunt trauma patients. Ann Emerg Med 2006;47(5):415–8.

41. Fitzgerald MT, Ashley DW, Abukhdeir H, et al. Rib fracture fixation in the 65 years and older population: a paradigm shift in management strategy at a level I trauma center. J Trauma 2017;82(3):524–7.

42. Bulger EM, Edwards T, Klotz P, et al. Epidural analgesia improves outcome after multiple rib fractures. Surgery 2004;136(2):426–30.

43. Teixeira PGR, Georgiou CC, Inaba K, et al. Blunt cardiac trauma: lessons learned from the medical examiner. J Trauma 2009;67:1259–64.

44. Legome E, Kadish H. Cardiac injury from blunt trauma. In: Moreira ME, Torrey SB, Grayzel J, Editors. UpToDate. 2016. Available at: http://www.uptodate.com/contents/cardiac-injury-from-blunt-trauma. Accessed December 17, 2016.

45. Salim A, Velmahos GC, Jindal A, et al. Clinically significant blunt cardiac trauma: role of serum troponin levels combined with electrocardiographic findings. J Trauma 2001;50:237–43.

46. Velmahos GC, Karaiskakis M, Salim A, et al. Normal electrocardiography and serum troponin I levels preclude the presence of clinically significant blunt cardiac injury. J Trauma 2003;54:45–51.
47. Clancy K, Velopulos C, Bilaniuk JW, et al. Screening for blunt cardiac injury: an Eastern Association for the Surgery of Trauma practice management guideline. J Trauma 2012;73:S301–6.
48. Mirakhur A, Cormack R, Eesa M, et al. Endovascular therapy for acute trauma: a pictorial review. Can Assoc Radiol J 2014;65:158–67.
49. Fox N, Schwartz D, Salazar JH, et al. Evaluation and management of blunt traumatic aortic injury: a practice management guideline from the Eastern Association for the Surgery of Trauma. J Trauma 2015;78:136–46.
50. Branco BC, DuBose JJ, Zhan LX, et al. Trends and outcomes of endovascular therapy in the management of civilian vascular injuries. J Vasc Surg 2014;60:1297–307.
51. Dente CJ, Feliciano DV. Torso vascular trauma at an urban level-I trauma center. Perspect Vasc Surg Endovasc Ther 2011;23(1):36–46.
52. Karmy-Jones R, Jurkovich GJ, Nathens AB, et al. Timing of urgent thoracotomy for hemorrhage after trauma. Arch Surg 2001;136:513–8.

Major Abdominal Trauma

Critical Decisions and New Frontiers in Management

 CrossMark

Megan Brenner, MD, MS, RPVI[a,b], Christopher Hicks, MD, MEd, FRCPC[c,*]

KEYWORDS

- Major abdominal trauma • Focused abdominal sonogram for trauma • FAST
- Resuscitative endovascular balloon occlusion of the aorta • REBOA

KEY POINTS

- Be on the lookout for patients with abdominal trauma who have an immediate indication for laparotomy. These patients should be aggressively resuscitated and prepared for transfer to the operating room in consultation with a trauma surgeon. Axial imaging is contraindicated in this patient population.
- The peritoneum can accommodate nearly all of a patient's circulating blood volume and, therefore, represents an uncontrollable and potentially catastrophic source of internal hemorrhage. In the unstable multisystem trauma patient, the priority is usually aggressive resuscitation and rapid surgical control of hemorrhage.
- Stable patients with serious injuries can deteriorate without warning. Isolated drops in blood pressure or significant base deficit predict recurrent episodes of hypotension and the need for early therapeutic intervention.
- In stable patients for whom immediate axial imaging is planned, abdominal focused abdominal sonogram for trauma (FAST) adds little additional clinical information and can be omitted. Assessment with FAST should not be used to determine the need for computed tomography (CT) imaging.
- Axial imaging is an excellent test for determining the specific anatomy and severity of injury but when used in the wrong population confers significant risk of harm. CT imaging should be avoided when indications for immediate trauma laparotomy are present.
- Local wound exploration is a safe an effective way to exclude intraabdominal injury in patients with anterior abdominal stab wounds.

Disclosures: The following authors has a conflict of interest: M. Brenner: Clinical Advisory Board Member, Prytime Medical Inc.
[a] Division of Trauma/Critical Care, RA Cowley Shock Trauma Center, 22 South Greene Street, T1R50, Baltimore, MD 21202, USA; [b] Division of Vascular Surgery, University of Maryland School of Medicine, 22 South Greene Street, T1R50, Baltimore, MD 21202, USA; [c] St. Michael's Hospital, University of Toronto, 30 Bond Street, 1st Floor Bond Wing Room 1008, Toronto M5B 1W8, Canada
* Corresponding author.
E-mail address: chrismikehicks@gmail.com

Emerg Med Clin N Am 36 (2018) 149–160
https://doi.org/10.1016/j.emc.2017.08.012
0733-8627/18/© 2017 Elsevier Inc. All rights reserved.
emed.theclinics.com

WHAT ARE THE IMMEDIATE MANAGEMENT PRIORITIES IN THE UNSTABLE PATIENT WITH ABDOMINAL TRAUMA?

The primary survey should proceed in a stepwise and systematic fashion for all trauma patients, regardless of injury pattern, and should address immediate threats to life. The Advanced Trauma Life Support program provides a preliminary framework that allows for a systematic and organized approach; however, when resources permit, multisystem assessment and resuscitation should proceed in parallel rather than in sequence. Specific to the abdomen, the key to efficient management is ruling in or out life-threatening hemorrhage, usually with a combination of mechanism of injury, physical examination, and bedside imaging. The patient who has suffered blunt or penetrating abdominal trauma and is hemodynamically unstable should be aggressively resuscitated and evaluated immediately for surgical exploration. Rapid transport to definitive surgical care is of paramount importance for those with abdominal injuries and ongoing hemodynamic instability. In hypotensive patients with gunshot wounds, delaying operative management by more than 10 minutes is associated with a 3-fold increase in mortality.[1]

Unlike thoracic trauma, hemodynamic instability from intraabdominal injuries arises exclusively from major hemorrhage; therefore, resuscitation should involve the early use of blood and blood products. Excessive crystalloid administration in this context disrupts the coagulation cascade, inhibits clot formation, and should be avoided. A damage control approach that includes permissive hypotension, early tranexamic acid, and a balanced ratio of blood products is preferred until definitive hemostasis can be achieved.[2] Massive or refractory hemodynamic instability should prompt consideration for massive solid organ or vascular injury. Patients with serious blunt abdominal trauma rarely have single-system injuries; other sources of obstructive or hemorrhagic shock should be actively sought and excluded. In general, large-bore peripheral intravenous cannula (14 or 16 gauge, placed in the bilateral antecubital fossae) provides excellent vascular access for the purpose of volume resuscitation. If major abdominal or pelvic trauma is suspected, peripheral and central lines should be placed above the diaphragm, in the subclavian or internal jugular veins. Temporary vascular access can be obtained via intraosseous placement in 1 or both humeral heads.

Intraabdominal hemorrhage resulting in hypotension requires definitive surgical treatment regardless of associated injuries. As a third space for hemorrhage, the peritoneum presents the dual dangers of a noncompressible source of bleeding that can accommodate nearly all of a patient's circulating blood volume, making it the priority for management even in the face of other serious injuries. Traumatic brain injury (TBI), contained blunt thoracic aortic injury, extremity injuries without severe hemorrhage, and ischemia to any extremity may be addressed once hemorrhage control occurs. Patients with both major abdominal hemorrhage and a significant pelvic fracture that remains unstable after resuscitation and application of a pelvic binder are best managed in the operating room (OR)[3] in the absence of a hybrid room. Compared with angiography, the OR is typically available immediately, and allows for management of both intraabdominal injuries and temporizing of pelvic bleeding with preperitoneal packing. Angiography can still proceed after laparotomy and preperitoneal packing if ongoing pelvic bleeding is suspected. The advent of the hybrid OR allows some institutions to bring the patient to a single location for all hemostatic procedures, including exploratory laparotomy, angiography, and orthopedic and neurosurgical interventions. This the most ideal place for the patient requiring multiple emergent procedures. TBI is often not fully characterized until a computerized tomography (CT) scan is performed, which usually occurs after hemorrhage control. If a patient has physical examination findings suggestive of severe TBI or imminent herniation, a neurosurgical team should be consulted early and ideally attend the trauma laparotomy so that emergency decompression maneuvers can be performed concurrent with laparotomy. In all situations of gross instability, the key is to achieve immediate hemostasis, often by way of a damage control laparotomy; associated injuries can be diagnosed and treated in conjunction with or immediately once early hemorrhage is stayed.

Diagnostic peritoneal aspirate (DPA) is valuable for a patient who is too unstable for CT, in whom an intraabdominal source of hemorrhage cannot be ruled out by mechanism of injury or bedside imaging. Specifically, DPA can assist in decision-making when suspicion of intraperitoneal hemorrhage remains high following an indeterminate or negative focused abdominal sonogram for trauma (FAST) examination. Similar to diagnostic peritoneal lavage (DPL), DPA involves entering the peritoneal cavity under direct visualization and placement of a DPL or central line catheter. Aspiration of 10 mL or more of frank blood in the presence of ongoing hemodynamic instability is an indication for immediate laparotomy. The lavage component can be used to detect red cells not visible on inspection or the presence of food fibers, although the utility of these findings for informing immediate surgical decision-making in grossly unstable patients is debatable.

CT imaging is contraindicated in unstable patients with an indication for laparotomy. Definitive surgical treatment should never be delayed in favor of additional imaging tests. Although well-intentioned, pursuing CT imaging in this population prolongs bleeding time without adding data to inform surgical decision-making. Similarly, transport to a trauma center should not be delayed in unstable patients in favor of CT imaging. Common indications for immediate laparotomy are listed in **Box 1**.

STABLE PATIENTS WITH ABDOMINAL INJURY: HOW DOES THE MANAGEMENT DIFFER?

The paradigm of classifying trauma patients as stable or unstable to determine the need for resuscitation or surgical intervention is problematic. The authors use the terms in the context of abdominal trauma with some reservation. Stability is assessed on a spectrum, can change at any moment, and needs to be considered in light of a patient's age, injury severity, and presence of comorbid illness. Hemodynamic status should be reassessed frequently, and reassuring vital signs should never be regarded as such in the face of serious clinical suspicion of major injury.

Box 1
Indications for laparotomy in abdominal trauma

Absolute: prepare for the operating room
- Ongoing or gross hemodynamic instability, with or without a positive FAST examination or DPA
- Generalized peritonitis
- Implement in situ
- Evisceration

Relative indications: discuss with a trauma surgeon
- Free air on plain films or CT imaging[a]
- Signs of gastrointestinal hemorrhage with a suspected traumatic source (frank blood in the nasogastric aspirate or on digital rectal examination)
- Penetrating abdominal trauma: gunshot wounds (most) and stab wounds (some)
- Multisystem trauma with ongoing hemodynamic instability, where the source of injury is not known

[a] Free air in the abdomen is not pathognomonic for intraabdominal injury because air may track from thoracic or external sources.

That said, a patient deemed to be hemodynamically stable (ie, whose vital signs on initial assessment and over time are in keeping with what would be considered normal physiology, given patient age, comorbid illness, and mechanism of injury) may benefit from additional diagnostic testing to help inform pattern of injury and next steps in management.

A stable patient with no findings on examination or imaging, and without significant mechanism of injury, may be observed or go on to have additional imaging, depending on local resources. Radiographs of the abdomen are of no value unless specifically for the purpose of evaluating trajectory in penetrating injury (bullets; indwelling missiles; or, in rare cases, free air). If used to detect free air, the yield of a portable chest radiograph may be improved by sitting the patient upright for 2 minutes before obtaining images.

THE EVOLVING ROLE OF POINT-OF-CARE ABDOMINAL ULTRASOUND

In the hands of an expert operator, a FAST examination of the abdomen is a specific (but not sensitive) test to detect hemoperitoneum, capable of detecting as little as 200 mL of free fluid.[4] Abdominal FAST examination is often included as part of the primary survey, even in patients who are clinically stable. This may be problematic because the ultrasound machine and the operator will occupy space within key operational real estate around the patient's upper extremities, chest, and abdomen. In turn, this may encumber intravenous access, phlebotomy, attaching monitors, and physical assessment. In a stable patient, positive free fluid detected on FAST may provide additional data for planning (eg, anticipating the need for blood products) and predicting potential clinical deterioration, but it does not immediately direct management. In stable patients with blunt injuries, the authors defer the FAST examination until after the primary survey is complete and more pressing assessment and management priorities have been addressed. In contrast, intraabdominal free fluid detected in the hypotensive patient should prompt a discussion about the need to proceed directly to the OR for laparotomy without further imaging.

In 2016, the National Institute for Health and Care Excellence (NICE) released guidelines on major trauma management that include recommendations to limit the use of FAST "to the minimum needed to direct intervention in patients with suspected haemorrhage and haemodynamic instability who are not responding to volume resuscitation." Furthermore, NICE recommends omitting the FAST examination entirely in patients who are about to undergo CT imaging because the latter is a more sensitive and specific test for intraabdominal injury. The guidelines further recommend against the use of FAST as a screening test to determine the need for axial imaging.[5]

WHAT SPECIFIC INJURIES ARE LIKELY TO BE ENCOUNTERED AND HOW SHOULD THEY BE MANAGED?

Axial CT imaging has a high sensitivity and specificity for intraabdominal injury and is an excellent test to clarify the presence and severity of injury, and to help determine disposition. A full discussion of organ-specific injury and management is beyond the scope of this article; however, some general principles should be kept in mind when reviewing axial images of the abdomen.

Grading systems for solid organ injury have evolved to help guide surgical treatment plans, although they typically do not inform initial disposition and management. Solid organ injury of any degree should prompt a discussion with a trauma surgeon to help determine next steps. Most low-grade solid organ injuries require no treatment, but observation should be at the discretion of the trauma team.[1,2] Hollow viscous injuries resulting in free intraabdominal air on radiograph or CT require exploration. Minor injuries (contusions or mesenteric hematomas) to the small and large bowel can be managed conservatively in some cases, or explored if patients develop clinical peritonitis. Small amounts of intraabdominal free fluid without evidence of solid organ or hollow viscous injury pose a specific challenge because this may indicate occult small bowel or mesenteric injury. Although these patients usually do not require immediate operative intervention, they should be admitted and observed closely, and a change in clinical status (peritonitis, pyrexia, leukocytosis, or hemodynamic instability) should prompt a surgical consultation.

Diaphragmatic injuries can usually be managed conservatively if right-sided, whereas left-sided injuries usually require operative intervention to prevent transdiaphragmatic herniation of intraabdominal organs, including stomach and bowel. The utility of CT in diagnosis of diaphragmatic injury has increased with improvements in technology: 64-slice helical CT has a sensitivity and specificity up to 90%.[3] When concern persists despite a negative CT (eg, with a penetrating injury to the left thoracoabdominal region), laparoscopic and open exploration may be indicated to ensure the diaphragm has not been violated.

PREDICTING THE CRASH: WHAT IS THE CRUMP FACTOR?

The most challenging patient is hemodynamically labile, with relatively unpredictable or unexpected variance in hemodynamic status. For these patients, the safest route is usually the most conservative, in which a worst case scenario approach is adopted at the first sign of demise. Specific to abdominal trauma, this approach involves the assumption that any significant deterioration is in part due to hemorrhage from intraabdominal injury. Management decisions in labile patients depend greatly on local resources. If interfacility transfer or the need for surgical intervention is anticipated, early planning and consultation can be life-saving. Similar to unstable patients, axial imaging should generally be deferred when local resources do not have the capacity to effectively manage the findings.

Transient hypotension in the prehospital setting that resolves spontaneously is an important sign associated with significant injury and the need for early therapeutic intervention. Several trauma-patient series have underscored the importance of a single drop in blood pressure (BP) for predicting hemodynamic deterioration (or crumping) and the need for early operative intervention. Patients with transient hypotension (systolic BP [SBP] <90 mm Hg) and a base deficit (BD) of less than or equal to −6 were more than twice as likely to experience repeated episodes of hypotension in the ED.[6] In a prospective observational study of 145 consecutive major trauma subjects, isolated prehospital hypotension less than 105 mm Hg was associated with a 4-fold increase in the need for immediate therapeutic intervention.[7] In the authors' practice, when abdominal or thoracoabdominal injuries are suspected, the presence of transient or isolated hypotension in the field, or BD less than or equal to −6, presents an opportunity to pause and reflect on management priorities. In some situations, this redirects the patient away from the CT suite in favor of operative exploration because these patients have a significant risk of rapidly and unexpectedly deteriorating. The authors' approach to imaging in abdominal trauma is summarized in **Table 1**.

BLUNT VERSUS PENETRATING INJURIES: GENERAL PRINCIPLES

The approach to the patient with blunt or penetrating injury differs in many respects. The primary and secondary surveys are of significant importance, but understanding the mechanism of injury can be of great value to diagnosis and treatment. Blunt abdominal trauma can result diffuse injury, whereas injuries secondary to penetrating mechanisms are along the trajectory of the projectiles. Gunshot wounds can cause

Table 1
Diagnostic imaging decision-making in abdominal trauma

Clinical Status	Recommendation
1. Rock solid Normal vital signs, nonconcerning mechanism of injury, reassuring clinical assessment	• Consider foregoing CT imaging • Consider foregoing transport to a trauma center
2. Stable No immediate concerns based on vital signs or primary survey, concerning mechanism of injury 3. Dynamic Transient drop in SBP <105 mm Hg or nonreassuring trend in vital signs or BD	• CT imaging may be useful to define nature and severity of injuries
4. Unstable Sustained blood pressure <105 mm Hg, loss of peripheral pulses, altered mental status 5. Prearrest Sustained blood pressure <70 mm Hg, loss of central pulses	• Resuscitate, early surgical consultation • Consider REBOA • Prep for transport to OR or trauma center • CT imaging contraindicated

Abbreviation: REBOA, resuscitative endovascular balloon occlusion of the aorta.

significant blast effect in the surrounding tissues, whereas a knife will only cause direct tissue injury to the locations it has traveled.

BLUNT ABDOMINAL TRAUMA

Blunt abdominal injury can be a significant challenge. Details of the mechanism of injury from prehospital providers are extremely useful in predicting specific patterns of injury and severity. For example, handlebar injuries can be associated with duodenal and pancreatic trauma, and a seatbelt sign can suggest possible injury to bowel. Injuries to the lower thorax or upper abdomen (the thoracoabdominal region) should prompt consideration of serious injury both above and below the diaphragm. Patients with TBI or altered mental status from drugs, alcohol, or metabolic disturbances cannot be clinically assessed to a satisfactory degree, and a CT scan of the abdomen is an important adjunct in their evaluation. Patients who can be clinically assessed and do not have any signs or symptoms of abdominal injury may be observed, although serial abdominal examinations (repeated physical assessment every 4 hours or less) must be performed by the same provider to detect subtle changes in status. Mechanism of injury should be used in the decision-making process to determine the utility of further imaging. Patients who have sustained low-velocity motor vehicle collision, falls from standing, and other minor mechanisms of injury without signs or symptoms can be managed expectantly.

PENETRATING ABDOMINAL TRAUMA

Penetrating anterior abdominal wounds can result in a range of injury, from superficial irritation to significant life-threatening hemorrhage and tissue destruction. Evisceration of bowel or omentum and bleeding from the wound are indications for surgical exploration, regardless of hemodynamic status. In the absence of the aforementioned signs, local wound exploration (LWE) can be extremely useful for diagnosis and triage. With LWE, the only relevant question that requires an answer is whether the missile has penetrated the abdominal fascia. This can be accomplished within a sterile field using instruments found on a standard suture tray and adequate lighting. Digital palpation of the wound track or probing with a swab stick or sterile instrument is not an effective way to confirm the depth of injury and this practice should be abandoned. The Western Trauma Association has published guidelines for decision-making using LWE that has been subsequently validated (**Fig. 1**).[8,9] Patients who have a definitely negative LWE can be discharged from the emergency department (ED) without CT imaging. Positive or equivocal LWE may involve admission and serial observation or surgical exploration. LWE is not appropriate for flank or

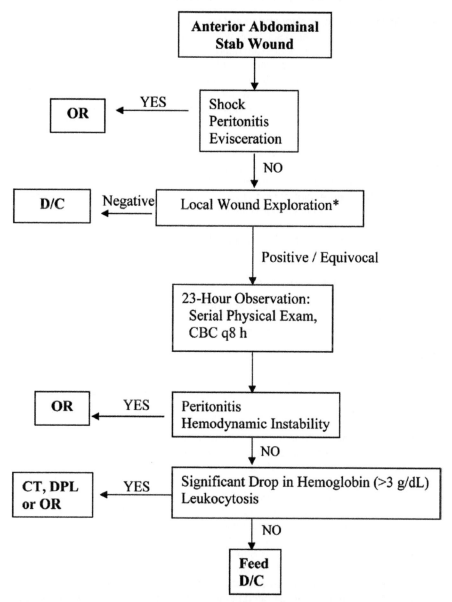

Fig. 1. The Western Trauma Association algorithm for LWE and anterior abdominal stab wounds. CBC, complete blood count. (*From* Biffl WL, Kaups KL, Cothren CC, et al. Management of patients with anterior abdominal stab wounds: a Western Trauma Association multicenter trial. J Trauma 2009;66(5):1294–301; with permission.)

back injuries, or when body habitus complicates the ability to assess the full depth of the injury. Although the OR is a preferred location for wound exploration, LWE for anterior abdominal wounds can be performed in the ED by a skilled operator, and is a safe and effective means for excluding peritoneal violation, provided proper technique is used.

COMPUTED TOMOGRAPHY IMAGING OF THE ABDOMEN: THE WHAT AND THE HOW

The specific imaging protocol for abdominal trauma varies depending on the nature of injures suspected. In general, discussion with a radiologist that includes the mechanism of injury, findings on physical examination, point-of-care imaging, and suspected injuries can help to refine the specific axial imaging protocol used. In most circumstances, images are enhanced with the use of intravenous contrast in the arterial phase. Oral contrast, once a mainstay for assessing injuries in the proximal gut, does not increase the yield of axial imaging, and results in unnecessary delays.[10] Run-off studies captured in the arterial phase are used when major vascular injury to the aorta and its distal tributaries is suspected, and typically involve imaging from the proximal aorta to the femoral vessels and beyond. If renal, ureteric, or bladder injuries are suspected, delay films can be obtained, whereby abdominal images are reacquired after a prespecified amount of time following intravenous contrast administration to capture contrast in the renal pelvis or collecting system. Penetrating injuries to the thoracoabdominal region, flank, or back may require the addition of rectal contrast to detect injuries to the rectum, sigmoid, and large bowel. It should be noted that there are no controlled studies to suggest that rectal contrast is useful in this regard, and patients should be managed according to local protocol and preference.

PITFALLS IN ASSESSMENT AND TRIAGE

Patients with a worrisome mechanism of injury, hemodynamic instability, or multiple obvious and severe injuries should be evaluated by the trauma team as soon as possible. Decisions to forego imaging in favor of operative management are at the discretion of the trauma team. In cases of hemodynamic instability, diagnosis should be limited to physical examination, bedside FAST examination, and radiograph imaging if time allows. Taking an unstable patient to the CT scan can result in catastrophe. Patients with free fluid on CT, without solid organ injury, should be evaluated by the trauma team and may require admission for serial examinations or exploration. The FAST examination may be falsely negative in cases of hemorrhage outside the abdominal cavity (retroperitoneum or pelvis), or in cases of small-volume hemorrhage. Repeating the FAST examination can be useful and may diagnose intraabdominal hemorrhage before the onset of hemodynamic instability. In patients who are combative with a consistent mechanism of injury, hemorrhagic shock should be ruled out before assuming the altered mental status is related to drugs or alcohol. Patients who are hemodynamically stable on presentation can also deteriorate rapidly if a contained hematoma ruptures or if there is no longer compensation for ongoing bleeding.

Finally, in blunt injury, abdominal trauma is often a marker of severe multisystem injury. Hemodynamic compromise is often multifactorial, resulting from a combination of injuries and causes of shock. Although identifying free fluid on abdominal FAST examination may point to the nature and cause of shock. A systematic assessment of injuries must be performed in all circumstances to avoid anchoring and premature diagnostic closure. Conversely, a negative or indeterminate abdominal FAST examination that does not fit with the clinical picture or suspicion of injury should be ignored or, at the very least, repeated.

THE ROLE OF RESUSCITATIVE ENDOVASCULAR BALLOON OCCLUSION OF THE AORTA IN ABDOMINAL TRAUMA

Traditional means of proximal aortic control for patients with exsanguinating abdominal hemorrhage include thoracotomy with aortic cross clamp. Dismal survival rates have resulted in a need to find a way to occlude the aorta another way. The advent of endovascular surgery resulted in technologic advancements making transfemoral aortic balloon occlusion the first step in the treatment of ruptured abdominal aortic aneurysms.[11] Although few case series using trauma subjects emerged prior to, and after the advent of endovascular surgery, the utility of this technique was demonstrated. Since then, the procedure has been adopted and modified by select trauma centers and is currently the standard of care for specific patients at these institutions. Current use of resuscitative endovascular balloon occlusion of the aorta (REBOA) is for hemorrhage below the diaphragm, in which case the balloon is inflated in the distal thoracic aorta (zone 1); in cases of hemorrhage from pelvic or junctional areas, the balloon is inflated at the distal abdominal aorta (zone 3).

REBOA is reserved for patients with blunt or penetrating injuries below the diaphragm who are unresponsive, or transiently responsive, to resuscitation. Translational and early case series have demonstrated improved physiologic measures and good outcomes from use of REBOA.[12,13] Institutional clinical algorithms have been developed for use in abdominal trauma (**Fig. 2**).[14] In patients who are persistently hypotensive (SBP <90 mm Hg) or transient responders to resuscitation with a negative chest radiograph and positive abdominal FAST examination, REBOA can be performed for aortic occlusion at the distal zone 1. This has been shown to significantly increase SBP,[15,16] allowing time for transport to definitive care. In situations of arrest from intraabdominal hemorrhage, some high-volume centers have replaced ED thoracotomy (EDT) with REBOA and high-quality cardiopulmonary resuscitation (CPR).[17] Recent data suggest that open cardiac massage in traumatic arrest offers no benefit to high-quality CPR.[18] EDT presents a viable means of proximal arterial control for noncompressible truncal hemorrhage, it carries a significant morbidity and is not without risk to the provider. The minimally invasive nature of REBOA makes this an attractive alternative to EDT.

Common femoral artery (CFA) access is a rate-limiting step for performance of REBOA. If percutaneous access, with or without ultrasound, is not possible, a groin cut down is required to cannulate the CFA. This may be due to a combination of low or no intravascular volume and lack of palpable pulse, the low threshold due to simple ability to open the groin. Approximately half of REBOAs performed in the Aortic Occlusion for Resuscitation in Trauma and Acute Care Surgery (AORTA) trial required cut-down regardless of the sheath size ultimately required; in most of these, the patients were in arrest.[16] Complications from REBOA have been reported and include arterial dissection, pseudoaneurysms, hematoma, thromboembolism, and extremity ischemia.[16] International data describe amputation in some cases,[19] which has not been reported in the United States, as a direct cause of REBOA. Interpretation of international data must come with an understanding of the differences in REBOA use abroad. Technology, indications, clinical algorithms, management of in-dwelling sheaths, providers and their training, and trauma resources must all be taken into account, and are not clearly delineated in some publications. Smaller catheters may be associated with fewer complications from REBOA.[20] Duration of balloon inflation has not been well defined, but translational studies are demonstrating partial REBOA may become an effective measure to decrease distal ischemia (Brenner M, Teeter W, Romagnoli A, et al. "Resuscitative

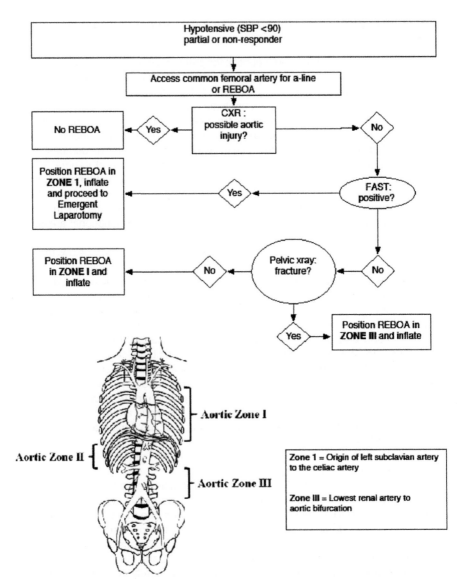

Fig. 2. Baltimore Shock Trauma REBOA algorithm. CXR, chest radiograph. (*From* Brenner M, Hoehn M, Pasley J, et al. Basic endovascular skills for trauma course: bridging the gap between endovascular techniques and the acute care surgeon. J Trauma Acute Care Surg 2014;77(2):286–91; with permission.)

endovascular balloon occlusion of the aorta [REBOA] is a feasible option for proximal aortic control in severe hemorrhage and arrest." Pacific Coast Surgical Association 2017, submitted to JAMA).[21,22] Clinical research demonstrates that survival and outcomes may or may not be affected, and definitive studies are lacking. However, data are demonstrating that Acute Care Surgeons are performing REBOA safely in the resuscitation area and, as a result, paradigm shifts in clinical practice have occurred in the 2 high-volume REBOA centers in the United States.[15–17] The most challenging aspects of REBOA are indications, CFA access, and management of the balloon and sheath, including troubleshooting. These represent current hurdles to nonsurgeon and prehospital provider use. Expansion is likely to occur with data, advancing skills, training, and technology. Recent and successful use in the battlefield has demonstrated transfer of skills by both acute care surgeons and Emergency Medicine military providers after a focused training course.[14]

SUMMARY

Initial evaluation, including attention to mechanism of injury, physical examination, and primary or secondary surveys all aid in triage of the trauma patient. Hemodynamic stability should be among the most significant determinants of patient disposition. Imaging modalities such as FAST and CT scan can aid in diagnosing abdominal injury. REBOA is an adjunct for patients in extremis from intraabdominal hemorrhage, and may allow time for transfer to definitive operation.

REFERENCES

1. Meizoso JP, Ray JJ, Karcutskie CA 4th, et al. Effect of time to operation on mortality for hypotensive patients with gunshot wounds to the torso: the golden 10 minutes. J Trauma Acute Care Surg 2016;81(4):685–91.
2. Ball CG. Damage control resuscitation: history, theory and technique. Can J Surg 2014;57(1):55–60.
3. Thorson CM, Ryan ML, Otero CA, et al. Operating room or angiography suite for hemodynamically unstable pelvic fractures? J Trauma Acute Care Surg 2012; 72(2):364–70 [discussion: 371–2].
4. Stengel D, Bauwens K, Sehouli J, et al. Systematic review and meta-analysis of emergency ultrasonography for blunt abdominal trauma. Br J Surg 2001;88(7): 901–12.
5. Glen J, Constanti M, Brohi K. Guideline development group. Assessment and initial management of major trauma: summary of NICE guidance. BMJ 2016; 353:i3051.
6. Bilello JF, Davis JW, Lemaster D, et al. Prehospital hypotension in blunt trauma: identifying the "crump factor". J Trauma 2011;70(5):1038–42.
7. Seamon MJ, Feather C, Smith BP, et al. Just one drop: the significance of a single hypotensive blood pressure reading during trauma resuscitations. J Trauma 2010;68(6):1289–94 [discussion: 1294–5].
8. Biffl WL, Kaups KL, Cothren CC, et al. Management of patients with anterior abdominal stab wounds: a Western Trauma Association multicenter trial. J Trauma 2009;66(5):1294–301.
9. Biffl WL, Kaups KL, Pham TN, et al. Validating the Western Trauma Association algorithm for managing patients with anterior abdominal stab wounds: a Western Trauma Association multicenter trial. J Trauma 2011;71(6):1494–502.
10. Ramirez RM, Cureton EL, Ereso AQ, et al. Single-contrast computed tomography for the triage of patients with penetrating torso trauma. J Trauma 2009;67(3): 583–8.
11. Malina M, Veith F, Ivancev K, et al. Balloon occlusion of the aorta during endovascular repair of ruptured abdominal aortic aneurysm. J Endovasc Ther 2005;12(5): 556–9.
12. White JM, Cannon JW, Stannard A, et al. Endovascular balloon occlusion of the aorta is superior to resuscitative thoracotomy with aortic clamping in a porcine model of hemorrhagic shock. Surgery 2011;150:400–9.

13. Avaro JP, Mardelle V, Roch A, et al. Forty minute endovascular aortic occlusion increases survival in an experimental model of uncontrolled hemorrhagic shock caused by abdominal trauma. J Trauma 2011;71:720–6.
14. Brenner M, Hoehn M, Pasley J, et al. Basic endovascular skills for trauma course©: bridging the gap between endovascular techniques and the acute care surgeon. J Trauma Acute Care Surg 2014;77(2):286–91.
15. Brenner ML, Moore LJ, DuBose JJ, et al. A clinical series of resuscitative endovascular balloon occlusion of the aorta for hemorrhage control and resuscitation. J Trauma Acute Care Surg 2013;75(3):506–11.
16. DuBose JJ, Scalea TM, Brenner M, et al, AAST AORTA Study Group. The AAST prospective Aortic Occlusion for Resuscitation in Trauma and Acute Care Surgery (AORTA) registry: Data on contemporary utilization and outcomes of aortic occlusion (REBOA). J Trauma Acute Care Surg 2016;81(3):409–19.
17. Moore LJ, Brenner M, Kozar RA, et al. Implementation of resuscitative endovascular balloon occlusion of the aorta as an alternative to resuscitative thoracotomy for noncompressible truncal hemorrhage. J Trauma Acute Care Surg 2015;79(4): 523–30.
18. Bradley M, Bonds B, Chang L, et al. Open chest cardiac massage offers no benefit over closed chest compressions in patients with traumatic cardiac arrest. J Trauma Acute Care Surg 2016;81(5):849–54.
19. Saito N, Matsumoto H, Yagi T, et al. Evaluation of the safety and feasibility of resuscitative endovascular balloon occlusion of the aorta. J Trauma Acute Care Surg 2015;78(5):897–903.
20. Teeter WA, Matsumoto J, Idoguchi K, et al. Smaller introducer sheaths for REBOA may be associated with fewer complications. JTACS 2016;81(6):1039–45.
21. Williams TK, Neff LP, Johnson MA, et al. Automated variable aortic control vs. complete aortic occlusion in a swine model of hemorrhage. J Trauma Acute Care Surg 2017;82(4):694–703.
22. Manley JD, Mitchell BJ, DuBose JJ, et al. A modern case series of resuscitative endovascular balloon occlusion of the aorta (REBOA) in an out-of-hospital, combat casualty care setting. J Spec Oper Med 2017;17(1):1–8.

Acute Management of the Traumatically Injured Pelvis

Steven Skitch, MD, PhD, RDMS[a,b], Paul T. Engels, MD, FRCSC[b,c],*

KEYWORDS

- Pelvis • Trauma • Hemorrhage control • Open fracture • REBOA

KEY POINTS

- Severe pelvic injury has a high mortality even in modern series.
- Exsanguination from blunt pelvic trauma is a common cause of preventable death.
- Initial treatment generally involves damage control resuscitation and external pelvic wrapping.
- Definitive hemorrhage control may require multiple modalities and multiple disciplines.
- Recognition of associated injuries, particularly the presence of compound fractures, is essential.

Managing patients with severe pelvic fractures is one of the most challenging aspects of trauma care. Pelvic fractures frequently result from high-energy mechanisms, often with associated multisystem injuries, and can lead to catastrophic hemorrhage. There is a high risk for serious morbidity and mortality with these injuries. Trauma registry studies from multiple countries report that unstable pelvic fractures are associated with mortalities ranging from 8% to 32%.[1–6] However, there has been a trend toward decreased mortality among patients with severe pelvic fractures as trauma care has evolved.[7] Despite advances in trauma care, mortality remains high for the subset of patients presenting with pelvic fractures complicated by hemorrhagic shock. Contemporary studies, using modern best management practices, report mortalities of 32% for these patients.[5]

Conflicts of Interest: All of the authors report no financial or professional conflict of interest.
[a] Department of Emergency Medicine, McMaster University, Hamilton General Hospital, 6 North Wing - Room 616, 237 Barton Street East, Hamilton, Ontario L8L 2X2, Canada; [b] Department of Critical Care, McMaster University, Hamilton General Hospital, 6 North Wing - Room 616, 237 Barton Street East, Hamilton, Ontario L8L 2X2, Canada; [c] Department of Surgery, McMaster University, Hamilton General Hospital, 6 North Wing - Room 616, 237 Barton Street East, Hamilton, Ontario L8L 2X2, Canada
* Corresponding author. Department of Surgery, McMaster University, Hamilton General Hospital, 6 North Wing - Room 616, 237 Barton Street East, Hamilton, Ontario L8L 2X2, Canada.
E-mail address: engelsp@mcmaster.ca

This article focuses on the current approach to severe pelvic injury, including diagnosis and classification, pelvic binding, angiography and embolization, operative stabilization, and treatment of associated injuries, as well as exploring emerging therapies, including resuscitative endovascular balloon occlusion of the aorta (REBOA) and hybrid operative and angiography suites.

ANATOMY AND CLASSIFICATION FOR EMERGENCY MEDICINE TRAUMA PRACTITIONERS

The bony anatomy of the pelvis can be conceptualized as a ring formed by the sacrum and right and left innominate bones, specifically the ischium, ilium, and pubis.[8] Viscera of the gastrointestinal and genitourinary system are housed within the bony pelvis. Paired internal iliac arteries and their related tributaries are the predominant arterial supply of the pelvis. The venous system follows a similar path but is arranged in a plexus adherent to the posterior pelvic wall. Pelvic fracture bleeding predominantly arises from the venous plexus or cancellous bone; however, arterial bleeding occurs in a significant number of cases and is associated with life-threatening hemorrhage.[9] Knowledge of pelvic fracture classification is useful in predicting likelihood of severe injury and to aid communication with consultants.

A variety of classification systems have been proposed; the 2 most commonly described in the emergency medicine (EM) literature are the Young-Burgess (YB) and Tile fracture classification systems. The YB system is mechanistically based with fractures classified as lateral compression, anteroposterior compression, vertical shear, or combination injuries with levels of gradation depending on the degree of disruption of the ligamentous and bony stabilizers of the pelvis.[10] The Tile classification system is based on the integrity of the posterior sacroiliac ligaments of the pelvis and associated mechanical instability (Tile A, stable; Tile B, rotationally unstable; Tile C, rotationally and vertically unstable).[11] Further details regarding these classification systems are available in EM and trauma textbooks[8] and review articles.[12] Several studies support the utility of both the YB and Tile systems to predict need for blood transfusion and associated injuries.[10,13–16] However, these results have not been consistently replicated across all studies and fracture classification cannot reliability predict mortality.[9,17–19] In the subset of patients with persistent shock after initial resuscitation (for the authors, this means an appropriately placed pelvic binder and administration of 2units packed red blood cells and tranexamic acid), the presence of a severe pelvic fracture does predict an increased probability of a pelvic source of hemorrhage and need for arterial embolization.[20] Fracture pattern should be considered as one component of determining the likelihood of an associated vascular or visceral injury but must be interpreted in the context of the patient's hemodynamic status and associated injuries.

APPROACH TO INITIAL ASSESSMENT AND MANAGEMENT OF PELVIC FRACTURES

The authors' approach to the assessment and management of the severely injured pelvis is outlined in **Fig. 1**. Further details and description are provided later, including exploration of areas of nonconsensus among trauma practitioners.

Initial Resuscitation

Resuscitation of severely injured patients with trauma is covered in depth elsewhere (see Tim Harris and colleagues article, "The Evolving Science of Trauma Resuscitation," in this issue). Specific to patients with severe pelvic fractures is the need to obtain meaningful supradiaphragmatic intravenous (IV) access. The potential

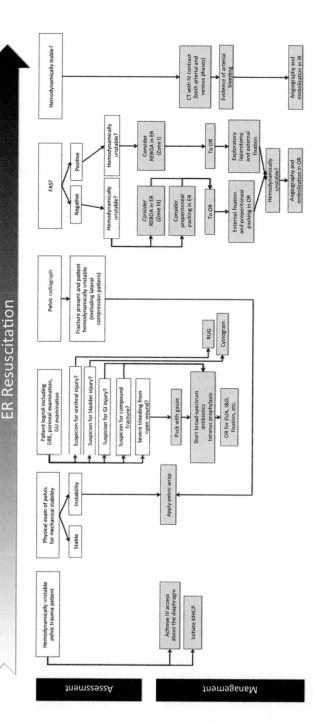

Fig. 1. Pelvic trauma assessment and management algorithm. CT, computed tomography; DRE, digital rectal examination; ER, emergency room; EUA, examination under anesthesia; FAST, focused assessment with sonography for trauma; GI, gastrointestinal; GU, genitourinary; I&D, incision and drainage; IR, interventional radiology; IV, intravenous; MHCP, massive hemorrhage control protocol (also known as massive transfusion protocol); OR, operating room; RUG, retrograde urethrogram.

for significant injury to the pelvic vasculature renders femoral venous access unreliable, because fluids infused through this location may never reach the right atrium. Two or more large-bore (14–18 gauge) IV catheters placed in the antecubital fossae or an 8-French or 9-French percutaneous introducer sheath placed in the subclavian vein are required to adequately resuscitate a patient with a severely injured pelvis. If initial attempts for peripheral IV catheterization are unsuccessful, then expedient placement of an intraosseous (IO) catheter in the proximal humerus should be sought as a bridge to obtaining adequate IV access. Fluid resuscitation should be consistent with damage control resuscitation principles as espoused in this issue.

The Role of Radiography

Pelvic radiography has traditionally been recommended as an adjunct to the primary survey in all patients with blunt trauma to the torso.[21] The dogma of routine pelvic radiography has recently been challenged by multiple lines of evidence. First, radiography has limited sensitivity for detection of pelvic fractures compared with computed tomography (CT), particularly for sacral and iliac fractures.[22–24] Second, in hemodynamically stable patients with blunt trauma receiving a CT scan as part of their work-up, the addition of pelvic radiographs does not lead to any significant changes in management.[25,26] Third, in awake and alert patient who sustain trauma, clinical examination has sufficient sensitivity to exclude significant pelvic fracture.[27–29] This evidence suggest that routine radiographs can be foregone in selected patients with blunt trauma. Radiographs should still be obtained in patients presenting with altered level of consciousness, abnormal clinical examination, or hemodynamic instability in whom pelvic radiographs can expedite diagnosis and definitive care.[30,31] Given the lethal risks of missing the diagnosis of a pelvic fracture and the simplicity and minimal risk of obtaining pelvic radiographs, the authors recommend both an examination of pelvic stability and a pelvic radiograph for all stable patients at risk of pelvic injury who will not have a pelvic CT scan performed as part of their trauma diagnostics.

The Role of Focused Assessment with Sonography for Trauma and Diagnostic Peritoneal Lavage

In hemodynamically unstable patients with pelvic fractures, the rapid exclusion of alternative sources of hemorrhage is imperative for making optimal management decisions. Specifically, the trauma provider needs to assess for the presence of significant thoracic and abdominal hemorrhage. The ubiquity of bedside ultrasonography has substantially changed trauma care with the FAST (focused assessment with sonography for trauma) examination frequently used in the work-up of unstable patients with trauma to assess for hemoperitoneum. In general, the presence of free intraperitoneal fluid on FAST and hemodynamic instability is an indication for emergent laparotomy. The presence of free fluid on the FAST examination of a patient with a pelvic fracture has excellent specificity for intra-abdominal lesions requiring surgical intervention.[32] However, this fluid is not always the cause of the patient's hemodynamic instability. Among a series of patients with pelvic fractures who had positive abdominal FAST examinations, in 19% of cases the free fluid was urine as a result of an intraperitoneal bladder rupture.[33] Interpretation of a negative FAST examination is even more challenging. In the setting of a pelvic fracture, the reported sensitivity of FAST for intraperitoneal fluid ranges from 23% to 80%.[33–35] This range may be caused by anatomic distortion by pelvic/retroperitoneal hematoma that confounds image interpretation. Although continual improvement in ultrasonography resolution and operator training may attenuate such effects, it must be remembered that the absence of free fluid on a FAST examination in a patient with pelvic fracture does not have sufficient sensitivity to rule out the presence of hemoperitoneum.

Diagnostic peritoneal aspirate (DPA) or diagnostic peritoneal lavage (DPL), first described in 1965,[36] is an alternative method for determining the presence of hemoperitoneum in unstable patients with blunt trauma with pelvic fracture. DPA is the aspiration of fluid from the peritoneal cavity once access to this cavity has been obtained (whether by open cut-down or percutaneous catheter placement). DPA should be performed in an open supraumbilical manner for patients with pelvic fracture.[21] Free aspiration with a syringe of greater than 10 mL of frank blood, gastrointestinal contents, vegetable fibers, or bile in patients with hemodynamic abnormalities mandates laparotomy.[21] In the absence of these findings, DPL is performed by infusing 1000 mL of warmed isotonic crystalloid solution into the peritoneal cavity, which is then mixed by compressing the abdomen and logrolling the patient to each side. The effluent is then drained either by sump action by dropping the IV crystalloid bag onto the floor and allowing the lavage fluid to drain via the infusion catheter, or by aspirating the lavage fluid with a syringe. The lavage fluid is sent for cell count and Gram stain analysis with positive thresholds of greater than 100,000 red blood cells/mm^3 or 500 white blood cells/mm^3, or presence of bacteria on Gram stain. DPL has excellent sensitivity for hemoperitoneum and is particularly sensitive among hemodynamically unstable patients with trauma.[37,38] In the investigators' practice, a positive DPA is viewed as a powerful signal localizing exsanguinating hemorrhage to the abdomen, whereas a nonpositive DPA that proceeds to a DPL requires significant time for the hospital laboratory to analyze the sample to determine the DPL positivity and therefore does not meaningfully inform management of hemodynamically unstable patients with pelvic fracture. In addition, contemporary trauma practitioners have less exposure to DPA/DPL, which limits its applicability.[39] Taking into account the potential difficulties with the pelvic view of the FAST, in the authors' experience, exsanguinating hemorrhage originating within the peritoneal cavity should have a positive FAST in the upper abdominal views and these are the easiest views to obtain. We reserve DPA for persistently hemodynamically unstable patients with pelvic fractures in whom FAST cannot yield interpretable upper abdominal views (eg, severe bilateral subcutaneous emphysema). The authors think that DPA should be performed by the surgeon who is going to operate on the abdomen if the aspirate is positive, and should not be performed outside of that context.

Pelvic Binding

Temporary stabilization of unstable pelvic fractures with noninvasive external compression (pelvic binding) is recommended as part of routine management. The benefits of this technique are posited through several mechanisms, including prevention of further pelvic motion, reduction of pelvic volume leading to decreased hemorrhage, and lessening patient discomfort.[40] Stabilization can be rapidly achieved through circumferential application of a bed sheet centered at the level of the greater trochanter. Accurate placement is important. Both cadaveric and clinical studies have shown that placement of circumferential binding at locations other than the greater trochanter leads to inadequate reduction.[41] Several commercial devices are also available for pelvic binding. There is insufficient evidence to indicate that any commercial device is superior to binding with a sheet. Certain commercial devices may be advantageous in terms of ease and consistency of application[42] but can impair access to the groin for percutaneous access to the femoral vessels for angiography or REBOA placement, whereas a bedsheet can easily have a defect cut over the vessels to facilitate access while maintaining integrity of the pelvic wrap. Bedsheet wraps can be secured with Kelly clamps to decrease the risk of skin necrosis compared with knots;

however, Kelly clamps may cause some CT scan artifact and this can be avoided by using commercially available zip ties (**Fig. 2**). Cadaveric studies have consistently shown that pelvic binding provides adequate reduction of anterior-posterior compression fractures.[43] Furthermore, pelvic binding has been shown to lead to improved hemodynamics and reduced requirement for blood transfusion.[40]

The utility of pelvic binding in patients with trauma with unstable lateral compression fractures is controversial. There is concern that excessive external compression in this subset of patients can worsen internal rotation deformity. Both clinical and cadaveric studies have confirmed that, when pelvic binders are applied to patients with lateral compression fractures, deformity can worsen.[43,44] Although no studies have shown a negative clinical impact of this effect, in patients with lateral compression fractures it is prudent to apply pelvic binders with caution, and the recent Western Trauma Association guideline recommends against application of a pelvic binder in this setting.[45] In these situations, the binder should be applied, if at all, with the aim of reducing further fracture displacement rather than correcting any rotational deformity. Trauma providers should be aware of case reports of skin breakdown with pelvic binding and avoid applying excessive traction.[46] A postbinding pelvic radiograph can be obtained to ensure reapproximation of the pelvic ring. As shown in **Fig. 1**, the authors place a pelvic binder immediately on diagnosing a mechanically unstable fracture on physical examination or in hemodynamically unstable patients with significant pelvic fractures on radiograph.

Resuscitative Endovascular Balloon Occlusion of the Aorta

REBOA is an endovascular or internal cross-clamp of the aorta. The creation of REBOA as a viable clinical tool in the twenty-first century is the result of the merger

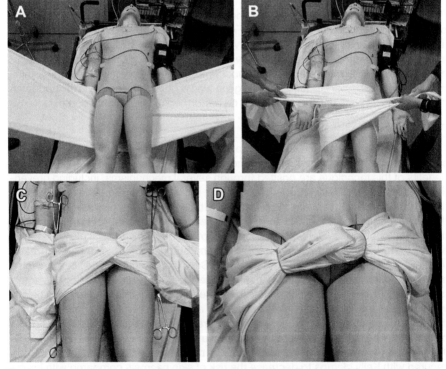

Fig. 2. Pelvic wrap being placed (*A, B*) and secured with Kelly clamps (*C*) or zip ties (*D*).

of endovascular technology with the trauma surgeon's knowledge and expertise in the principles of damage control resuscitation. The emergence of REBOA is in many ways in response to the difficulty of controlling bleeding from a severely injured pelvis and the lack of universal efficacy of other hemorrhage control measures. First described in 1954 by Col. Hughes[47] during the Korean War, the technique has undergone several variations in the trauma setting[48,49] and benefitted from advances made in endovascular aortic aneurysm repair.[50,51] The informal use of the intra-aortic balloon pump, most conventionally used for cardiogenic shock, to control gastrointestinal hemorrhage has been reported,[52] as has several other such case reports.[53–55] Involvement of the United States and its allies in armed conflicts in Iraq and Afghanistan in the first decade of the twenty-first century generated significant research relating to the battlefield deaths and injuries sustained by military personnel.[56] Out of this research, the need for a technique to treat noncompressible torso hemorrhage was identified and in 2014 the Joint Theater Trauma System clinical practice guideline for the use of REBOA for hemorrhagic shock was released.[57] This practice guideline included the use of REBOA in the algorithm for traumatic arrest and in the management of profound shock. In 2013, Brenner and colleagues[58] published their clinical series using REBOA in 6 patients. Following this clinical breakthrough, the American Association for the Surgery of Trauma (AAST) multi-institutional study entitled Aortic Occlusion for Resuscitation in Trauma and Acute Care Surgery (AORTA) was initiated to compare resuscitative thoracotomy with REBOA in participating US trauma centers. Results published from this registry have shown the clinical efficacy of this resuscitative tool in the treatment of profound hemorrhagic shock.[59] Note that the use of aortic balloon occlusion has also been reported in France,[60] the United Kingdom,[61] Australia,[62] and most notably in Japan.[63,64] The reported experiences in Japan of more than 450 cases of REBOA use have not shown improved mortality[64] and have reported significant complications, such as limb loss.[63] However, the clinical context of REBOA deployment and use seem to differ significantly from North American deployment[58] and experience,[59] and thus cannot be directly compared.

As a clinical tool in the treatment of severe hemorrhage from pelvic fractures, the REBOA balloon is typically deployed in zone III of the aorta, or just above the aortic bifurcation (see Megan Brenner and Christopher Hicks article, "Major Abdominal Trauma: Critical Decisions and New Frontiers in Management," in this issue). First-generation technology involves obtaining arterial access to the common femoral artery and placement of a 12-French sheath, then placement of an endovascular guidewire within the descending aorta, and then positioning and inflation of a Coda balloon (Cook Medical Inc, Bloomington IN). Although ideally performed under real-time fluoroscopy, the often dire circumstances of its placement as well as the results of the AORTA registry support its placement using radiographs and sometimes only anatomic landmarks.[59] Successful placement using ultrasonography has also been reported.[65,66]

Second-generation technology, in the form of the ER-REBOA Catheter (Prytime Medical Devices, Boerne TX), has now become available with approval by the US Food and Drug Administration in October 2015 and achievement of the CE (Conformité Européene) mark of approval (European Union) in December 2016. This device is a single stiff balloon occlusion catheter with integrated arterial pressure monitoring that is placed through a 7-French arterial access sheath, thereby removing the requirement for common femoral artery placement and mandatory arterial vascular repair as was the case with the use of 12-French sheath equipment. Data regarding the performance of this specific catheter are not yet available but it is in use at major trauma centers across the United States at the time of writing.

Where available, REBOA is currently recommend to be placed in aorta zone III in the setting of a patient with pelvic trauma who continues to be hemodynamically unstable despite pelvic wrapping and appropriate resuscitation.[45] Successful placement of REBOA in this setting is a temporizing maneuver and involves creating total lower-body ischemia. Minimizing the duration of balloon inflation is therefore critical, and such a patient should be taken emergently to the operating room (OR) or angiographic suite as dictated by their other injuries and institutional capabilities. The authors consider REBOA deployment for patients who are persistently hemodynamically unstable after pelvic binding and initial resuscitation (see **Fig. 1**). REBOA deployment may be considered in the setting of traumatic cardiac arrest as an alternative to resuscitative thoracotomy in certain settings (see Chris Evans and colleagues article, "Reanimating the Traumatic Cardiac Arrest Patient: A Practical Approach Informed by Best Evidence," in this issue). Most recent available data from US trauma centers on REBOA use indicate the necessity for arterial cutdown in 50%, radiographic guidance being used in 50%, mean procedure times of approximately 6 minutes, and no reports of limb ischemia or amputation.[59] However, data regarding the impact of second-generation REBOA technology on these parameters are not yet available.

The ultimate role for this evolving technique remains to be determined, as does the type of practitioner who may safely use it. However, its future may include use not only at high-level trauma centers but conceivably at rural and remote hospitals without surgical capabilities or meaningful blood product stocks that are forced to manage patients exsanguinating from a lower-body source.

HEMORRHAGE CONTROL

Following initial trauma bay resuscitation, patients with pelvic fractures and ongoing hemodynamic instability require further intervention to achieve hemorrhage control. Potential options include (1) external pelvic fixation, (2) extraperitoneal packing, and (3) angiographic embolization. REBOA, as described earlier, may be placed in the emergency department (ED) as a temporizing bridge to obtaining definitive hemorrhage control. These treatment options and their combined application and sequencing are discussed in further detail later.

External Pelvic Fixation

Compared with pelvic binding, external percutaneous fixation provides more definitive control of a mechanically unstable pelvis and reduces pelvic volume to tamponade venous bleeding. There are 2 general approaches for external fixation described in the literature.[67] For rotationally unstable anterior-posterior compression and lateral compression fractures an anterior external fixation approach is preferred. In the case of vertically unstable pelvic fractures a C-clamp device is used to stabilize posterior pelvic elements (**Fig. 3**). Case series of patients managed with percutaneous external fixation suggest that this technique is effective in reducing hemorrhage and may have a mortality benefit.[68–71] Application of external pelvic fixation devices has been described in both the trauma bay and the OR settings.[70] In the modern era, given the efficacy and easy of applicability of external pelvic binding techniques, percutaneous fixation is best reserved for the OR. Provider experience with this technique is crucial because reported complications include neurovascular injury caused by screw malposition, fixation failure, and infection.[68]

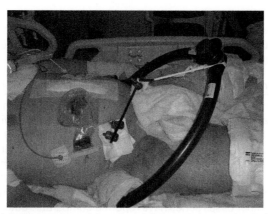

Fig. 3. Patient with both anterior pelvic external fixator and posterior C-clamp pelvic fixator.

Extraperitoneal Packing

Extraperitoneal packing both as a stand-alone procedure and in combination with percutaneous external fixation has been described as an effective method for achieving hemorrhage control in unstable patients with pelvic fractures. Historical experiences with pelvic packing, when the procedure was combined with a laparotomy, peritoneal violation, and resultant retroperitoneal decompression, were disappointing because this often worsened pelvic hemorrhage.[72] Contemporary approaches to packing involve a direct preperitoneal approach to the pelvis that allows access to the retroperitoneal space without violating the peritoneum, as described and illustrated by Smith and colleagues.[73] In this approach, packing is used as a stabilizing procedure before more definitive management and packing must subsequently be removed. There are no published randomized controlled trials examining the efficacy of extraperitoneal packing; however, cases series have shown that this technique is associated with improved blood pressure[74] and reduced blood transfusion requirements.[75,76] A recently published study, which used propensity score analysis to compare patients who received extraperitoneal packing with those who did not, reported a significant mortality benefit (20% vs 52%).[77] Although preferably performed in the OR, extraperitoneal packing can be accomplished in the ED with appropriate surgical equipment and a trained practitioner. As such, the authors do not recommend it to be performed by nonexperienced EM practitioners; obtaining the skillset for safe REBOA placement may be more appropriate for such practitioners.

Angiography and Embolization

Most hemorrhage related to pelvic fractures is venous in origin; however, when arterial bleeding occurs it frequently leads to significant hemodynamic instability and a high risk of exsanguination. Transcatheter arterial embolization (TAE) has been found to be the optimal treatment modality for pelvic fractures complicated by arterial hemorrhage. A recent systematic review of TAE for pelvic fracture reported an efficacy rate between 81% and 100% in controlling arterial hemorrhage with a reduction in need for blood product transfusion and reduced mortality caused by pelvic bleeding.[78] Risk factors for requiring TAE include ongoing hemodynamic instability after initial resuscitation and pelvic binding, presence of a contrast blush on CT, large pelvic hematoma on CT, and older age.[42] Delay in provision of TAE has been associated with increased risk for mortality[79,80] and reducing time to angiography is a major challenge even in busy trauma centers with substantial resources.[81] There is significant interest in determining the optimal approach to sequencing hemorrhage control interventions in hemodynamically unstable patients with pelvic fractures.

Optimal Sequencing on Interventions for Hemorrhage Control in Pelvic Fractures

Following initial resuscitation in the ED, the decision of where to transport hemodynamically unstable patients for further intervention can be fraught with difficulty (see **Fig. 1**). Incorrect choice can delay time to definitive hemorrhage control and increases the risk of patient mortality.[82] In a registry study of 558 consecutive trauma deaths, the most common preventable cause of death was exsanguination from blunt pelvic injuries.[83] In most of these cases, patients were initially taken to the OR for a laparotomy and percutaneous external fixation and subsequently died before receiving angiography. In contrast, other cases series have reported comparable outcomes regardless of whether patients are initially taken for laparotomy before angioembolization.[84,85] Ultimately, the optimal approach may depend on local resource availability and practice patterns. Several centers have adopted an approach combining extraperitoneal packing with TAE to provide improved outcomes for severe pelvic fractures. Owing to the reality that interventional radiology capabilities are often not immediately available, these protocols most often involve extraperitoneal packing to reduce hemorrhage before TAE. Multiple centers have shown that an approach of packing before TAE reduces time to intervention[86,87] and reduced hemorrhage-related mortality compared with historical controls.[87–89] In unstable patients for whom there will be an excessive delay (>45 minutes)[87] in TAE or who require operative intervention for intra-abdominal injuries, extraperitoneal packing should be strongly considered as part of their management.

Ultimately, the optimal approach to managing patients with blunt trauma with refractory hemodynamic instability after initial resuscitation may be transfer to a setting that can provide combined operative and interventional radiology interventions. Such an approach has recently been described in the literature as hybrid operating suites that combine capacity for diagnostic radiology investigations, percutaneous vascular interventions, and open operative techniques in a single location.[90] A recent retrospective study of patients with severe traumatic injuries and persistent hypotension found that 7% of this cohort required emergent operative and angiographic interventions and would benefit from a hybrid operating suite.[91] Severely injured patients with unstable pelvic fractures are a subgroup of patients who are likely to derive particular benefit from a hybrid operating suite that can minimize delays in hemorrhage control. There are currently a handful of centers that have capacity for this approach and studies assessing their clinical impact are sorely needed.

COMPOUND PELVIC FRACTURES AND ASSOCIATED INJURIES

Compound or open (not to be confused with open-book) fractures comprise only 2% to 4% of all pelvic fractures but have a severe morbidity rate of more than 50% and carry a significant mortality of up to 23% even in modern series.[92] An open pelvic fracture is present when there is a direct communication between a skin, rectal, or vaginal wound and the fracture. Open pelvic fractures usually occur from high-energy trauma with resultant pelvic bone disruption and subsequent laceration of the pelvic tissues thereby creating associated injuries. Anorectal injuries are reported to be present in 18% to 64% of cases and urogenital tract injuries in 24% to 57%.[93] Early diagnosis is essential because delayed diagnosis is associated with infective complications and increased mortality.[93]

The clinical spectrum of an open pelvic fracture can encompass everything from an iliac wing fracture with a small puncture wound to massive perineal disruptions with gross fecal contamination and exsanguinating hemorrhage. Regardless of the magnitude of injury, the foundation of management is still hemodynamic stabilization, as discussed previously, but should also include careful physical examination with subsequent diagnostic procedures when indicated and appropriate for the patient's condition. It is also important to note that any potential tamponade effect from controlling pelvic volume may be lost with larger wounds and hemorrhage can be significant.[94] Examination of the patient includes a meticulous inspection of the perianal, vulvar, and perineal tissues, including a digital rectal examination (DRE) and digital vaginal examination (DVE). Anorectal injuries should be suspected if blood is found on rectal examination or rectal wall weakness is detected (the presence of palpable bony fragments on DRE or DVE is diagnostic of an open pelvic fracture). Urogenital injuries should be suspected if blood is present at the external urethral meatus; the prostate is superiorly displaced on DRE; or there is significant perineal ecchymosis, gross hematuria, or vaginal bleeding and lacerations. Anorectal injuries should be more thoroughly assessed by a surgeon in the OR under anesthesia to appropriately diagnose and treat any injury or perform fecal diversion if indicated; although specific when positive (**Fig. 4**), rectal contrast studies do not adequately assess the lower rectum or the sphincter complex. Vaginal lacerations usually result from direct penetration by bony fragments, are often combined with larger lacerations involving the perineum and rectum, and are best assessed and repaired in the operating theater. Injuries to the uterus, cervix, or ovaries caused by pelvic fractures are rare.[95,96]

The American Urological Association urotrauma guidelines[97] and American College of Surgeons[21] endorse clinicians to perform retrograde urethrography as a diagnostic procedure in patients with blood at the urethral meatus after pelvic trauma (**Box 1, Fig. 5**), and recommend that clinicians should establish prompt urinary drainage in patients with pelvic fracture–associated urethral injury. An update to these guidelines clarifies that a single passage of a urethral catheter can be attempted by an expert

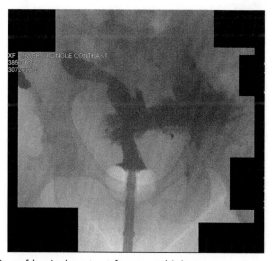

Fig. 4. Extravasation of luminal contrast from rectal injury.

Box 1
Retrograde urethrogram

- Obtain a small-bore urethral catheter (14 F) and catheterization setup, radiopaque contrast (such as that used for a cystogram), personal lead apron, portable x-ray machine, and technician

- Position patient with hips rotated 30°; for patients in spinal precautions, this can be accomplished by logroll or use of appropriate bolstering

- Under sterile conditions, place catheter 1 to 2 cm into the fossa navicularis

- Inflate the balloon with 1 to 2 mL of water to achieve a snug fit

- Take an initial scout radiograph to confirm appropriate field of view

- Fill syringe with 30 mL of contrast and gently inject, taking radiograph as last 10 mL are injected

practitioner to allow immediate urinary drainage in the acute trauma setting, followed by a pericatheter urethrogram to rule out significant urethral injury when the patient is stable.[98] On occasion, a Foley catheter may already have been placed before evaluation of the urethra. Further imaging is not warranted if no meatal blood is present and suspicion of injury is low. If blood is present a pericatheter retrograde urethrogram should be performed to identify potential missed urethral injury.[97] Suprapubic catheter drainage can be placed in the operating theater or potentially at the bedside under ultrasonography guidance[99] (**Box 2**).

Injury to the bladder may occur in cases of pelvic trauma and its appropriate management requires early diagnosis: intraperitoneal bladder injuries require operative repair, whereas uncomplicated extraperitoneal injuries can generally be managed with catheter drainage alone.[97] As noted earlier, urethral injury must first be ruled out as a source of meatal blood. However, once a catheter is successfully placed, the presence of hematuria necessitates further investigation. Gross hematuria in the setting of a pelvic fracture or mechanism concerning for bladder injury requires a

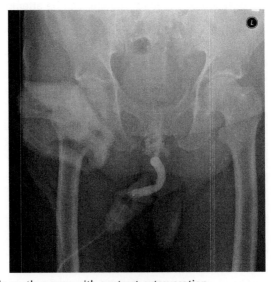

Fig. 5. Retrograde urethrogram with contrast extravasation.

Box 2
Ultrasonography-guided suprapubic cystostomy

- Prepare sterile field, including sterile-draped ultrasound probe
- Visualize distended bladder in both longitudinal and transverse axes
- After infiltrating local anesthesia, make a vertical skin incision of 5 to 10 mm with scalpel in suprapubic region in the midline
- Using a percutaneous suprapubic catheter set, insert trocar through skin into the bladder with real-time ultrasonography guidance
- Once urine is aspirated, advance catheter 3 to 5 cm, then remove trocar
- Secure catheter in place with suture

---

cystogram,[97] and the authors exclusively use retrograde CT cystograms performed during the same sequence of trauma CT scans as part of the secondary survey.[21] Note that clamping the Foley catheter to allow IV-administered contrast to accumulate in the bladder is not appropriate. Instillation of a minimum of 300 mL of dilute water-soluble contrast to distend the bladder is required to exclude injury.[97]

Although the definitive management of open pelvic fractures is often complicated, requires multidisciplinary surgical care, and may require a prolonged hospital stay, emergent management focuses on hemodynamic stabilization and identification of the compound fracture and any associated injuries. Once an open pelvic fracture is identified, immediate administration of IV broad-spectrum antimicrobials is indicated and urgent surgical consultation should be sought. Patients with open pelvic fractures should be transferred to a center with the expertise to provide definitive care, which in most cases is a regional trauma referral center.[100]

SUMMARY

The severely injured pelvis continues to challenge even the most experienced trauma practitioners. With a record of excessive morbidity and mortality, even in contemporary series with modern technologies, severe pelvic fractures remain a primary cause of preventable traumatic death. The conundrum is its ability, when suitably injured, to create multifocal venous and arterial hemorrhage that is noncompressible; there is no large vessel to tie off or organ to remove, and thus its injury is treated in a largely supportive fashion to facilitate intrinsic hemostasis. The advent of new technologies, such as REBOA and hybrid OR suites, will increase trauma practitioners' ability to temporize bleeding in the ED and minimize the interval from ED arrival to definitive hemorrhage control by providing multimodality treatment in a single location. Nevertheless, many trauma patients are not transported directly from the scene of injury to a trauma center and/or may require transport that lasts hours. For the severely injured pelvic patients with trauma, damage control resuscitation and pelvic binding should start as early as possible (ie, with emergency medical services and/or first treating hospital), followed by expeditious multimodality hemorrhage control at the trauma center in order to provide optimal management of these vexing injuries.

REFERENCES

1. Giannoudis PV, Grotz MRW, Tzioupis C, et al. Prevalence of pelvic fractures, associated injuries, and mortality: the United Kingdom perspective. J Trauma 2007;63(4):875–83.

2. Hauschild O, Strohm PC, Culemann U, et al. Mortality in patients with pelvic fractures: results from the German pelvic injury register. J Trauma 2008;64(2): 449–55.

3. Yoshihara H, Yoneoka D. Demographic epidemiology of unstable pelvic fracture in the United States from 2000 to 2009: trends and in-hospital mortality. J Trauma Acute Care Surg 2014;76(2):380–5.

4. Vaidya R, Scott AN, Tonnos F, et al. Patients with pelvic fractures from blunt trauma. What is the cause of mortality and when? Am J Surg 2016;211(3): 495–500.

5. Costantini TW, Coimbra R, Holcomb JB, et al. Current management of hemorrhage from severe pelvic fractures. J Trauma Acute Care Surg 2016;80(5): 717–25.

6. Inaba K, Sharkey PW, Stephen DJG, et al. The increasing incidence of severe pelvic injury in motor vehicle collisions. Injury 2004;35(8):759–65.

7. Black SR, Sathy AK, Jo C, et al. Improved survival after pelvic fracture: 13-year experience at a single trauma center using a multidisciplinary institutional protocol. J Orthop Trauma 2016;30(1):22–8.

8. Choi SB, Cwinn AA. Chapter 55 – Pelvic trauma. In: Marx J, Walls R, Hockberger R, editors. Rosen's emergency medicine - concepts and clinical practice. 2014. p. 656–71.

9. Cook RE, Keating JF, Gillespie I. The role of angiography in the management of haemorrhage from major fractures of the pelvis. J Bone Joint Surg Br 2002; 84(2):178–82.

10. Dalal SA, Burgess AR, Siegel JH, et al. Pelvic fracture in multiple trauma: classification by mechanism is key to pattern of organ injury, resuscitative requirements, and outcome. J Trauma 1989;29:981–1000.

11. Tile M. Acute pelvic fractures: I. causation and classification. J Am Acad Orthop Surg 1996;4(3):143–51.

12. Alton TB, Gee AO. Classifications in brief: young and burgess classification of pelvic ring injuries. Clin Orthop Relat Res 2014;472:2338–42.

13. Ohmori T, Matsumoto T, Kitamura T, et al. Scoring system to predict hemorrhage in pelvic ring fracture. Orthop Traumatol Surg Res 2016;102(8):1023–8.

14. Ruatti S, Guillot S, Brun J, et al. Which pelvic ring fractures are potentially lethal? Injury 2015;46(6):1059–63.

15. Osterhoff G, Scheyerer MJ, Fritz Y, et al. Comparing the predictive value of the pelvic ring injury classification systems by Tile and by Young and Burgess. Injury 2014;45(4):742–7.

16. Manson T, O'Toole RV, Whitney A, et al. Young-Burgess classification of pelvic ring fractures: does it predict mortality, transfusion requirements, and non-orthopaedic injuries? J Orthop Trauma 2010;24(10):603–8.

17. Brun J, Guillot S, Bouzat P, et al. Detecting active pelvic arterial haemorrhage on admission following serious pelvic fracture in multiple trauma patients. Injury 2014;45(1):101–6.

18. Cortina Gualdo J, Barastegui Fernandez D, Teixidor Serra J, et al. Pelvic fractures in polytrauma: which classification system better predicts hemodynamic instability? Eur Orthop Traumatol 2013;4(1):35–9.

19. Sarin EL, Moore JB, Moore EE, et al. Pelvic fracture pattern does not always predict the need for urgent embolization. J Trauma 2005;58(5):973–7.

20. Eastridge BJ, Starr A, Minei JP, et al. The importance of fracture pattern in guiding therapeutic decision-making in patients with hemorrhagic shock and pelvic ring disruptions. J Trauma 2002;53(3):446–50, 1.

21. American College of Surgeons. Advanced trauma life support: ATLS instructor manual. 9th edition. Chicago: American College of Surgeons; 2012.
22. Obaid AK, Barleben A, Porral D, et al. Utility of plain film pelvic radiographs in blunt trauma patients in the emergency department. Am Surg 2006;72(10): 951–4.
23. Reilly PM, Schwab CW. Pelvic radiography in blunt trauma resuscitation: a diminishing role. J Trauma 2002;53(6):1043–7.
24. Obaid KA, Barleben A, Porral D, et al. Pelvic trauma imaging: a blinded comparison of computed tomography roentgenograms. J Trauma Inj Infect Crit Care 1996;41(6):994–8.
25. Barleben A, Jafari F, Rose J, et al. Implementation of a cost-saving algorithm for pelvic radiographs in blunt trauma patients. J Trauma 2011;71(3):582–4.
26. Kessel B, Sevi R, Jeroukhimov I, et al. Is routine portable pelvic X-ray in stable multiple trauma patients always justified in a high technology era? Injury 2007; 38(5):559–63.
27. Gonzalez RP, Fried PQ, Bukhalo M. The utility of clinical examination in screening for pelvic fracture in blunt trauma. J Am Coll Surg 2002;194(2):121–5.
28. Duane TM, Cole FJ, Weireter LJ, et al. Blunt trauma and the role of routine pelvic radiographs. Am Surg 2001;67(9):849–52.
29. Civil ID, Ross SE, Botehlo G, et al. Routine pelvic radiography in severe trauma: is it necessary? Ann Emerg Med 1988;17(5):488–90.
30. Fu CY, Wang SY, Hsu YP, et al. The diminishing role of pelvic x-rays in the management of patients with major torso injuries. Am J Emerg Med 2014;32(1): 18–23.
31. Verbeek DO, Burgess AR. Importance of pelvic radiography for initial trauma assessment: an orthopedic perspective. J Emerg Med 2016;50(6):852–8.
32. Ruchholtz S, Waydhas C, Lewan U, et al. Free abdominal fluid on ultrasound in unstable pelvic ring fracture: is laparotomy always necessary? J Trauma 2004; 57(2):278–85, 287.
33. Tayal VS, Nielsen A, Jones AE, et al. Accuracy of trauma ultrasound in major pelvic injury. J Trauma 2006;61(6):1453–7.
34. Friese RS, Malekzadeh S, Shafi S, et al. Abdominal ultrasound is an unreliable modality for the detection of hemoperitoneum in patients with pelvic fracture. J Trauma 2007;63(1):97–102.
35. Ballard RB, Rozycki GS, Newman PG, et al. An algorithm to reduce the incidence of false-negative FAST examinations in patients at high risk for occult injury. J Am Coll Surg 1999;189(2):145–51.
36. Root HD, Hauser CW, Mckinley CR, et al. Diagnostic peritoneal lavage. Surgery 1965;57:633–7.
37. Biffl WL, Moore EE. Diagnostic peritoneal lavage remains a valuable adjunct to modern imaging techniques. J Trauma 2009;67(2):330–4 [discussion: 334–6].
38. Nagy KK, Roberts RR, Joseph KT, et al. Experience with over 2500 diagnostic peritoneal lavages. Injury 2000;31:479–82.
39. Fakhry SM, Watts DD, Michetti C. The resident experience on trauma: declining surgical opportunities and career incentives? Analysis of data from a large multi-institutional study. J Trauma 2003;54(1):1–7 [discussion: 7–8].
40. Bakhshayesh P, Boutefnouchet T, Tötterman A. Effectiveness of non invasive external pelvic compression: a systematic review of the literature. Scand J Trauma Resusc Emerg Med 2016;24:73.

41. Bonner TJ, Eardley WGP, Newell N, et al. Accurate placement of a pelvic binder improves reduction of unstable fractures of the pelvic ring. J Bone Joint Surg Br 2011;93 B(11):1524–8.
42. Cullinane DC, Schiller HJ, Zielinski MD, et al. Eastern Association for the Surgery of Trauma practice management guidelines for hemorrhage in pelvic fracture–update and systematic review. J Trauma 2011;71(6):1850–68.
43. Bottlang M, Krieg JC, Mohr M, et al. Emergent management of pelvic ring fractures with use of circumferential compression. J Bone Joint Surg Am 2002;84:43–7.
44. Toth L, King KL, McGrath B, et al. Efficacy and safety of emergency non-invasive pelvic ring stabilisation. Injury 2012;43(8):1330–4.
45. Shatz DV, Mitchell J. Western Trauma Association Critical Decisions in Trauma: management of pelvic fracture with hemodynamic instability — 2016 updates. J Trauma Acute Care Surg 2016;81(7):1171–4.
46. Schaller TM, Sims S, Maxian T. Skin breakdown following circumferential pelvic antishock sheeting: a case report. J Orthop Trauma 2005;19(9):661–5.
47. Hughes CW. Use of an intra-aortic balloon catheter tamponade for controlling intra-abdominal hemorrhage in man. Surgery 1954;36(1):65–8.
48. Low RB, Longmore W, Rubinstein R, et al. Preliminary report on the use of the Percluder occluding aortic balloon in human beings. Ann Emerg Med 1986;15(12):1466–9.
49. Gupta BK, Khaneja SC, Flores L, et al. The role of intra-aortic balloon occlusion in penetrating abdominal trauma. J Trauma 1989;29(6):861–5.
50. Hesse FG, Kletschka HD. Rupture of abdominal aortic aneurysm: control of hemorrhage by intraluminal balloon tamponade. Ann Surg 1962;155(2):320–2.
51. Greenberg RK, Srivastava SD, Ouriel K, et al. An endoluminal method of hemorrhage control and repair of ruptured abdominal aortic aneurysms. J Endovasc Ther 2000;7(1):1–7.
52. Karkos CD, Bruce IA, Lambert ME. Use of the intra-aortic balloon pump to stop gastrointestinal bleeding. Ann Emerg Med 2001;38(3):328–31.
53. Harma M, Harma M, Kunt AS, et al. Balloon occlusion of the descending aorta in the treatment of severe post-partum haemorrhage. Aust N Z J Obstet Gynaecol 2004;44(2):170–1.
54. Matsuoka S, Uchiyama K, Shima H, et al. Temporary percutaneous aortic balloon occlusion to enhance fluid resuscitation prior to definitive embolization of posttraumatic liver hemorrhage. Cardiovasc Intervent Radiol 2001;24(4):274–6.
55. Søvik E, Stokkeland P, Storm BS, et al. The use of aortic occlusion balloon catheter without fluoroscopy for life-threatening post-partum haemorrhage. Acta Anaesthesiol Scand 2012;56(3):388–93.
56. Stannard A, Morrison JJ, Scott DJ, et al. The epidemiology of noncompressible torso hemorrhage in the wars in Iraq and Afghanistan. J Trauma Acute Care Surg 2013;74(3):830–4.
57. US Department of Defense. CENTCOM Joint Theater Trauma System (JTTS) clinical practice guidelines. Resuscitative endovascular balloon occlusion of the aorta (REBOA) for hemorrhagic shock. 2014. Available at: http://www.usaisr.amedd.army.mil/cpgs/REBOA_for_Hemorrhagic_Shock_16Jun2014.pdf. Accessed February 15, 2017.
58. Brenner ML, Moore LJ, DuBose JJ, et al. A clinical series of resuscitative endovascular balloon occlusion of the aorta for hemorrhage control and resuscitation. J Trauma Acute Care Surg 2013;75(3):506–11.

59. DuBose JJ, Scalea TM, Brenner M, et al, AAST AORTA Study Group. The AAST prospective Aortic Occlusion for Resuscitation in Trauma and Acute Care Surgery (AORTA) registry: data on contemporary utilization and outcomes of aortic occlusion and resuscitative balloon occlusion of the aorta (REBOA). J Trauma Acute Care Surg 2016;81(3):409–19.

60. Martinelli T, Thony F, Declety P, et al. Intra-aortic balloon occlusion to salvage patients with life threatening hemorrhagic shock from pelvic fractures. J Trauma 2010;68(4):942–8.

61. World's first prehospital REBOA performed. London's Air Ambulance Website. 2014. Available at: https://londonsairambulance.co.uk/our-service/news/2014/06/we-perform-worlds-first-pre-hospital-reboa. Accessed February 15, 2017.

62. O'Leary C. Simple gadget stops injured people from bleeding to death. The West Australian. 2015. Available at: http://health.thewest.com.au/news/1811/simple-gadget-stops-injured-people-from-bleeding-to-death. Accessed February 15, 2017.

63. Saito N, Matsumoto H, Yagi T, et al. Evaluation of the safety and feasibility of resuscitative endovascular balloon occlusion of the aorta. J Trauma Acute Care Surg 2015;78(5):409–19.

64. Nori T, Crandall C, Terasaka Y. Survival of severe blunt trauma patients treated with resuscitative endovascular balloon occlusion of the aorta compared with propensity score-adjusted untreated patients. J Trauma Acute Care Surg 2015;78(4):721–8.

65. Guliani S, Amendola M, Strife B, et al. Central aortic wire confirmation for emergent endovascular procedures: as fast as surgeon-performed ultrasound. J Trauma Acute Care Surg 2015;79(4):549–54.

66. Chaudery M, Clark J, Morrison JJ, et al. Can contrast-enhanced ultrasonography improve Zone III REBOA placement for prehospital care? J Trauma Acute Care Surg 2016;80(1):89–94.

67. Stahel PF, Mauffrey C, Smith WR, et al. External fixation for acute pelvic ring injuries: decision making and technical options. J Trauma Acute Care Surg 2013;75(5):882–7.

68. Barei DP, Bellabarba C, Mills WJ, et al. Percutaneous management of unstable pelvic ring disruptions. Injury 2001;32(Suppl 1):SA33–44.

69. Heini PF, Witt J, Ganz R. The pelvic C-clamp for the emergency treatment of unstable pelvic ring injuries. A report on clinical experience of 30 cases. Injury 1996;27(Supp 1):SA38–45.

70. Henry SM, Tometta P, Scalea TM. Damage control for devastating pelvic and extremity injuries. Surg Clin North Am 1997;77(4):879–95.

71. Riemer BL, Butterfield SL, Diamond DL, et al. Acute mortality associated with injuries to the pelvic ring: the role of early patient mobilization and external fixation. J Trauma 1993;35(5):671–7.

72. Lustenberger T, Wutzler S, Störmann P, et al. The role of pelvic packing for hemodynamically unstable pelvic ring injuries. Clin Med Insights Trauma Intensive Med 2015;6:1–8.

73. Smith WR, Moore EE, Osborn P, et al. Retroperitoneal packing as a resuscitation technique for hemodynamically unstable patients with pelvic fractures. J Trauma 2005;59(6):1510–4.

74. Tötterman A, Madsen JE, Skaga NO, et al. Extraperitoneal pelvic packing: a salvage procedure to control massive traumatic pelvic hemorrhage. J Trauma Acute Care Surg 2007;62(4):843–52.

75. Burlew CC, Moore EE, Smith WR, et al. Preperitoneal pelvic packing/external fixation with secondary angioembolization: optimal care for life-threatening hemorrhage from unstable pelvic fractures. J Am Coll Surg 2011;212(4):628–35.

76. Cothren CC, Osborn PM, Moore EE, et al. Preperitonal pelvic packing for hemodynamically unstable pelvic fractures: a paradigm shift. J Trauma 2007;62(4): 834–9.

77. Chiara O, di Fratta E, Mariani A, et al. Efficacy of extra-peritoneal pelvic packing in hemodynamically unstable pelvic fractures, a propensity score analysis. World J Emerg Surg 2016;11:22.

78. Papakostidis C, Kanakaris N, Dimitriou R, et al. The role of arterial embolization in controlling pelvic fracture haemorrhage: a systematic review of the literature. Eur J Radiol 2012;81(5):897–904.

79. Schwartz DA, Medina M, Cotton BA, et al. Are we delivering two standards of care for pelvic trauma? Availability of angioembolization after hours and on weekends increases time to therapeutic intervention. J Trauma Acute Care Surg 2014;76(1):134–9.

80. Tanizaki S, Maeda S, Matano H, et al. Time to pelvic embolization for hemodynamically unstable pelvic fractures may affect the survival for delays up to 60 min. Injury 2014;45(4):738–41.

81. Tesoriero R, Bruns B, Narayan M, et al. Angiographic embolization for hemorrhage following pelvic fracture: is it "time" for a paradigm shift? J Trauma Acute Care Surg 2017;82(1):18–26.

82. Holcomb JB, Fox EE, Scalea TM, et al. Current opinion on catheter-based hemorrhage control in trauma patients. J Trauma Acute Care Surg 2014;76(3): 888–93.

83. Tien HC, Spencer F, Tremblay LN, et al. Preventable deaths from hemorrhage at a level I Canadian trauma center. J Trauma 2007;62(1):142–6.

84. Katsura M, Yamazaki S, Fukuma S, et al. Comparison between laparotomy first versus angiographic embolization first in patients with pelvic fracture and hemoperitoneum: a nationwide observational study from the Japan Trauma Data Bank. Scand J Trauma Resusc Emerg Med 2013;21:82.

85. Thorson CM, Ryan ML, Otero CA, et al. Operating room or angiography suite for hemodynamically unstable pelvic fractures? J Trauma Acute Care Surg 2012; 72(2):364–70.

86. Li Q, Dong J, Yang Y, et al. Retroperitoneal packing or angioembolization for haemorrhage control of pelvic fractures–Quasi-randomized clinical trial of 56 haemodynamically unstable patients with Injury Severity Score ≥33. Injury 2016;47(2):395–401.

87. Burlew CC, Moore EE, Stahel PF, et al. Preperitoneal pelvic packing reduces mortality in patients with life-threatening hemorrhage due to unstable pelvic fractures. J Trauma Acute Care Surg 2017;82(2):233–42.

88. Osborn PM, Smith WR, Moore EE, et al. Direct retroperitoneal pelvic packing versus pelvic angiography: a comparison of two management protocols for haemodynamically unstable pelvic fractures. Injury 2009;40(1):54–60.

89. Tai DKC, Li WH, Lee KYKB, et al. Retroperitoneal pelvic packing in the management of hemodynamically unstable pelvic fractures: a level I trauma center experience. J Trauma Acute Care Surg 2011;71(4):E79–86.

90. D'Amours SK, Rastogi P, Ball CG. Utility of simultaneous interventional radiology and operative surgery in a dedicated suite for seriously injured patients. Curr Opin Crit Care 2013;19(6):587–93.

91. Fehr A, Beveridge J, D'Amours SD, et al. The potential benefit of a hybrid operating environment among severely injured patients with persistent hemorrhage: how often could we get it right? J Trauma Acute Care Surg 2016;80(3):457–60.
92. Cannada LK, Taylor RM, Reddix R, et al, Southeastern Fracture Consortium. The Jones-Powell Classification of open pelvic fractures: a multicenter study evaluating mortality rates. J Trauma Acute Care Surg 2013;74(3):901–6.
93. Grotz MR, Allami MK, Harwood P, et al. Open pelvic fractures: epidemiology, current concepts of management and outcome. Injury 2005;36(1):1–13.
94. Langford JR, Burgess AR, Liporace FA, et al. Pelvic fractures: part 1. Evaluation, classification, and resuscitation. J Am Acad Orthop Surg 2013;21(8):448–57.
95. Govender S, Sham A, Singh B. Open pelvic fractures. Injury 1990;21(6):373–6.
96. Smith RJ. Avulsion of the nongravid uterus due to pelvic fracture. South Med J 1989;82(1):70–3.
97. Morey AF, Brandes S, Dugi DD 3rd, et al. Urotrauma: AUA guideline. J Urol 2014;192(2):327–35.
98. Stein DM, Santucci RA. An update on urotrauma. Curr Opin Urol 2015;25(4): 323–30.
99. Aguilera PA, Choi T, Durham BA. Ultrasound-guided suprapubic cystostomy catheter placement in the emergency department. J Emerg Med 2004;26(3): 319–21.
100. Sinnott R, Rhodes M, Brader A. Open pelvic fracture: an injury for trauma centers. Am J Surg 1992;163(3):283–7.

Management of Major Vascular Injuries

Neck, Extremities, and Other Things that Bleed

Chris Evans, MD, MSc, FRCPC[a],*, Tim Chaplin, MD, FRCPC[b],
David Zelt, MD, MSc, FRCSC[c]

KEYWORDS

- Neck trauma • Vascular injury • Vascular trauma • Blunt cerebrovascular
- Computed tomography angiography • Tourniquet

KEY POINTS

- Clinical guidelines from the Western Trauma Association should be used to screen for blunt cerebrovascular injuries in patients at risk so that antiplatelet, antithrombotic, or endovascular treatments can be initiated to reduce the risk of stroke.
- Patients with deep penetrating neck injuries and no indications for immediate surgery can be worked up with a careful physical examination and computed tomography–based angiography regardless of the zone of injury.
- Because the time to reperfusion is the major determinant of limb salvage in patients with extremity arterial injuries, emergency physicians' primary responsibility is to make the diagnosis.
- The arterial pressure index is a highly sensitive and specific physical examination maneuver for diagnosing extremity arterial injuries and should be performed in all patients with high-risk injuries or clinical concern for vascular injury.
- Appropriately applied tourniquets are a useful means of temporarily controlling peripheral arterial hemorrhage when direct pressure and wound packing have failed.

INTRODUCTION

Patients with major vascular injuries represent a significant clinical challenge to emergency physicians whether in a small community hospital, a high-volume urban trauma center, or n the battlefield. Such injuries may be clinically obvious and dramatic or

Disclosure: None of the authors have any conflicts of interest or funding sources to declare.
[a] Trauma Services, Department of Emergency Medicine, Kingston General Hospital, Queen's University, Kingston, Ontario K7L 2V7, Canada; [b] Department of Emergency Medicine, Queen's University, Kingston, Ontario K7L 2V7, Canada; [c] Division of Vascular Surgery, Kingston General Hospital, Queen's University, Kingston, Ontario K7L 2V7, Canada
* Corresponding author.
E-mail address: c.evans@queensu.ca

Emerg Med Clin N Am 36 (2018) 181–202
https://doi.org/10.1016/j.emc.2017.08.013
emed.theclinics.com

present with minimal initial clinical findings and subsequently progress to limb-threatening ischemia if not identified. Several types of vascular injuries have been described in the settings of blunt or penetrating trauma (**Box 1**).[1-3]

There have been numerous advances in the management of vascular trauma over the past several decades, including the advent of computed tomography (CT) with angiography (CT-A),[4,5] the resurgence of prehospital tourniquets,[6,7] the establishment of damage control resuscitation principles,[8,9] as well as greater reliance on endovascular therapies.[5,10] This article discusses practical and, wherever possible, evidence-based strategies for managing patients with significant vascular injuries. Potential pitfalls and opportunities are highlighted throughout, as are areas of clinical equipoise and controversy. Because it is not possible to cover the full spectrum of vascular trauma in this short article, the authors have chosen to focus on the resuscitation, diagnosis, and definitive management of those vascular injuries that are common, rapidly lethal, or associated with significant morbidity. This article comprises 3 parts:

1. The diagnosis and management of blunt and penetrating injuries to the neck vessels.
2. Diagnostic issues in extremity vascular injuries.
3. The perspective of vascular surgeons in managing peripheral vascular injuries.

PART I: VASCULAR INJURIES IN THE NECK

Injuries to the major neck vessels (the carotid and vertebral arteries) are among the most common injuries of all major vessels.[3] Whether caused by blunt or penetrating mechanisms, these injuries can cause severe neurologic sequelae or lead to rapid exsanguination.

Pathophysiology of Blunt Cerebrovascular Injuries

Blunt injuries to the carotid arteries tend to be caused by the application of shear forces via one of 4 mechanisms (**Box 2**).

In contrast, vertebral artery injuries are caused by variable directions and patterns of shear force, including hyperextension and hyperflexion.[11] Fractures of the upper cervical spine (C1 to C3), especially to the foramen transversarium,[12] and facet joint dislocations are particularly associated with blunt injuries to the vertebral vessels.[11]

Most blunt cerebrovascular injuries are caused by motor vehicle collisions,[11,13] but there is a diversity of causes, including sporting injuries, falls, and even trivial-appearing trauma such as chiropractic manipulation or shaving.[14]

Box 1
Types of vascular injury

Vasospasm

External compression

Contusion

Intimal disruption

Subintimal or intimal hematoma

Focal wall defects with pseudoaneurysm or hemorrhage

Laceration

Transection

Box 2
Fundamental mechanisms of blunt trauma to the carotid arteries

1. Hyperextension and contralateral rotation of the head and neck with stretching of the internal carotid over the lateral processes of the upper cervical spine

2. Direct application trauma to the vessel (eg, strangulation, seatbelt)

3. Intraoral trauma (eg, toddler who falls with foreign body in mouth)

4. Basilar skull fracture in proximity to the carotid canal

Data from Crissey MM, Bernstein EF. Delayed presentation of carotid intimal tear following blunt craniocervical trauma. Surgery 1974;75(4):543–9.

Once the vessel has been injured, a dissection flap forms and this acts as a nidus for platelet aggregation and thrombus formation, followed by either distal embolization or vessel occlusion. Less frequently, the vessel tears either incompletely and creates a pseudoaneurysm, or, least frequently, it ruptures altogether.[15] If untreated, cerebral ischemia and infarction subsequently ensue.

A grading scale for injuries to the carotid and vertebral arteries (based on imaging findings) has been developed and is helpful in both understanding the pathophysiologic spectrum of injury and in guiding management (**Box 3**).

Pathophysiology of Penetrating Injuries to the Neck Vessels

In contrast with the shear forces involved in blunt cerebrovascular injuries, penetrating injuries cause local tissue destruction as the penetrating object crushes and separates tissue planes, and, in the case of gunshot wounds, secondary to the concussive shockwave.[16] The tight and complex anatomic confines of the deep neck spaces, coupled with localized energy dissipation associated with penetrating neck injuries (PNIs), creates a much greater potential for associated injuries to the aerodigestive, endocrine, and neurologic systems than is found with blunt neck trauma.

Diagnosis and Management of Blunt Cerebrovascular Injuries

Making the diagnosis of a blunt cerebrovascular injury (BCVI) is challenging because of the infrequency of the problem, the multitude of mechanisms of injury, and the frequently delayed development of neurologic injury. Unless there is immediate complete arterial occlusion, the development of stroke symptoms typically takes many hours to even days to develop as thrombus and/or distal embolization evolves.[17] As

---

Box 3
Blunt carotid and vertebral artery injury grading scale

Grade	Description
I	Luminal irregularity or dissection with 25% luminal narrowing
II	Dissection or intramural hematoma with 25% luminal narrowing, intraluminal thrombus, or raised intimal flap
III	Pseudoaneurysm
IV	Occlusion
V	Transection with free extravasation

Data from Biffl WL, Moore EE, Offner PJ, et al. Blunt carotid arterial injuries: implications of a new grading scale. J Trauma 1999;47(5):845–53.

a consequence, rates of severe neurologic disability with these injuries can approach 50%.[18] Given the difficulty in establishing the diagnosis and the potential for significant morbidity and mortality, there has been great interest in the past 2 decades in developing criteria for screening patients at high risk for BCVI.[17–19] Use of these screening criteria is supported by clinical practice guidelines[17,19] and has been shown to be effective in preventing strokes by allowing earlier initiation of anticoagulation or antiplatelet therapies.[20] One small, retrospective study found that the sensitivity and specificity for these screening criteria were 97% (95% confidence interval [CI], 83%–100%) and 42% (95% CI, 20%–67%), respectively.[21]

Patients with symptoms compatible with a blunt cerebrovascular injury

Patients with the following signs and symptoms are presumed to have a BCVI and should undergo emergent multidetector CT-A from the aortic arch through the neck and cerebral vessels (**Box 4**).

Patients who are neurologically normal and lack any symptoms listed in **Box 4**, but are classified as high risk for a BCVI because of either their mechanism of injury or concurrently identified injuries (**Box 5**), should undergo screening CT-A.

How accurate is computed tomography angiography in identifying blunt cerebrovascular injury?

At most trauma centers, CT-A has largely replaced digital subtraction angiography (DSA) as the primary screening test for BCVI because of several factors, including the greater availability of this imaging modality; its noninvasive nature; the concurrent need to obtain CT images of the head, neck, and other body regions in patients with blunt trauma; and the reduced contrast dye burden.

As a screening test, CT-A is not perfect and the diagnostic accuracy varies greatly depending on the number of slices obtained in the scan, as well as the patient population selected and the interpreting radiologist.[22] The largest meta-analysis on the topic found that the pooled sensitivity and specificity for CT-A compared with DSA were 66% (95% CI, 49%–79) and 97% (95% CI, 91%–99), respectively.[22] In general, to have even moderate sensitivity, a 16-slice CT-A scan must be obtained. The limited sensitivity of CT-A implies that, for patients with a high pretest probability of BCVI, a negative CT-A scan should be followed by DSA to definitely exclude an injury but a positive CT-A scan is sufficient to confirm the diagnosis. Patients with clinical

---

Box 4
Symptoms suggestive of blunt cerebrovascular injury warranting emergent computed tomography angiography

Suspected arterial hemorrhage from nose, mouth, or neck

Expanding cervical hematoma

Cervical bruit in patient less than 50 years old

Focal neurologic deficit

Neurologic deficit inconsistent with findings on CT or MRI

Stroke identified on CT or MRI

Data from Biffl WL, Cothren CC, Moore EE, et al. Western Trauma Association critical decisions in trauma: screening for and treatment of blunt cerebrovascular injuries. J Trauma Inj Infect Crit Care 2009;67(6):1150–3; and Bromberg WJ, Collier BC, Diebel LN, et al. Blunt cerebrovascular injury practice management guidelines: the Eastern Association for the Surgery of Trauma. J Trauma 2010;68(2):471–7.

Box 5
Injury mechanisms and patterns associated with blunt cerebrovascular injury that warrant screening computed tomography angiography

Mechanisms
  Any mechanism consistent with severe cervical hyperextension, hyperflexion, or rotation
  Near-hanging with ischemic brain injury
  Clothesline-type injury or seat belt abrasion with altered mental status, significant pain, or swelling

Associated injuries
  Any cervical spine fracture at the C1 to C3 level
  Cervical vertebral body or transverse foramen fracture, subluxation, or ligamentous injury, regardless of level
  Severe facial fractures (eg, Le Fort fractures)
  Basilar skull fracture in proximity to carotid canal
  Diffuse axonal injury pattern with Glasgow Coma Scale score less than 6

Data from Biffl WL, Cothren CC, Moore EE, et al. Western Trauma Association critical decisions in trauma: screening for and treatment of blunt cerebrovascular injuries. J Trauma Inj Infect Crit Care 2009;67(6):1150–3; and Bromberg WJ, Collier BC, Diebel LN, et al. Blunt cerebrovascular injury practice management guidelines: the Eastern Association for the Surgery of Trauma. J Trauma 2010;68(2):471–7.

---

features consistent with a BCVI and a negative CT-A scan can be difficult to manage outside a trauma center and transfer for DSA and/or assessment by clinicians with expertise in trauma, cerebrovascular surgery, and interventional radiology should be considered. Similarly, patients with equivocal CT-A findings should proceed to formal DSA.[17]

Treatment of Blunt Cerebrovascular Injury

The treatment of BCVI remains controversial and several factors contribute to the management option undertaken, including the grade of injury, the patient's concurrent injuries, the location of the injury, local resource availability, and clinical expertise (see **Box 3**). In general, the options are antiplatelet agents, anticoagulation, endovascular therapy, and surgery.[17,19] Overall, there is a very limited evidence base to guide decision making.

Most injuries (grades I–IV) are treated with systematic anticoagulation using either unfractionated heparin (no bolus; 10 U/kg/h to target partial thromboplastin time of 40–50 s)[17] or antiplatelet agents (aspirin or clopidogrel).[19] The Western Trauma Association guidelines suggest unfractionated heparin for patients without contraindications because it is reversible, has proven efficacy in reducing neurologic disability, and may be more effective than antiplatelet agents.[17] In contrast, the Eastern Association for the Surgery of Trauma (EAST) suggests that either therapy would be reasonable.[19] For patients with contraindications to systemic anticoagulation, antiplatelet therapy is suggested. The optimal duration of treatment is unknown and guidelines suggest continuing until the injured vessel has healed on follow-up imaging,[17] which may be as early as 7 to 10 days after injury but may be many months. In some cases, patients require lifelong antiplatelet or anticoagulation therapy.[17]

Patients with a transection of the carotid or vertebral artery (grade V injury) have very high rates of morbidity and mortality. These patients require emergent hemorrhage control, usually via angioembolization, because the lesion is typically not surgically accessible.[15,17,19]

Diagnosis and Management of Penetrating Vascular Injuries of the Neck

PNIs represent about 1% of trauma admissions to trauma centers in the United States and are associated with a 5% rate of mortality. Almost all deaths (~80%) relate to cerebral infarctions, with the remainder relating to uncontrolled hemorrhage.[23]

The initial resuscitation efforts are directed at the most likely causes of early death after a PNI: exsanguination and asphyxiation caused by airway obstruction. Additional considerations in patients with low-neck injuries or associated wounds include tension pneumothorax, massive hemothorax, and cardiac tamponade.

A patient with a PNI must be considered a difficult airway and approached carefully. Patients with so-called hard signs of significant injury to vascular or aerodigestive structures require immediate airway control (**Fig. 1**). In general, hard signs of injury should be identified during the typical primary survey component of the assessment of patients with trauma.

It is important to be able to distinguish hard from soft signs in PNI (**Box 6**). The former are essentially diagnostic of a serious injury (approximately 90% rate of significant injury[24]) and require immediate surgical consultation, whereas the latter are nonspecific features that warrant further work-up with at least CT-A. Soft signs of injury are identified during a systemic examination after immediate life threats have been managed.

Concurrent with digital pressure to sites of hemorrhage, the patient should be passively preoxygenated with a nonrebreather oxygen mask and nasal cannula, placed on continuous cardiorespiratory monitoring devices, have large-bore intravenous access obtained, and the difficult airway equipment at the bedside.

Whenever possible, bag-mask ventilation should be avoided because there is a risk of the positive pressure displacing air into violated soft tissue spaces of the neck and

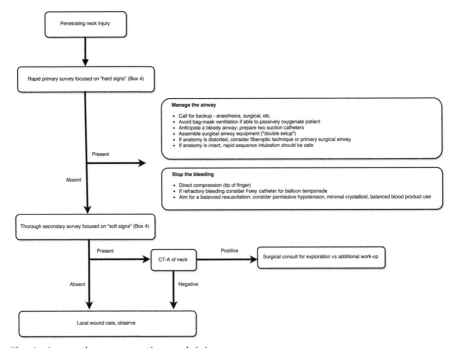

Fig. 1. Approach to penetrating neck injury.

Box 6		
Hard and soft signs of vascular and aerodigestive tract injuries in penetrating neck trauma		
	Hard Signs	**Soft Signs**
Vascular Injury	Severe uncontrolled hemorrhage	Minor bleeding
	Refractory shock/hypotension	Small, nonexpanding hematoma
	Large, expanding, or pulsatile hematoma	Proximity wound
	Unilateral extremity pulse deficit	
	Bruit or thrill	
	Neurologic deficit consistent with stroke	
Aerodigestive	Airway compromise	Mild hemoptysis
Tract Injury	Bubbling through wound	Mild hematemesis
	Extensive subcutaneous emphysema	Dysphonia
	Stridor	Dysphagia
	Hoarse voice	Mild subcutaneous emphysema

further distorting the airway anatomy. Two suction catheters should be prepared to manage significant bleeding. The authors agree with EAST guidelines for the management of PNIs, which indicate that, if the patient is conscious and has no overt neurologic deficits, cervical spine immobilization is unnecessary[25] and risks obscuring wounds, increasing patient agitation, and complicating airway management. This recommendation applies to both gunshot wounds and stab wounds, because, in these populations, neurologic deficits are established and final at the time of presentation to the emergency department.[26] Overall, the incidence of cervical spinal cord injury among patients with penetrating trauma is less than 1%.[26]

If bleeding persists despite direct digital pressure to the wound, an 18-F Foley catheter may be inserted with a finger into the wound and directed to the palpated or estimated location of bleeding before inflating the balloon with sterile water until the bleeding stops or moderate resistance is felt (**Fig. 2**).[27] A hemostat can then be applied to the distal end of the catheter to prevent it from migrating into the wound.[27] In some cases a second catheter is required to occlude both proximal and distal ends of the vascular defect.[27] Once inflated within the wound (not the vascular lumen), the balloon exerts extrinsic tamponade on the vessel.

Airway management in penetrating neck injuries: is the anatomy intact or distorted?
Patients with clearly distorted airway anatomy require a multidisciplinary team approach, including the emergency physician, anesthesia, respiratory therapist, and locally available surgical consultants (trauma/general surgery, otolaryngology, and so forth). In general, it should be anticipated that patients with PNI and distorted airway anatomy will require a surgical airway. Even if the anatomy initially appears intact, clinicians should be vigilant for changes in the patient's airway status and be prepared for all possible scenarios, including the performance of a surgical airway.

If the larynx or trachea has been lacerated and is open to the skin, the preferred approach is to place the endotracheal tube directly through the wound and into the larynx or trachea (**Fig. 3**).[28]

If the airway is not accessible externally, the next best option is awake fiberoptic intubation so that any airway injury can be directly visualized and the tube clearly advanced past the lesion with the assurance that no false tract will be created.[28]

Awake fiberoptic intubation[29] requires a cooperative patient and is very challenging if there are significant amounts of blood in the airway. If fiberoptic intubation is not an option, then awake direct or video laryngoscopy is the next best. The limitation of these techniques is that they are blind techniques in that the operator is unable to

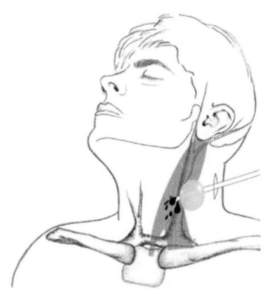

Fig. 2. Foley catheter balloon tamponade of hemorrhage from penetrating neck injury. (*From* Weppner J. Improved mortality from penetrating neck and maxillofacial trauma using Foley catheter balloon tamponade in combat. J Trauma acute Care Surg 2013;75(2):221; with permission.)

visualize the airway distally and risks introducing the tube into a tract leading to subcutaneous tissues or converting a partial tracheal laceration into a complete laceration.[30] There is little research on this scenario but common sense suggests that a gentle, bougie-guided intubation strategy using a smaller-than-normal endotracheal tube may be helpful in reducing the risk of creating a false passage.

Whether fiberoptic or direct techniques are used, a double setup approach is essential. In this case, the double setup includes having the skin prepped, landmarks

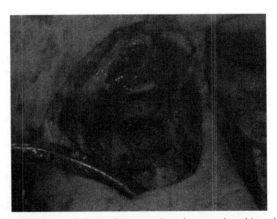

Fig. 3. Endotracheal tube passed through external neck wound and into larynx. (a) thyroid cartilage, (b) epiglottis, (c) posterior pharyngeal wall, (d) endotracheal tube. (*From* Youssef N, Raymer KE. Airway management of an open penetrating neck injury. Can J Emerg Med 2015;17(1):90; with permission.)

identified, local anesthesia administered, and all equipment and personnel set up to proceed immediately to cricothyroidotomy (tracheostomy if transected larynx) if intubation is unsuccessful.

If the airway anatomy appears externally intact, then rapid sequence intubation (RSI) is generally considered to be safe and effective in the setting of PNIs.[31,32] If an RSI is the initial technique chosen, clinicians should still consider the possibility of an occult airway injury and have a clear backup plan in place, including a surgical airway kit assembled and supraglottic airway devices prepared for rescue oxygenation.

What is the current approach to working up a penetrating neck injury?

Historically, PNIs were approached from the diagnostic and therapeutic perspectives using a zone-based system that classified injuries according to the anatomic location of the injury: zone I injuries in the region bounded by the clavicles/sternum up to the cricoid cartilage; zone II injuries between the cricoid cartilage and the angle of mandible; and zone III injuries superior to the angle of the mandible.[33,34]

The zone-based approach is useful for identifying patients with zone II injuries for whom operative exploration would be pursued, without further investigation. However, reports indicating that roughly half of all neck explorations were nontherapeutic[34,35] led to interest in identifying noninvasive testing methods that could better discern patients who could be managed nonoperatively.

Concurrently, several limitations of the zone-based approach to PNI became apparent, including (1) the limited correlation between external wound location and internal injury site,[36] (2) the exclusion of injuries to the posterior neck from the classification scheme, (3) problem of wounds traversing more than 1 zone, and (4) the issue of patients often having more than 1 wound.[23] As a consequence of these challenges as well as the advent of CT-A, the zone-based approach has largely fallen out of favor in preference to the no-zone approach. The latter approach is based on timely resuscitation, triage of patients with hard signs directly to the operating room, the use CT-A to work up patients with soft signs of injury, and observation for asymptomatic patients (see **Fig. 1**).

The no-zone approach to penetrating neck injuries

Once the patient has been resuscitated, found to have no concerning signs of vascular or aerodigestive tract injury (hard signs), and confirmed to have a deep neck wound (ie, platysma violating) to any area of the neck, the next step is to conduct a focused examination looking for soft signs of injury that would require further assessment with CT-A.[24,33,37] CT-A has been found in numerous studies to have very favorable diagnostic test characteristics in the context of PNI, and most recently in a prospective, multicenter study was shown to have 100% sensitivity and 97.5% specificity in identifying clinically significant injuries.[33] If there is any doubt regarding the depth of the wound (ie, whether it violates the platysma), the physician should consult with a trauma specialist and/or proceed to CT-A.

Patients with CT-A findings consistent with injury to the vascular or aerodigestive structures undergo either immediate operative exploration or further investigations (eg, catheter-directed angiography, endoscopy, bronchoscopy) at the discretion of the treating clinician. Those patients who are asymptomatic (no hard signs or soft signs of injury) and have negative CT-A do not require further work-up but should be considered for a period of observation (see **Fig. 1**).[24]

PART II: DIAGNOSIS OF EXTREMITY VASCULAR INJURIES

Peripheral vascular injuries are the most common types of vascular injuries encountered at civilian trauma centers.[2] Unlike junctional or thoracoabdominal vascular injuries, peripheral vascular trauma involves smaller vessels that are amenable to direct pressure and tourniquet control. These features explain the low incidence of mortality from peripheral vascular injuries. Advances over the last 50 years in diagnostics and operative techniques, and improvements in resuscitation, have resulted in a decreased rate of amputation following peripheral vascular trauma and an increased rate of functional limb recovery.[1]

Like injuries to the neck vessels, extremity vascular injuries can range from subtle intimal tears to complete transection of the vessel (see **Box 1**) and can occur following either a blunt or a penetrating injury mechanism.

What is the Current Diagnostic Approach to Extremity Vascular Injuries?

The approach to patients with peripheral vascular trauma is similar to any patient with trauma and should begin with a brief primary survey for immediate threats to life or limb. In patients with polytrauma with peripheral vascular injuries, there may be concomitant injuries that take priority. However, if there is obvious external hemorrhage, this should be managed immediately with direct pressure or a tourniquet, either before or in conjunction with efforts to manage airway or ventilatory problems.

The peripheral vascular examination: hard signs, soft signs, and the arterial pressure index

Time to revascularization is the variable most strongly correlated with the functional outcome in vascular trauma. As such, it is important to consider and evaluate for vascular injuries in all patients with trauma because delays to diagnosis frequently occur when signs of injury are present but go unrecognized early in the care of these patients.[38] Patients with certain injuries should be approached with a high index of suspicion for peripheral vascular injury (**Box 7**).

The most important diagnostic tool in extremity arterial trauma is the physical examination.[38] Specifically, searching for (and documenting) the presence or absence of hard and/or soft signs (**Box 8**) of peripheral vascular injury is the most crucial part of the diagnostic work-up of any trauma case, but in particular those with high-risk orthopedic injuries (see **Box 7**). Note that although there is some overlap, there are differences in what is considered a hard sign of vascular injury in the neck (see **Box 6**) versus the extremity (see **Box 8**).

Hard signs of extremity arterial injury (see **Box 8**) are not subtle and should lead to emergent vascular surgery consultation because they are associated with a very high (>90%) likelihood of arterial injury requiring operative repair.[38] However, patients more

---

Box 7
High-risk orthopedic injuries

Orthopedic Injury	Arterial Injury
Shoulder dislocation	Axillary
Supracondylar humerus fracture	Brachial
Femur fracture	Popliteal
	Superficial femoral
Knee dislocation	Popliteal
Tibial plateau fracture	Popliteal
The floating joint: long bone fractures on either side of a major joint (eg, humerus and ulna, femur and tibia fractures)	Brachial or popliteal

Data from Callcut RA, Mell MW. Modern advances in vascular trauma. Surg Clin North Am 2013;93(4):941–61, ix.

Box 8	
Hard and soft signs of extremity arterial injury	
Hard Signs	**Soft Signs**
Absent distal pulse	History of significant blood loss at the scene
Active/pulsatile bleeding	Proximity of a penetrating wound or blunt
Rapidly expanding hematoma	trauma to an artery
Classic signs of distal ischemia, 5Ps: pallor,	Nonpulsatile hematoma
pain, paresthesias, paralysis, pulseless	Neurologic deficit attributed to a nerve
Palpable thrill or audible bruit over the	adjacent to a named artery
injured area	Delayed capillary refill
	Diminished pulse compared with
	contralateral extremity

Data from Callcut RA, Mell MW. Modern advances in vascular trauma. Surg Clin North Am 2013;93(4):941–61, ix.

often present with soft signs of arterial injury. The management of these patients requires careful consideration. For instance, a single soft sign may be associated with only a 3% risk of arterial injury[38] but, when several soft signs are present, or one is present in combination with a high-risk orthopedic injury (see **Box 8**), the risk of arterial injury increases substantially.

The arterial pressure index

More helpful than the soft signs of arterial injury is the arterial pressure index (API). The API (also known as injured extremity index, ankle-brachial index, or ankle-arm index) is a noninvasive screening tool that can be used at the bedside and involves measuring the systolic pressure at the ankle or wrist (ie, distal to the injury) using a blood pressure cuff and a Doppler probe (not palpation).[39] The Doppler systolic blood pressure of the injured limb is divided by the Doppler systolic blood pressure of the contralateral uninjured upper limb as shown in **Box 9**.

For example, patients with right knee dislocation would have their blood pressure measured using a Doppler probe at the right ankle (dorsalis pedis or posterior tibial pulse) first and this would then be divided by the blood pressure measured in the left arm (brachial pulse). This test is analogous to the ankle-brachial index used for the detection of peripheral vascular disease, which has been described in detail elsewhere.[40]

There are a limited number of studies that have assessed the diagnostic accuracy of the API. However, an API less than 0.9 seems to be both highly sensitive (95%–100%) and specific (97%–100%) for arterial injury compared with arteriography.[39,41] However, these two studies included a small number of patients (total of 138) from a single trauma center and the possibility of exaggerated diagnostic test performance characteristics (spectrum bias)[42] needs to be considered.

In the patient with a normal clinical examination and an API greater than 0.9, significant vascular injury has been ruled out and the patient can be discharged and

Box 9	
Formula for calculating the arterial pressure index	

API = Doppler systolic pressure distal to injury (radial/ulnar artery for arm injury, or dorsalis pedis/posterior tibial artery for leg injury)/Doppler systolic pressure of uninjured upper extremity (typically brachial artery).

followed according to local practice, assuming the patient has no other injuries requiring admission.[2,43,44] However, if the API is abnormal (<0.9 in a healthy patient or a difference of >0.1 compared with the contralateral extremity in patients with pre-existing vascular disease), then surgical consultation and additional imaging are warranted (**Fig. 4**). This approach can be applied to high-risk injuries, including knee dislocations (see **Box 7**), and is consistent with recent guidelines from the Western Trauma Association.[2]

Limitations of the arterial pressure index

Certain limitations of the API should be kept in mind. First, the API does not detect venous injuries. This test is focused on arterial vessels. The API also does not detect

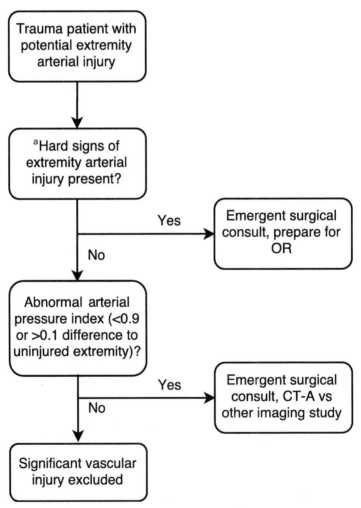

Fig. 4. Diagnostic approach to extremity arterial injury. [a]Hard signs: absent distal pulse, active/pulsatile bleeding, rapidly expanding hematoma, "classic" signs of distal ischemia (pallor, pain, paresthesias, paralysis, pulseless, bruit or thrill over injured area). OR, operating room.

injuries to the profunda brachii, profunda femoris, or peroneal arteries because no direct flow from these arteries is measured distally. Next, minor luminal injuries, such as small intimal flaps, that do not affect flow may not be detected. The API is also less sensitive in hypotensive and/or hypothermic patients and should be used with caution in these groups.[43]

The proximity soft sign

The soft sign of proximity of a penetrating or blunt injury to an artery deserves special mention. There is abundant literature to suggest that this sign is not helpful when evaluating patients for potential vascular injury. For example, Weaver and colleagues[45] evaluated 373 patients with a penetrating extremity injury. They performed angiography for the sole indication of proximity to a neurovascular bundle in 157 patients and found an arterial injury in less than 10% of patients and only 1 that required repair. They concluded that arteriography for proximity alone rarely identifies a significant injury and should be abandoned.[45] This conclusion was corroborated by a study by Conrad and colleagues[46] (2002) in which 300 patients with penetrating injury and a normal examination (API>1.0) were sent home. Follow-up at 10 months involved 154 patients and found no clinically significant missed injuries.

What is the preferred imaging test for a suspected peripheral vascular injury?

There are several imaging modalities that can be used to interrogate the vascular system. The 3 most common are catheter-based angiography, duplex ultrasonography, and CT-A.

Catheter-based angiography was developed in the 1970s as a less-invasive option, compared with surgical exploration, for arterial imaging in patients with presumed vascular injury. However, this test carries a 1% to 2% risk of morbidity (pseudoaneurysm, renal contrast toxicity), as well as significant costs related to the interventional radiology team required for the procedure.[43] Direct angiography remains a helpful tool in certain situations; specifically, intraoperative angiography for patients with a high pretest probability of arterial injury who are undergoing an unrelated operation, or those with hard signs of vascular trauma and uncertain location of injury (eg, shotgun wounds).

Duplex ultrasonography uses gray-scale ultrasonography to evaluate the anatomy of the injured area as well as color Doppler-ultrasonography to assess blood flow. It has the advantages of speed, low cost, portability, and being noninvasive. However, it is highly operator dependent and requires a trained vascular technologist, it can also be technically difficult because of patient habitus or location of the injury. The reported sensitivity and specificity range from between 50% and 100% and more than 95%, respectively.[2,47]

CT-A has become the investigation of choice for the diagnosis of peripheral vascular injuries.[5] It is noninvasive, rapid, accurate, and can simultaneously assess for associated injuries. It has been shown to have equal sensitivity and specificity compared with traditional catheter-based angiography.[4,5] Although CT-A has proved to be the initial diagnostic test of choice for peripheral arterial injury, a few pitfalls should be kept in mind (**Box 10**).

In general, it is prudent to involve the vascular or trauma surgeon when considering a vascular imaging study for a suspected arterial injury. Doing so confirms that testing is indicated, ensures that the most appropriate study is performed, and facilitates timely definitive management of any injuries that are identified.

> **Box 10**
> **Pitfalls in using computed tomography angiography as a diagnostic test for peripheral vascular injury**
>
> Decreased sensitivity in patients with shock/low-cardiac-output states
>
> Decreased sensitivity in distal arterial injuries (ie, peroneal, tibial arteries)
>
> Foreign bodies (eg, shrapnel) and/or patient movement artifact can affect image quality

PART III: MANAGEMENT OF EXTREMITY ARTERIAL INJURIES

Successful management of any vascular injury relies on the early recognition of its presence. Failure to do so can risk limb loss or loss of life. Over the last 5 decades since the first arterial repair of popliteal injuries in the Korean War,[48] refinements in surgical repair of peripheral arterial injuries have progressed significantly, with amputation rates now less than 10%.[49] However, long-term disability from concomitant skeletal and nerve injuries persists.[50]

A rapid and thorough examination of the patient should be performed to determine the extent of the injury, with documentation of any associated musculoskeletal injury or peripheral nerve deficits. The priority of an arterial injury should be established early in the management of the patient, and this is critical because any substantive delay in arterial repair increases the risk of major amputation. Irreversible neuromuscular changes can be seen in patients presenting with significant ischemia who have a delay in arterial repair in as little as 8 hours.

Initial Hemorrhage Control: Digital Pressure, Tourniquets, and Wound Packing

Tourniquets are increasingly being used in civilian trauma for the management of extremity trauma with significant hemorrhage. Many emergency medical services now carry tourniquets for this indication. However, on arrival at the emergency department, firm direct digital pressure on the bleeding vessel is the preferred initial approach because it does not result in complete limb ischemia and is often successful in hemorrhage control.[2] Only with failure to control bleeding with direct pressure should a tourniquet be used. In these circumstances, a properly applied tourniquet can be very effective in controlling peripheral arterial hemorrhage until definitive control can be obtained.[51]

If a tourniquet is applied it is important to use a commercially available device with a windlass to ensure it is applied tightly enough to stop arterial hemorrhage. Improvised tourniquets (belts, shirts, and so forth) or commercially available tourniquets that are not applied properly have the potential to worsen hypovolemia by decreasing venous return while concurrently allowing ongoing arterial hemorrhage.[52] In cases of severe peripheral arterial hemorrhage a second, more proximally applied tourniquet may be required.[52]

There is the potential for substantial morbidity with tourniquets, including amputation, fasciotomy, and nerve palsy.[53] The risk of these complications increases if the tourniquet has been applied for greater than 1 to 2 hours.[54] Some practical aspects of using a tourniquet are listed in **Box 11**.

Injuries to the junctional areas of the body (neck, axillae, groins) are not amenable to tourniquet application and are particularly challenging to manage. These wounds are best managed initially with direct digital pressure.[55] If this fails, the next step is to pack the wound tightly. Tips for wound packing for hemorrhage control are provided in

---

Box 11
Practical aspects of tourniquet use

Apply direct firm digital pressure initially to control hemorrhage

Record the time of application on the tourniquet as well as the patient's chart

Watch the clock: complication rates increase after 1 to 2 hours of occlusion

Use the lowest pressure that effectively stems bleeding

Apply the tourniquet early (before the development of shock) in the setting of significant extremity hemorrhage

Data from Callcut RA, Mell MW. Modern advances in vascular trauma. Surg Clin North Am 2013;93(4):941–61, ix; and Sambasivan CN, Schreiber MA. Emerging therapies in traumatic hemorrhage control. Curr Opin Crit Care 2009;15(6):560–8.

Box 12. These techniques should be applied in conjunction with efforts to coordinate transfer to the operating theater for definitive hemostasis.

Resuscitation

Concurrent with hemorrhage control, resuscitation of patients with significant extremity arterial hemorrhage should follow established guidelines[56] (**Box 13**). The patient should be managed as expeditiously as possible at a center with vascular and endovascular expertise.

Definitive Management

Endovascular management: principles

Over the last decade there have been significant technological advances in endovascular interventions for the management of traumatic vascular injuries, ranging from applications for reconstructing vessels with stents to controlling bleeding vessels with coil embolization. Endovascular treatment should always be considered and is especially well suited for patients with (1) multiple comorbidities, (2) concurrent severe injuries, or (3) distal arterial injuries that are difficult to isolate and identify surgically.

Endovascular coiling and embolization

Intra-arterial coiling is best suited for selected distal arterial injuries such as false aneurysms, low-flow arteriovenous fistulae, and active bleeding in the small distal arterial

---

Box 12
Tips for packing a wound to control hemorrhage

1. Apply and maintain continuous firm digital pressure to the wound with your nondominant hand

2. Use rolls of standard gauze bandage (25-mm, 50-mm, 100-mm [1, 2, 4 inch] sizes, as appropriate) with or without an approved topical hemostatic gauze base[55]

3. Pack the gauze into the wound in small increments going under and around your finger

4. Keep packing until the wound is full to its depth and bleeding has ceased

5. Once packing is completed, continue to maintain pressure on the wound to allow clot formation

---

Box 13
Resuscitation of patients with bleeding trauma

1. Minimize the time elapsed from injury to definitive hemorrhage control.

2. Use a restricted volume replacement strategy with an isotonic crystalloid solution to target a systolic blood pressure of 80 to 90 mm Hg until major bleeding has been controlled (assuming no traumatic brain injury).

3. Transfuse blood products using either a fixed-ratio strategy of fresh frozen plasma to packed red blood cells of at least 1:2 or transfuse packed red blood cells and fibrinogen concentrate based on laboratory parameters.

4. Administer tranexamic acid to bleeding patients who are within 3 hours of the time of injury.

5. Monitor for traumatic coagulopathy with traditional laboratory measures (prothrombin time, activated partial thromboplastin time, platelet counts, and fibrinogen) and/or a viscoelastic method.

6. Identify and treat hypothermia early.

---

tree. Coils generally consist of a metal frame (stainless steel, superalloy, or platinum) and have a coating of synthetic material. Available in a variety of diameters and sizes, once deployed into a vessel, the coil expands and lodges at the site of extrusion and the synthetic tuff promotes thrombosis of the artery. Other materials available to control bleeding are vascular plugs, Gelfoam pledgets, particles, liquids (eg, N-butyl cyanoacrylate), or a combination of these. Many case studies have shown an advantage to management of distal arterial bleeding, false aneurysms, and arteriovenous fistulae with endovascular techniques.[57,58]

Endovascular stenting

There are no large series to clearly delineate the role of stenting in management of peripheral arterial trauma.[59–61] However, stenting should be considered in multitraumatized patients or unstable patients not suitable for major reconstruction. The approach combines a stent with a synthetic covering. Although studies report excellent technical success, the long-term effectiveness remains unknown.[62] Ongoing surveillance for stent stenosis, migration, or endoleak is required, especially if being considered in a young patient.[62]

Surgical management principles

Operative intervention remains the standard of care and is mandatory if the vascular injury is associated with soft tissue injury that requires debridement. Once the decision to operate is made, the patient should be moved expeditiously to the operating room. Preoperative antibiotics and tetanus immunization should be provided, especially in patients with blunt trauma and associated bony injuries.

The surgeon's initial approach is to attain proximal and distal control before exploring the site of injury. In some circumstances, such as with axillary or subclavian injuries, proximal control is best attained with a fluoroscopically placed endoluminal balloon occlusion (**Fig. 5**). A sterile pneumatic tourniquet can also be used to minimize intraoperative blood loss in managing extremity injuries.

The type of arterial repair chosen depends on the extent of the arterial injury and gap in the artery after debridement to healthy tissue. Repair usually requires an interposition vein graft (typically using the greater saphenous vein), although on occasions patch angioplasty or a direct end-to-end arterial repair is feasible. It is paramount

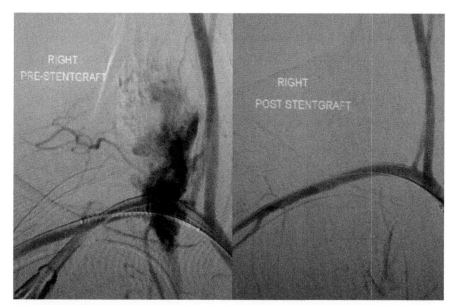

Fig. 5. Right subclavian artery transection with active contrast extravasation on angiography (*left*). Injury was treated with proximal balloon occlusion for hemorrhage control followed by stent graft placement (*right*). (*From* Branco BC, Boutrous ML, DuBose JJ, et al. Outcome comparison between open and endovascular management of axillosubclavian arterial injuries. J Vasc Surg 2016;63(3):702–9.)

that the graft is covered by healthy tissue to avoid deterioration of the graft and subsequent rupture.

A summary of the management considerations for major peripheral arterial injuries is provided in **Box 14**.

Vascular injuries associated with musculoskeletal trauma

Although arterial injuries of the lower extremity associated with orthopedic injury are uncommon, the surgical treatment of combined vascular and orthopedic injuries can be challenging.[64–66] Arterial repair to reestablish distal perfusion should generally always proceed before orthopedic stabilization or reconstruction. Infrequently with massive injuries, external fixation must be performed first to stabilize the limb to enable the vascular repair. The use of temporary intra-arterial shunting to quickly establish flow to the distal limb then enables an unhurried orthopedic and vascular repair.[67] Temporary intravascular shunts have been used aggressively in military zones until definitive reconstruction is possible, as a component of damage control surgery.

The mangled limb: primary amputation versus reconstruction

The vascular injury itself is rarely the deciding factor in determining the ability to salvage a limb affected by massive injury involving musculoskeletal, soft tissue, and nerve damage. A multidisciplinary approach to the decision making is necessary, involving orthopedic surgeon and plastic surgeon in addition to the vascular surgeon. From the vascular standpoint, the salvage rate of the ischemic limb decreases as time progresses. Limbs revascularized within 6 hours of ischemia can have a salvage rate of 90%. Rates decrease dramatically beyond this time (50% for 12–18 hours; 20% for 24 hours or longer).[68] These timelines are guidelines only. The decision to proceed with amputation is based on an extensive physical examination. In severely

---

Box 14
Clinical points and definitive management considerations for extremity arterial injuries

Injured Artery	Clinical Points	Preferred Management
Axillary	Critical ischemia attributable to this artery is uncommon because of extensive collateral circulation High index of suspicion is required for diagnosis	Endovascular repair with covered stent is often preferred because access for surgical repair is challenging
Brachial	Often associated with humerus fractures Anticipate concomitant injuries to median, ulnar, or radial nerves	Surgical repair
Radial or ulnar	Confirm integrity of complete palmar arch with Allen test	Single-vessel injuries are ligated if palmar arch intact If injuries to both vessels, ulnar is preferentially repaired because it is dominant
Common or superficial femoral	Delayed diagnosis/repair critical to poor outcome	Surgical repair
Popliteal	Most serious and challenging lower extremity injury to manage	Traditionally surgical repair, but endovascular repairs being increasingly reported[63]
Peroneal, posterior, or anterior tibial	Similar considerations to forearm arterial injuries	Single-vessel injury can often be ligated or can be embolized angiographically Two-vessel injuries or peroneal trunk injuries require surgical repair

---

traumatized limbs, vascular reconstruction can almost always be performed. It is the associated injuries that invariably determine whether the limb should be considered for reconstruction. Permanent disability, especially with significant nerve injury, is common and ultimately requires amputation.[69–71]

SUMMARY

Major vascular injuries remain a clinical challenge for emergency physicians. The current approach to diagnosing these injuries involves a high index of suspicion, a careful examination focused on hard and soft signs of injury, and the use of CT-A for patients without indications for immediate surgical exploration. The mainstays of therapy for emergency physicians include controlling hemorrhage with direct digital pressure, wound packing, tourniquets, and resuscitation with a balanced blood product strategy.

REFERENCES

1. Callcut RA, Mell MW. Modern advances in vascular trauma. Surg Clin North Am 2013;93(4):941–61, ix.

2. Feliciano DV, Moore FA, Moore EE, et al. Evaluation and management of peripheral vascular injury. Part 1. Western Trauma Association/critical decisions in trauma. J Trauma 2011;70(6):1551–6.

3. DuBose JJ, Savage SA, Fabian TC, et al. The American Association for the Surgery of Trauma PROspective Observational Vascular Injury Treatment (PROOVIT) registry. J Trauma Acute Care Surg 2015;78(2):215–23.

4. Inaba K, Branco BC, Reddy S, et al. Prospective evaluation of multidetector computed tomography for extremity vascular trauma. J Trauma 2011;70(4):808–15.

5. Patterson BO, Holt PJ, Cleanthis M, et al. Imaging vascular trauma. Br J Surg 2012;99(4):494–505.

6. Schroll R, Smith A, McSwain NE, et al. A multi-institutional analysis of prehospital tourniquet use. J Trauma Acute Care Surg 2015;79(1):10–4.

7. Inaba K, Siboni S, Resnick S, et al. Tourniquet use for civilian extremity trauma. J Trauma Acute Care Surg 2015;79(2):232–7.

8. Bellanova G, Motta A, Mazzetti C, et al. Damage control strategy and aggressive resuscitation in polytraumatized patient with severe hypothermia. Importance of multidisciplinary management from the territory to the operating room. Case report. Ann Ital Chir 2013;84(4):445–9.

9. Schreiber MA. Damage control surgery. Crit Care Clin 2004;20(1):101–18.

10. Johnson CA. Endovascular management of peripheral vascular trauma. Semin Interv Radiol 2010;27(1):38–43.

11. deSouza RM, Crocker MJ, Haliasos N, et al. Blunt traumatic vertebral artery injury: a clinical review. Eur Spine J 2011;20(9):1405–16.

12. Biffl WL, Moore EE, Elliott JP, et al. The devastating potential of blunt vertebral arterial injuries. Ann Surg 2000;231(5):672–81.

13. Cogbill TH, Moore EE, Meissner M, et al. The spectrum of blunt injury to the carotid artery: a multicenter perspective. J Trauma 1994;37(3):473–9.

14. Biffl WL, Moore EE, Elliott JP, et al. Blunt cerebrovascular injuries. Curr Probl Surg 1999;36(7):505–99.

15. Biffl WL, Moore EE, Offner PJ, et al. Blunt carotid arterial injuries: implications of a new grading scale. J Trauma 1999;47(5):845–53.

16. Bietz GJ, Bobadilla JL. Overview of vascular trauma. In: Dua A, Desai SS, Holcomb JB, et al, editors. Clinical review of vascular trauma. Heidelberg (Germany): Springer; 2014.

17. Biffl WL, Cothren CC, Moore EE, et al. Western Trauma Association critical decisions in trauma: screening for and treatment of blunt cerebrovascular injuries. J Trauma Inj Infect Crit Care 2009;67(6):1150–3.

18. Biffl WL, Moore EE, Ryu RK, et al. The unrecognized epidemic of blunt carotid arterial injuries: early diagnosis improves neurologic outcome. Ann Surg 1998;228(4):462–70.

19. Bromberg WJ, Collier BC, Diebel LN, et al. Blunt cerebrovascular injury practice management guidelines: the Eastern Association for the Surgery of Trauma. J Trauma 2010;68(2):471–7.

20. Kaye D, Brasel KJ, Neideen T, et al. Screening for blunt cerebrovascular injuries is cost-effective. J Trauma Inj Infect Crit Care 2011;70(5):1051–7.

21. Beliaev AM, Barber PA, Marshall RJ, et al. Denver screening protocol for blunt cerebrovascular injury reduces the use of multi-detector computed tomography angiography. ANZ J Surg 2014;84(6):429–32.

22. Roberts DJ, Chaubey VP, Zygun DA, et al. Diagnostic accuracy of computed tomographic angiography for blunt cerebrovascular injury detection in trauma patients. Ann Surg 2013;257(4):621–32.
23. O'Brien PJ, Cox MW. A modern approach to cervical vascular trauma. Perspect Vasc Surg Endovasc Ther 2011;23(2):90–7.
24. Inaba K, Branco BC, Menaker J, et al. Evaluation of multidetector computed to-mography for penetrating neck injury: a prospective multicenter study. J Trauma acute Care Surg 2012;72(3):576–83.
25. Tisherman SA, Bokhari F, Collier B, et al. Clinical practice guideline: penetrating zone II neck trauma. J Trauma 2008;64(5):1392–405.
26. Rhee P, Kuncir EJ, Johnson L, et al. Cervical spine injury is highly dependent on the mechanism of injury following blunt and penetrating assault. J Trauma 2006; 61(5):1166–70.
27. Weppner J. Improved mortality from penetrating neck and maxillofacial trauma using Foley catheter balloon tamponade in combat. J Trauma acute Care Surg 2013;75(2):220–4.
28. Youssef N, Raymer KE. Airway management of an open penetrating neck injury. Can J Emerg Med 2015;17(1):89–93.
29. Peiris K, Frerk C. Awake intubation. J Perioper Pract 2008;18(3):96–104.
30. Roepke C, Benjamin E, Jhun P, et al. Penetrating neck injury: what's in and what's out? Ann Emerg Med 2016;67(5):578–80.
31. Tallon JM, Ahmed JM, Sealy B. Airway management in penetrating neck trauma at a Canadian tertiary trauma centre. Can J Emerg Med 2007;9(2):101–4.
32. Mandavia DP, Qualls S, Rokos I. Emergency airway management in penetrating neck injury. Ann Emerg Med 2000;35(3):221–5.
33. Sperry JL, Moore EE, Coimbra R, et al. Western Trauma Association critical de-cisions in trauma: penetrating neck trauma. J Trauma acute Care Surg 2013; 75(6):936–40.
34. Roon AJ, Christensen N. Evaluation and treatment of penetrating cervical injuries. J Trauma 1979;19(6):391–7.
35. Apffelstaedt JP, Muller R. Results of mandatory exploration for penetrating neck trauma. World J Surg 1994;18(6):917–9 [discussion: 920].
36. Low GM, Inaba K, Chouliaras K, et al. The use of the anatomic 'zones' of the neck in the assessment of penetrating neck injury. Am Surg 2014;80(10):970–4.
37. Shiroff AM, Gale SC, Martin ND, et al. Penetrating neck trauma: a review of man-agement strategies and discussion of the 'No Zone' approach. Am Surg 2013; 79(1):23–9.
38. Frykberg ER, Dennis JW, Bishop K, et al. The reliability of physical examination in the evaluation of penetrating extremity trauma for vascular injury: results at one year. J Trauma 1991;31(4):502–11.
39. Lynch K, Johansen K. Can Doppler pressure measurement replace "exclusion" arteriography in the diagnosis of occult extremity arterial trauma? Ann Surg 1991;214(6):737–41.
40. Grenon SM, Gagnon J, Hsiang Y. Video in clinical medicine. Ankle-brachial index for assessment of peripheral arterial disease. N Engl J Med 2009;361(19):e40.
41. Mills WJ, Barei DP, McNair P. The value of the ankle-brachial index for diagnosing arterial injury after knee dislocation: a prospective study. J Trauma 2004;56(6): 1261–5.
42. Montori VM, Wyer P, Newman TB, et al. Tips for learners of evidence-based med-icine: 5. The effect of spectrum of disease on the performance of diagnostic tests. Can Med Assoc J 2005;173(4):385–90.

43. Levy BA, Zlowodzki MP, Graves M, et al. Screening for extermity arterial injury with the arterial pressure index. Am J Emerg Med 2005;23(5):689–95.

44. Compton C, Rhee R. Peripheral vascular trauma. Perspect Vasc Surg Endovasc Ther 2005;17(4):297–307.

45. Weaver FA, Yellin AE, Bauer M, et al. Is arterial proximity a valid indication for arteriography in penetrating extremity trauma? A prospective analysis. Arch Surg 1990;125(10):1256–60.

46. Conrad MF, Patton JH Jr, Parikshak M, et al. Evaluation of vascular injury in penetrating extremity trauma: angiographers stay home. Am Surg 2002;68(3):269–74.

47. Fry WR, Smith RS, Sayers DV, et al. The success of duplex ultrasonographic scanning in diagnosis of extremity vascular proximity trauma. Arch Surg 1993; 128(12):1368–72.

48. Hughes CW. Arterial repair during the Korean war. Ann Surg 1958;147(4):555–61.

49. Wagner WH, Calkins ER, Weaver FA, et al. Blunt popliteal artery trauma: one hundred consecutive injuries. J Vasc Surg 1988;7(5):736–43.

50. Weaver FA, Papanicolaou G, Yellin AE. Difficult peripheral vascular injuries. Surg Clin North Am 1996;76(4):843–59.

51. Sambasivan CN, Schreiber MA. Emerging therapies in traumatic hemorrhage control. Curr Opin Crit Care 2009;15(6):560–8.

52. Eikermann M, Velmahos G, Abbara S, et al. Case records of the Massachusetts General Hospital. Case 11-2014. A man with traumatic injuries after a bomb explosion at the Boston Marathon. N Engl J Med 2014;370(15):1441–51.

53. Dayan L, Zinmann C, Stahl S, et al. Complications associated with prolonged tourniquet application on the battlefield. Mil Med 2008;173(1):63–6.

54. Welling DR, Burris DG, Hutton JE, et al. A balanced approach to tourniquet use: lessons learned and relearned. J Am Coll Surg 2006;203(1):106–15.

55. Bulger EM, Snyder D, Schoelles K, et al. An evidence-based prehospital guideline for external hemorrhage control: American College of Surgeons Committee on Trauma. Prehosp Emerg Care 2014;18(2):163–73.

56. Rossaint R, Bouillon B, Cerny V, et al. The European guideline on management of major bleeding and coagulopathy following trauma: fourth edition. Crit Care 2016;20:100.

57. Moramarco LP, Fiorina I, Quaretti P. Endovascular management of upper and lower extremity vascular trauma. Endovascular Today 2014;53–8.

58. Fox N, Rajani RR, Bokhari F, et al. Evaluation and management of penetrating lower extremity arterial trauma: an Eastern Association for the Surgery of Trauma practice management guideline. J Trauma acute Care Surg 2012;73(5 Suppl 4): S315–20.

59. Marin ML, Veith FJ, Panetta TF, et al. Transluminally placed endovascular stented graft repair for arterial trauma. J Vasc Surg 1994;20(3):466–72 [discussion: 472–3].

60. Hanson MM, Itoga NK, Schneider P. Stent placement to treat popliteal artery injury after knee dislocation in a surfing accident. Vascular Disease Management 2013;10(5):E92–5.

61. DuBose JJ, Rajani R, Gilani R, et al. Endovascular management of axillo-subclavian arterial injury: a review of published experience. Injury 2012;43(11): 1785–92.

62. Rossi PJ, Southard NM. Endovascular considerations in vascular trauma. In: Dua A, Desai SS, Holcomb JB, et al, editors. Clinical review of vascular trauma. New York: Springer; 2014. p. 75–89.

63. Zhong S, Zhang X, Chen Z, et al. Endovascular repair of blunt popliteal arterial injuries. Korean J Radiol 2016;17(5):789–96.
64. Weaver FA, Rosenthal RE, Waterhouse G, et al. Combined skeletal and vascular injuries of the lower extremities. Am Surg 1984;50(4):189–97.
65. Cone JB. Vascular injury associated with fracture-dislocations of the lower extremity. Clin Orthop Relat Res 1989;(243):30–5.
66. Coleman JJ, Tavoosi S, Zarzaur BL, et al. Arterial injuries associated with blunt fractures in the lower extremity. Am Surg 2016;82(9):820–4.
67. Inaba K, Aksoy H, Seamon MJ, et al. Multicenter evaluation of temporary intravascular shunt use in vascular trauma. J Trauma acute Care Surg 2016;80(3): 359–64.
68. Miller HH, Welch CS. Quantitative studies on the time factor in arterial injuries. Ann Surg 1949;130(3):428–38.
69. Alexander JJ, Piotrowski JJ, Graham D, et al. Outcome of complex vascular and orthopedic injuries of the lower extremity. Am J Surg 1991;162(2):111–6.
70. Manord JD, Garrard CL, Kline DG, et al. Management of severe proximal vascular and neural injury of the upper extremity. J Vasc Surg 1998;27(1):43–7.
71. Liang NL, Alarcon LH, Jeyabalan G, et al. Contemporary outcomes of civilian lower extremity arterial trauma. J Vasc Surg 2016;64(3):731–6.

Major Trauma Outside a Trauma Center

Prehospital, Emergency Department, and Retrieval Considerations

Preston J. Fedor, MD, FACEP[a],*, Brian Burns, DipRTM, MSc, MD, FACEM[b,c],
Michael Lauria, BA, NRP, FP-C[d],
Clare Richmond, FACEM, MBBS, BSci (Med Sci), Dip IMC[b,e]

KEYWORDS

- Trauma resuscitation • Prehospital trauma • Retrieval medicine
- Resource-limited environment • Rural hospital • Ultrasound

KEY POINTS

- Incoming Emergency Medical Services crews often have crucial information about trauma mechanism, contributing factors, specific injuries, effect of treatment, key timings, personal details, and more. They also can be an essential extra set of hands in settings with limited resources.
- Set up the resuscitation area for success and know the equipment and team capabilities. Create and rehearse emergency department and hospital procedures for quickly obtaining additional personnel and resources as needed.
- Extensive radiological and laboratory evaluation is often unnecessary and may delay access to definitive care. Only obtain studies that may provide actionable results and improve the course of management. Targeted bedside ultrasound can provide rapid and useful answers with appropriate training.
- An emergency physician must be prepared to provide immediate life, limb, and sight saving interventions when indicated, regardless of the clinical environment.
- Request transfer/retrieval as soon as the need for higher level of trauma care is presumed. A standard preretrieval process (with checklist) can make the transition of the patient out of the emergency department safer and more efficient.

---

[a] Department of Emergency Medicine, Division of Prehospital, Austere and Disaster Medicine, University of New Mexico, 1 University of New Mexico, MSC11 6025, Albuquerque, NM 87131-0001, USA; [b] Greater Sydney Area HEMS, NSW Ambulance, NSW 2200, Australia; [c] Sydney University, Sydney, NSW, Australia; [d] Dartmouth-Hitchcock Advanced Response Team (DHART), Dartmouth-Hitchcock Medical Center, Lebanon, NH, USA; [e] Royal Prince Alfred Hospital, Sydney, Australia
* Corresponding author.
E-mail address: pfedor@salud.unm.edu

Emerg Med Clin N Am 36 (2018) 203–218
https://doi.org/10.1016/j.emc.2017.08.010
0733-8627/18/© 2017 Elsevier Inc. All rights reserved.

emed.theclinics.com

PART ONE: PREHOSPITAL TRAUMA: CUTTING-EDGE CARE IN THE FIELD
Evolving Practices in Prehospital Care

Prehospital care has evolved significantly from its origins in military conflicts to today's complex Emergency Medical Services (EMS) systems. Highly specialized providers, structured protocols, and a broad scope of practice have contributed to prehospital medicine as a recognized medical specialty.[1] High-quality trauma care begins from the point of first medical contact and continues during transport to local hospitals and ultimately to designated trauma centers. Prehospital medicine is now an area of significant and substantive research that has led to important, patient-centered improvements in processes of care.

Thoughtful use of rigid cervical collars and backboards
Recent evidence suggests there is little benefit for the routine use of either backboard or cervical spine immobilization in trauma. In fact, neither technique provides effective spine immobilization and may result in patient harm through pain, skin breakdown, and complicating airway management.[2–9] Spinal immobilization in penetrating trauma is associated with increased mortality.[9,10]

Position statements by the National Association of EMS Physicians and the American College of Surgeons Committee on Trauma both recommend attention to spinal protection via "application of a cervical collar, adequate security to a stretcher, minimal movement/transfers, and maintenance of in-line stabilization during any necessary movement/transfer." Additionally, both groups recommend against immobilization for penetrating trauma.[11] We anticipate that a selective, rather than "routine" approach to spinal immobilization, will result in fewer patients immobilized without benefit during EMS transport.

Increasing use of ultrasound
Point-of-care ultrasound improves the diagnostic capability of prehospital physicians.[12] Non-physician providers can be trained to accurately obtain and interpret ultrasound examinations, such as the Focused Assessment with Sonography for Trauma (FAST) or examination of the abdominal aorta.[13] This skill set may improve the ability of EMS teams to assess trauma patients, triage a mass casualty incident, and direct patients to the most appropriate facility.[14] In some EMS systems, FAST examination findings directly impact patient care. For example, a shocked trauma patient with a positive prehospital FAST examination may trigger the administration of prehospital blood administration and be directly transported to the operating room of the receiving institution. Prehospital ultrasound is still in its infancy, and further studies will guide its use and establish its impact on patient outcomes.

Focus on hemorrhage control using strategies derived from combat medicine
Lessons learned from military conflicts have led to substantial developments in trauma management for civilian prehospital practice. Damage control resuscitation (DCR), a treatment paradigm that combines rapid hemorrhage control, minimal crystalloid, and permissive hypotension has become the standard for patients with serious injuries and presumed hemorrhage.[15,16] Prehospital clinicians can apply DCR principles by limited crystalloid administration, tourniquet application for extremity bleeding, and massive transfusion protocol initiation.[17] The use of blood products in the field is feasible and may improve survival.[18,19] Many advanced care EMS organizations now carry blood products, including both packed red blood cells and fresh frozen plasma.[20] A more detailed review of DCR principles is outlined in the trauma resuscitation sections of this issue.

A growing number of air and ground EMS organizations administer tranexamic acid (TXA) for select trauma patients.[21] TXA represents a feasible therapeutic adjunct for the bleeding patient, particularly for prehospital programs that lack the capability or logistical infrastructure to safely maintain and deliver blood products.

Limb tourniquets popularized in military conflicts are now a standard part of civilian EMS practice. They are safe and effective means for controlling hemorrhage from extremity wounds, as demonstrated in both military and civilian prehospital care.[22] Similarly, hemostatic dressings were developed from combat medicine, and many civilian EMS organizations include them in their hemorrhage control algorithms when pressure dressings fail, or in situations not amenable to tourniquet placement.

What Are Unique Aspects of Providing Medical Care Outside of a Hospital?

The defining characteristic of prehospital medical care is that it occurs outside of an established medical facility. It is inherently an austere environment spanning situations by the side of a road, the top of a mountain, or the back of a helicopter. Geography does not limit the care prehospital teams provide, but this does result in unique environmental challenges.

EMS providers assess and treat patients in extremes of weather, under threat, and without optimal medical facilities. These challenges may impact what interventions are completed before arrival in the emergency department (ED).

What Information Is Critical to Obtain from Prehospital Teams?

Prehospital personnel can provide critical information to the team on arrival in the ED.[23] In patients with an altered level of consciousness or intubated, the EMS team may be the only source of information regarding the mechanism of injury and prehospital clinical course. The speed of the vehicle before impact, the immediate clinical status of the patient after injury, and other scene factors can often only be provided by the prehospital team. Several studies highlight the importance of prehospital hypotension in predicting clinical course, a finding reliably associated with increased morbidity and mortality.[24–26] These findings suggest that the EMS-ED handover include mention of the lowest recorded blood pressure (BP, or if a BP could not be recorded). A structured rapid handover process can lead to a safer and more efficient transition of patient care.[27,28]

How Should Patient Information from the Field Be Communicated to the Emergency Department Team?

EMS reports provide important information to help prioritize and plan care before patient arrival. Key patient data need to be communicated clearly and concisely, and are often relayed remotely by radio, phone, or smart device to an ED charge nurse or physician. Several structured prehospital handover tools have been designed for this purpose, including the MIST report (Mechanism, Injury, Signs and Symptoms, Treatment, and Estimated time of arrival; **Box 1**).[29]

The downstream effect of prehospital notification can be lifesaving, allowing trauma teams to prepare equipment, free up operating room resources, call in off-site consultants (eg, neurosurgery, interventional radiology), or notify the blood bank.[17] EDs should work with their local EMS providers to develop protocols and standard operating procedures for communication with the prehospital team, emphasizing the importance of standardized language and concise, structured reporting.

Box 1
Sample radio call: MIST (Mechanism, Injury, Signs and Symptoms, Treatment, and Estimated time of arrival) report

Car 222 is coming in with a 37-year-old male

Mechanism
  High-speed motor vehicle accident

Injury
  Head, chest, and pelvic injuries

Signs and Symptoms
  GCS 8, HR 120, O2 saturation 90% on non-rebreather, BP 90/60, RR 30, decreased air entry on left, pupils equal and reactive.

Treatment
  IV, 20 mg ketamine, cervical spine collar, pelvic binder, IV fluids 250-mL bolus.

Estimated time of arrival
  5 minutes

Abbreviations: BP, blood pressure; GCS, Glasgow Coma Scale; HR, heart rate; IV, intravenous; RR, respiratory rate.

Controversies in Prehospital Trauma Management

Is there a role for physicians in prehospital trauma care?

Globally, prehospital teams vary tremendously in composition. In Europe and Australia, it is common for a physician to be part of the prehospital helicopter EMS (HEMS) team. In contrast, similar team composition is rare in the United States. Some studies suggest that physician-based HEMS teams may improve survival to hospital discharge and decrease mortality.[30,31] The generalizability of these findings is difficult, given confounders related to provider skill sets, care pathways, and deployment protocols.

Based on existing evidence and personal experience, we believe that physician-based prehospital teams are valuable to improve patient outcomes in trauma. In circumstances when trauma patients require immediate critical care interventions (eg, rapid sequence intubation, finger thoracostomy, extremity amputation), physician-led teams offer the best opportunity for success. Recent data support that physician prehospital involvement in complex battlefield trauma is beneficial.[32] These physician-led teams provided critical interventions, such as advanced airway management and pediatric resuscitation, that required advance skill sets not possessed by less-experienced military medics.[33] Heroic measures performed by highly trained prehospital physicians, such as resuscitative thoracotomy and Resuscitative Endovascular Balloon Occlusion of the Aorta (REBOA) are both possible and successful.[34,35]

The inclusion of physicians in prehospital teams offers benefits in clinical and procedural decision making, trauma system knowledge, and integration of EMS-initiated protocols on arrival in the ED (eg, prehospital activation of a massive transfusion protocol). Additionally, there are system-level benefits to physician involvement in EMS, including education and quality assurance opportunities, improved interprofessional relationships, and identifiable opportunities to improve care.[36]

Should endotracheal intubation be performed in the field on trauma patients?

There is conflicting evidence about the utility and patient-oriented outcomes of prehospital intubation. In large metropolitan areas, studies suggest that in the setting of head injury or severe trauma, prehospital intubation confers worse outcomes or equivocal benefit to mortality or morbidity.[37–40] Most notably, the Ontario Prehospital Advanced Life Support (OPALS) Major Trauma study found increased mortality with intubation of trauma patients in a before-after trial, compared with a group receiving basic life support care.[40] Other largely retrospective studies suggest that patients who undergo prehospital intubation following traumatic brain injury had improved outcomes compared with those for whom airway management was deferred until hospital arrival.[41,42]

Not surprisingly, success rates for endotracheal intubation are highly dependent on operator experience. Prehospital intubation performed by prehospital physicians or specially trained air medical teams with frequent intubation experience and airway governance may yield mortality benefit, but this has not been conclusively demonstrated. Physician teams can bring critical care skills refined from in-hospital experience to the prehospital setting, including airway management with first-pass success rates similar to those reported in the ED.[43,44]

Intubation in the prehospital setting can be accomplished safely and effectively by nonphysician providers in high-functioning EMS systems.[45] The procedure itself is well within the scope of practice of paramedics in North America; however, the expertise is variable across jurisdictions and agencies.[46] Airway management is a major focus of initial and ongoing training, as well as quality improvement initiatives. More studies are needed to better identify which patients require prehospital intubation and what degree of training is required to optimize success.

PART TWO: MAJOR TRAUMA AT A NONTRAUMA CENTER

Most modern, regionalized trauma systems in Europe, North America, and Australia involve set protocols that establish under what circumstances EMS providers can bypass a local hospital and proceed directly to a level 1 trauma center. This strategy, paired with regional systems that concentrate trauma expertise and resources in a select number of hospitals, is associated with a 25% reduction in injury-related mortality.[47] In situations involving prolonged transport times or in the presence of immediately life-threatening injuries, trauma patients may still be transported to a local hospital for initial assessment and stabilization. Although immediate priorities remain the same regardless of the initial point of contact, the nature, extent, and timing of diagnostic testing and therapeutic interventions will vary depending on local resources and access to interfacility transport.

How Should Ad Hoc Trauma Teams Prepare and Assemble?

Team members and composition
A dedicated trauma team with specific roles is essential to improve team performance and patient safety.[48,49] The team should be equipped and adequately skilled to effectively manage life-threatening conditions and be able to facilitate definitive care. Preparation should include space, staff, equipment, medications, and agents to assist hemostatic resuscitation.

The composition of trauma teams varies based on local resources: in remote locations, initial care may be undertaken at a nursing outpost, with or without access to an in-house physician.[50] In better resourced facilities, professionals from several distinct disciplines (emergency medicine, anesthesia, surgery, respiratory therapy) are often called on to form ad hoc teams, with the expectation that they will be able to perform as a cohesive unit, despite having few opportunities to practice team-based skills. The trauma team leader (TTL) must balance both operational (resuscitation logistics, procedures) and executive (planning, resource utilization) tasks, particularly when team composition is small. An emergency physician is often best positioned to assume the TTL role, although in some situations this role may be best delegated to another physician team member or senior nurse (registered nurse [RN]). For example, in 2-member MD/RN teams, an RN may be better positioned to maintain overall situation awareness, monitoring, and oversight, particularly at times when the physician is intently and appropriately task-focused. Designating specific roles, specifically team leader and team members, should be based on the skill set of the individual, not that individual's discipline of training. When teams must assemble ad hoc, institutional guidelines that prespecify roles and expectations for various team members can help improve cohesion, although it should be understood that role assignment is dynamic and depends on the nature of teamwork and task work being undertaken.

What is the best way to prepare the resuscitation space?

In an ideal circumstance, the resuscitation area should be located in close proximity to the ambulance bay, diagnostic imaging, and the operating room. A large resuscitation space with 360-degree access to the patient facilitates a pit crew–like approach whereby each member of the team has a defined role and physical position.[51] EMS prenotification allows the team to anticipate injuries and interventions required. The decision to open the equipment packaging before EMS arrival will depend on the anticipated need, preparation time, and urgency of the planned intervention. In limited resource settings, specifically those without surgical support, preparation should focus on lifesaving interventions and anticipating the need for rapid transfer to a regional trauma center. Early forward communication with the trauma center will aid this process.

The Emergency Medical Services Crew Has Arrived with the Patient: Now What?

To ensure critical information is communicated, a "hands-off, eyes on" approach to the EMS-ED clinical handover is suggested. The patient *remains on the EMS stretcher* during handover, which should typically be between 30 and 60 seconds. The astute TTL will observe the patient while listening intently to the EMS handover. A whiteboard can serve as a visible repository of patient information that can be referred to periodically as the case progresses,[52] or as new team members enter the resuscitation environment.

A structured, uninterrupted handover will allow the team to hear the required information in a succinct manner. In Australia, it is common for EMS to use the format I-MIST-AMBO (**Box 2**). A common structure reduces the overall time to handover, and increases retention of the information. Minimal interruptions during handover ensure that the EMS team can complete the transfer of care efficiently and without missing information. If immediate patient interventions are required, the handover can be limited to the crucial I-MIST, with AMBO being delayed until later.

In an ED in which resources and expertise are limited, it may be prudent for the EMS team to remain and continue to assist in managing the patient in the ED (eg, administer medications, splint fractures, assist with critical procedures).

Trauma in Austere or Under-Resourced Settings: An Efficient Approach

The primary goal of trauma in under-resourced settings is to identify, manage, and treat or temporize life-threatening conditions. Particularly when resources are limited, it is of crucial importance to focus exclusively on life or limb-preserving interventions, and defer the remainder. Standard Advanced Trauma Life Support (ATLS) algorithms provide a structured and systematic heuristic to guide a team through the primary survey, placing a heavy emphasis on completing assessment of airway before moving on to breathing, and so on. This can be advantageous when teams are unfamiliar or lack

---

Box 2
I-MIST-AMBO for trauma patient handover

I: Introduction (self, patient)

M: Mechanism of injury

I: Injuries (head to toe)

S: Signs and symptoms

T: Treatments given (Stop here if patient is critically unwell or immediate intervention is required; remaining details can be shared with the team once resuscitation priorities have been addressed.)

A: Allergies (if known)

M: Medications (if known or suspected)

B: Background (medical history if known)

O: Other (anything not given above important for hospital teams to know, such as family member contacts, police involvement, and so forth)

---

experience with assessing complex or multiply-injured trauma patients. It should be noted that hemorrhage is the leading cause of early preventable deaths in trauma, and it follows that control of major bleeding should be the most immediate priority in any setting, and in under-resourced settings in particular, where therapeutic interventions happen in series rather than in parallel. CABCDE and MARCH (**Table 1**) reorganize the traditional ABCDE approach espoused by ATLS in an effort to shift focus to early hemorrhage control.[53–56]

When does the airway get managed?
The threshold to perform definitive airway maneuvers may be lower for patients requiring transport to definitive care than among those already at a trauma center. Retrieval teams can contribute to airway management decision making, incorporating the patient's current clinical condition and projected course (see Part 3, later in this article). It is significantly more challenging to intubate a patient during transport than in a resuscitation room. We suggest that checklists for preintubation and postintubation be used for all trauma airways, as they help reinforce habit, routine, and familiarity during nonstandard operations, with the downstream goal of improving patient safety and reducing medical error.[57]

How Can Team Performance and Communication Be Optimized?

In resource-limited settings, the traditional approach of the physician leader, positioned at the foot of the bed, may require modification based on the availability of other skilled clinicians. The TTL may be required to perform critical interventions, such as

---

Table 1
CABDE and MARCH approaches to initial trauma assessment

CABCDE	MARCH
Catastrophic hemorrhage	Massive hemorrhage
Airway (with cervical spine control)	Airway
Breathing	Respirations
Circulation (with hemorrhage control)	Circulation
Disability	Hypothermia/head injury
Exposure	

airway management, when other skilled providers are lacking. The delegation of team leadership roles, including situational awareness and communication, is encouraged when the TTL is task-focused. When resources allow, we suggest that one team member be in charge of resuscitation safety, a hands-off role that focuses on potential harms to the patient or team.[58]

Clear communication and frequent "pause and reassess" summaries coordinated by the TTL can contribute to an effective shared mental model among team members. A team-oriented approach includes verbalizing changes in management goals and explicitly asking for team suggestions when uncertainty exists.

Once the resuscitation is complete and the patient is transferred to definitive care, we suggest a team debriefing with participation from all team members, to identify or clarify issues relating to clinical care (eg, critical procedures) or team performance (eg, leadership, communication).

Should Every Trauma Patient Have Imaging and Labs?

Investigations such as blood tests, radiographs, and computed tomography (CT) scans should be limited to those that may alter the clinical management of the patient in the short to medium term. The management of a critically ill trauma patient, and the decision to transfer, frequently does not require any blood tests or formal imaging. In fact, transfer to CT scan for the purpose of confirming clinically suspected injuries is not without significant risk for unstable patients.

In our experience, imaging is frequently repeated at the receiving trauma center, regardless of whether images are sent with the patient. As the decision to transfer to a trauma center is made primarily on clinical grounds, we strongly advise against delaying the transfer process to obtain laboratory results or imaging interpretations. Ideally, images are available to the receiving team through electronic medical records, as this aids in prearrival operative planning.

Point-of-care ultrasound (POCUS) is particularly beneficial in centers in which formal radiology is not readily available. Extended-FAST (e-FAST) provides real-time answers to binary clinical questions. In trauma, it can be used to identify a pneumothorax, pericardial tamponade, and intra-abdominal free fluid. POCUS improves success during procedures including venous access, nerve blocks, and to verify endotracheal tube placement.[59,60] Telemedicine technology allows remote guidance of ultrasound image acquisition and evaluation of images obtained by the novice.[61,62]

What if the Patient Needs a Massive Transfusion?

Most EDs have an established massive transfusion protocol for the coordinated management of major hemorrhage. In hospitals with limited or no blood products on site, a protocol to transfer blood products, via EMS or highway patrol, from a nearby hospital is a viable alternative.

Optimal management of bleeding trauma patients includes administration of blood products and TXA. A ratio-based approach, using either 2:1:1 or 1:1:1 (packed red blood cells, fresh frozen plasma, and platelets) is ideal.[63] Results from CRASH-2 suggest that TXA, given within 3 hours after injury, improves survival.[64] Before, and during transport, notification to the receiving trauma center of ongoing transfusion requirements is important to ensure continued blood product administration on patient arrival.

Beyond the emergency department: local operating theater and interventional radiology

In some instances, a trauma patient is simply too unstable for transfer despite DCR. These patients may require immediate surgical intervention. Most community hospitals have a surgeon who is trained to perform a laparotomy for hemorrhage control if alternative options are not available. High-level facilitated discussions among the ED, surgery, and interventional radiology (if available) should occur to discuss the best management for bleeding trauma patients presenting to the ED. Institutional trauma protocols and interdepartmental memorandums of understanding are extremely helpful products of these discussions.

Beyond the emergency department: hospital and health system

Trauma care is optimized when the ED functions in coordination with resources in the hospital and beyond, including the regional trauma center and the local EMS transport system. Hospitals, EMS providers, and retrieval organizations should develop trauma protocols and systems to provide coordinated trauma care for all major trauma patients presenting within local networks.

PART THREE: GETTING READY TO MOVE: PREPARING THE TRAUMA PATIENT FOR INTERFACILITY TRANSPORT

The emergency physician is essential in the efficient and safe transfer of the trauma patient. This represents a high-risk time during the patient's clinical course. It is subject to many potential pitfalls that can be mitigated with careful planning to expedite a safe departure to definitive care.

What Are the Legal Responsibilities of the Treating Emergency Physician?

Each country approaches the regulation of emergency access, stabilization, and transfer differently. In Australia and Canada, universal health care entitles citizens and legal residents to emergency care, and the duty of care for physicians is based on ethical constructs and, to a lesser extent, limited case law.[65] These large health care systems have established trauma referral networks, as well as centralized transfer and retrieval coordination centers.[66]

The Emergency Treatment and Active Labor Act (EMTALA) is a strict federal mandate that is familiar to most US emergency physicians; however, the details as they apply to the transfer of an unstable trauma patient may be uncertain. EMTALA requires a medical screening examination to determine if an emergency medical condition exists, but also to stabilize it within the capabilities of the physician, department, and the hospital as a whole. If the unstable patient's condition is beyond these capabilities, an appropriate transfer must be arranged.

Does the Law Allow the Transfer of an Unstable Trauma Patient?

An unstable trauma patient may be transferred only if the benefits of transfer outweigh the risks, or if the patient requests a transfer (after the risks are explained). EMTALA spells out what constitutes an appropriate transfer, which are as follows:

1. Initial stabilizing care is provided to minimize the risk of transfer.
2. The patient is sent to a hospital with qualified personnel and space, from which overt permission to transfer is obtained.
3. All relevant medical records must travel with the patient.
4. The transport must be conducted by qualified personnel, and life-supporting measures should continue en route.

Interestingly, no Medicare-participating hospital with specialized staff and facilities (ie, a level 1 trauma center) can refuse transfer of an unstable trauma patient, assuming they have the capacity to treat the patient. EMTALA does not apply to the transfer of stable patients (as listed previously), or inpatients.[67]

Which Patients Should Be Transferred, and When?

This is a clinical decision that depends on several factors:

- Clinical capabilities of the sending institution
- Current hemodynamic status of the patient
- Anticipated clinical course
- Expertise of the transport team
- Distance to receiving institution, mode of transport, and transport logistics

It is essential to recognize that the transfer process should be initiated when clinical demands have already or are expected to exceed local resources. The transfer request can be made without laboratory tests, imaging, or even a detailed history. The trauma center and retrieval team can be alerted after receiving a radio report from the incoming ambulance for a patient who has yet to arrive. Minimum information to initiate a transfer request is the mechanism of injury, potential threats to life, and basic patient demographics (age and weight). As further information becomes available, this can be transmitted to the transfer team and receiving institution.

What Is the Process for Transfer?

The process to transfer a critically injured patient is specific to each institution. The high-risk nature of trauma transfers calls for pre-established protocols to guide the process, rather than ad hoc decision making left to the transferring team. Transfer protocols should be readily available for the clinical team to reference but it is advisable that the TTL and other team members have familiarity with the process.

What Are the Options for Transport of the Trauma Patient?

It is the sending physician's responsibility to determine the appropriate mode of transportation (air vs ground) and the EMS skill level (BLS, ALS, Critical Care Transport) best suited to ensure optimal patient outcome.[26] These decisions can be complicated. Careful consideration of the risks and benefits of the transfer may require input from the retrieval service or transfer center.

Transport crew skill level

Selecting an appropriate transport team may at times impose a trade-off between skill level of the team and the time-sensitive nature of the transport. Most critical care transport teams are based out of larger centers, and summoning their services is typically associated with a significant delay in the arrival of the team. Contrastingly, a local ambulance with a combination of paramedics or emergency medical technicians is more readily available, but often more restricted in scope of care and clinical skill.

There are 2 important questions to ask when selecting a trauma transport team:

1. What meaningful interventions are anticipated during the transfer process?
2. What are the time-critical or lifesaving interventions this patient needs at the destination center?

Addressing these questions will help determine the level of clinical and procedural skill required to safely complete an interfacility transfer. In some situations, it may be appropriate to transfer the patient with a less skilled but readily available crew, if no advanced care interventions can be performed at the sending hospital, or during the transfer phase. The key principle of transfer medicine is to transfer the patient to the right place, in the right time, with the right level of care.

If a patient has significant and complex needs, and a critical care transport team is not available, it is not uncommon for a physician or nurse from the sending hospital to accompany the patient in the ambulance. This is a high-risk situation: working in an unfamiliar setting, with inadequate equipment, and an ad hoc team. Developing protocols, equipment, and training processes will reduce risks in settings in which these circumstances are unavoidable. Furthermore, subtracting a physician from an under-resourced environment places significant strain on the delivery of care for other patients. This should be weighed against the benefits of of having a physician present during transport, a decision that is primarily dependent on the patient's current and anticipated needs.

Air versus ground transport platform

In the United States, the choice of aeromedical versus ground transport is often dictated by geography. Long distances to the nearest trauma center mandate the use of aeromedical options. Air transport is also frequently staffed by advanced care prehospital teams, which may impact transport decision making. Fixed-wing aircraft are useful for movement outside of the typical helicopter range; however, this mode of transport will require a secondary transfer by ambulance at the airport.

Aeromedical transport is often perceived to be a panacea, a one-size-fits-all solution to issues of distance that plague rural hospitals. Helicopters are frequently called to transport stable patients to save a long drive to the referral center, which is inappropriate. Air transport is inherently dangerous: between 2006 and 2015 there were 90 deaths as 93 helicopters were lost in the HEMS industry.[68] As such, it is important to fly only those patients who have time-dependent injuries and/or critical care needs.

What about bringing the higher level of care to the patient?

Teams composed of trained clinicians may travel to peripheral hospitals to initiate time-dependent and lifesaving interventions that would not otherwise be available, including extracorporeal membrane oxygenation for critically ill medical patients.[69] It is possible that in the future, a helicopter team will transport a highly specialized team, including expert physicians, to perform advanced procedures at under-resourced institutions; for trauma, this could include REBOA catheter placement, evacuation of an epidural hematoma, or damage control surgery. The model of bringing the team to the patient to support clinical work at smaller institutions already exists in the United Kingdom and Australia, where specially trained intensive care, anesthesia, or emergency medicine physicians, along with a highly skilled paramedic or nurse, bring advanced equipment and experience to stabilize a patient before and during transport.[70] Telemedicine also holds promise as a simple and cost-effective way to virtually "export" trauma expertise, improve pretransport trauma care, and reduce the incidence of unnecessary interfacility patient transfers.

How Can an Emergency Department Best Prepare for an Efficient and Safe Transfer?

We suggest the first step be the creation of a structured and standardized approach to transfer preparation. A checklist attached to the transfer packet is ideal. Our approach is based on adaptation of a checklist developed by a retrieval service in South Australia (**Table 2**).[71]

What Is the Emergency Physician's Role When the Retrieval Team Arrives?

The treating physician should be present when the retrieval team arrives to provide a structured handover. A description of the clinical findings, treatment provided, outstanding issues, and expected clinical course are vital components of the verbal and documented handover. Following this, the retrieval team will perform a clinical assessment to establish a baseline, and ensure security of lines and tubes. The transport environment is a challenging one in which to undertake these clinical

Table 2
Transport checklist

Checklist	Transfer Preparation and Handover
AIRWAY	Self-maintained or protected. Difficulty of intubation. Tube size, depth. Cuff filled with air. Tube secured. Verified location on chest radiograph.
BREATHING	Sats. Evaluation for pneumothorax done. Finger thoracostomy vs chest tube. Vent settings and recent changes. ETCO2 correlated with ABG.
CIRCULATION	Recent heart rate and blood pressure. Any massive hemorrhage, obvious or suspected occult. Timing of tourniquets. Volume/type of blood products, need for additional. Pelvic binder if suspect pelvic injury.
DISABILITY	Initial/current GCS, pupils. Neurological examination before paralysis. Time of last paralytic.
EXPOSURE	Other injuries found or suspected. Splint fractures. Dress oozing wounds. Keep patient covered, warm, dry.
FLUIDS	Crystalloid volume given. Foley placed. Urine output. Empty urine bag, chest drains. If no catheter, patient should urinate before team arrival.
GUT/GIRTH	Last oral intake. Nasogastric tube placed and confirmed. Accurate weight and width of patient at widest point.
HEME	H/H trend, international normalized ratio. Tranexamic acid or PCC given.
INFUSIONS	Ongoing infusions for sedation and analgesia. Extra medications drawn up for transport team. Discontinue nonessential infusions.
JVP	Signs of tension pneumothorax, tamponade. Evaluated with ultrasound.
KELVIN	Initial and current temperature. Continued need for active warming. Foley or esophageal temperature probe.
LINES	Current access and lines. Two lines larger than 18G for transfer. Central or arterial line if indicated.
MICRO	Antibiotics and tetanus given.
NOTES/NEXT OF KIN	Documentation copied and in an envelope. Extra stickers. Imaging on disks or electronic. Next of kin aware of plan, contact information available.

Abbreviations: ABG, arterial blood gas; GCS, Glasgow Coma Scale; PCC, prothrombin complex concentrate.

Courtesy of MedSTAR Emergency Medical Retrieval Service, South Australia; with permission.

assessments, interventions, and troubleshoot equipment failures or patient deteriorations. During the assessment and transfer phase within the ED, local staff should assist the retrieval team in the preparation of the patient to facilitate the timely departure of the critically ill patient. The emergency physician should continue to communicate with the receiving center with a clinical update and the estimated time of arrival. The retrieval team may have reduced capacity to perform this task en route, limited by the competing roles in safe transportation and provision of clinical care.

SUMMARY AND RECOMMENDATIONS

Level 1 trauma centers do not have a monopoly on excellence in trauma resuscitation. The advantage these centers have over smaller EDs is a locus of in-house specialists and resources, and most importantly, a significant volume of trauma by which to gain experience. To achieve proficiency and (ultimately) excellence in the stabilization and transfer of trauma patients, a combination of personal training with ATLS, Emergency Trauma Management, or homegrown courses, coupled with a focus on team-based interdisciplinary training is recommended.[72,73] It is essential to have trauma champions in the ED who remain up to date with the latest literature, encourage training, guide quality and care reviews, and inspire others.

Regardless of the environment in which care is rendered, a thoughtful, active, and proactive approach to planning, preparation, evaluation, management, and transfer is required for optimal performance and outcomes. Prehospital, ED, and transfer and retrieval teams possess overlapping but nonidentical skill sets that can be leveraged when both time and local resources are constrained. The emergency physician plays a critical role in the coordination and execution of excellent clinical care for trauma patients, and is uniquely positioned to facilitate linkages in the continuum of care between prehospital, emergency department, retrieval, and trauma center environments.

REFERENCES

1. Williamson K, Ramesh R, Grabinsky A. Advances in prehospital trauma care. Int J Crit Illn Inj Sci 2011;1(1):44–50.
2. Podolsky S, Baraff LJ, Simon RR, et al. Efficacy of cervical spine immobilization methods. J Trauma 1983;23:461–4.
3. Perry SD, McLellan B, McIlroy WE, et al. The efficacy of head immobilization techniques during simulated vehicle motion. Spine 1999;24:1839–44.
4. Hauswald M, Ong G, Tandberg D, et al. Out-of-hospital spinal immobilization: its effect on neurologic injury. Acad Emerg Med 1998;5:214–9.
5. Chan D, Goldberg RM, Mason J, et al. Backboard versus mattress splint immobilization: a comparison of symptoms generated. J Emerg Med 1996;14:293–8.
6. Luscombe MD, Williams JL. Comparison of a long spinal board and vacuum mattress for spinal immobilisation. Emerg Med J 2003;20:476–8.
7. Goutcher CM, Lochhead V. Reduction in mouth opening with semi-rigid cervical collars. Br J Anaesth 2005;95:344–8.
8. Kwan I, Bunn F, Roberts I. Spinal immobilisation for trauma patients. Cochrane Database Syst Rev 2001;(2). CDC002803.
9. Sundstrøm T, Asbjørnsen H, Habiba S, et al. Prehospital use of cervical collars in trauma patients: a critical review. J Neurotrauma 2014;31(6):531–40.
10. Vanderlan WB, Tew BE, McSwain NE. Increased risk of death with cervical spine immobilisation in penetrating cervical trauma. Injury 2009;40:880–3.
11. White CC, Domeier RM, Millin MG, Standards and Clinical Practice Committee, National Association of EMS Physicians. EMS spinal precautions and the use of the long backboard—resource document to the position statement of the National Association of EMS Physicians and the American College of Surgeons Committee on Trauma. Prehosp Emerg Care 2014;18(2):306–14.
12. Noble VE, Lamhaut L, Capp R, et al. Evaluation of a thoracic ultrasound training module for the detection of pneumothorax and pulmonary edema by prehospital physician care providers. BMC Med Educ 2009;9(1):1.
13. Heegaard W, Hildebrandt D, Spear D, et al. Prehospital ultrasound by paramedics: results of field trial. Acad Emerg Med 2010;17(6):624–30.
14. Walcher F, Weinlich M, Conrad G, et al. Prehospital ultrasound imaging improves management of abdominal trauma. Br J Surg 2006;93(2):238–42.
15. Holcomb JB, Jenkins D, Rhee P, et al. Damage control resuscitation: directly addressing the early coagulopathy of trauma. J Trauma 2007;62(2):307–10.
16. Hodgetts TJ, Mahoney PF, Kirkman E. Damage control resuscitation. J R Army Med Corps 2007;153(4):299.

17. Weaver AE, Hunter-Dunn C, Lyon RM, et al. The effectiveness of a 'Code Red' transfusion request policy initiated by pre-hospital physicians. Injury 2016; 47(1):3–6.
18. O'Reilly DJ, Morrison JJ, Jansen JO, et al. Initial UK experience of prehospital blood transfusion in combat casualties. J Trauma 2014;77(3):S66–70.
19. Holcomb JB, Donathan DP, Cotton BA, et al. Prehospital transfusion of plasma and red blood cells in trauma patients. Prehosp Emerg Care 2015;19(1):1–9.
20. Lyon RM, de Sausmarez E, McWhirter E, et al. Pre-hospital transfusion of packed red blood cells in 147 patients from a UK helicopter emergency medical service. Scand J Trauma Resusc Emerg Med 2017;25(1):12.
21. Wafaisade A, Lefering R, Bouillon B, et al. Prehospital administration of tranexamic acid in trauma patients. Crit Care 2016;20(1):143.
22. Kue RC, Temin ES, Weiner SG, et al. Tourniquet use in a civilian emergency medical services setting: a descriptive analysis of the Boston EMS experience. Prehosp Emerg Care 2015;19(3):399–404.
23. Carter AJ, Davis KA, Evans LV, et al. Information loss in emergency medical services handover of trauma patients. Prehosp Emerg Care 2009;13(3):280–5.
24. Codner P, Obaid A, Porral D, et al. Is field hypotension a reliable indicator of significant injury in trauma patients who are normotensive on arrival to the emergency department? Am Surg 2005;71(9):768–71.
25. Shapiro NI, Kociszewski C, Harrison T, et al. Isolated prehospital hypotension after traumatic injuries: a predictor of mortality? J Emerg Med 2003;25(2):175–9.
26. Lipsky AM, Gausche-Hill M, Henneman PL, et al. Prehospital hypotension is a predictor of the need for an emergent, therapeutic operation in trauma patients with normal systolic blood pressure in the emergency department. J Trauma 2006;61(5):1228–33.
27. Dawson S, King L, Grantham H. Review article: improving the hospital clinical handover between paramedics and emergency department staff in the deteriorating patient. Emerg Med Australas 2013;25(5):393–405.
28. Meisel ZF, Shea JA, Peacock NJ, et al. Optimizing the patient handoff between emergency medical services and the emergency department. Ann Emerg Med 2015;65(3):310–7.
29. Iedema R, Ball C, Daly B, et al. Design and trial of a new ambulance-to-emergency department handover protocol: 'IMIST-AMBO'. BMJ Qual Saf 2012; 21:627–33.
30. Baxt WG, Moody P. The impact of a physician as part of the aeromedical prehospital team in patients with blunt trauma. JAMA 1987;257(23):3246–50.
31. Bøtker MT, Bakke SA, Christensen EF. A systematic review of controlled studies: do physicians increase survival with prehospital treatment? Scand J Trauma Resusc Emerg Med 2009;17:12.
32. Davis P, Rickards AC, Ollerton JE. Determining the composition and benefit of the pre-hospital medical response team in the conflict setting. J R Army Med Corps 2007;153(4):269–73.
33. Haldane A. Advanced airway management–a medical emergency response team perspective. J R Army Med Corps 2010;156(3):159–61.
34. Davies GE, Lockey DJ. Thirteen survivors of prehospital thoracotomy for penetrating trauma: a prehospital physician-performed resuscitation procedure that can yield good results. J Trauma 2011;70(5):E75–8.
35. Sadek S, Lockey DJ, Lendrum RA, et al. Resuscitative endovascular balloon occlusion of the aorta (REBOA) in the pre-hospital setting: an additional

resuscitation option for uncontrolled catastrophic haemorrhage. Resuscitation 2016;107:135–8.

36. Pepe PE, Stewart RD. Role of the physician in the prehospital setting. Ann Emerg Med 1986;15(12):1480–3.

37. Irvin CB, Szpunar S, Cindrich LA, et al. Should trauma patients with a Glasgow Coma Scale score of 3 be intubated prior to hospital arrival? Prehosp Disaster Med 2010;25(6):541–6.

38. Haltmeier T, Benjamin E, Siboni S, et al. Prehospital intubation for isolated severe blunt traumatic brain injury: worse outcomes and higher mortality. Eur J Trauma Emerg Surg 2016. [Epub ahead of print].

39. Cobas MA, De la Pena MA, Manning R, et al. Prehospital intubations and mortality: a level 1 trauma center perspective. Anesth Analg 2009;109(2):489–93.

40. Stiell IG, Nesbitt LP, Pickett W, et al. The OPALS Major Trauma Study: impact of advanced life-support on survival and morbidity. CMAJ 2008;178(9):1141–52.

41. Winchell RJ, Hoyt DB. Endotracheal intubation in the field improves survival in patients with severe head injury. Arch Surg 1997;132:592–7.

42. Davis DP, Peay J, Serrano JA, et al. The impact of aeromedical response to patients with moderate to severe traumatic brain injury. Ann Emerg Med 2005;46: 115–22.

43. Sunde GA, Heltne JK, Lockey D, et al. Airway management by physician-staffed Helicopter Emergency Medical Services—a prospective, multicentre, observational study of 2,327 patients. Scand J Trauma Resusc Emerg Med 2015;23:57.

44. Lockey DJ, Crewdson K, Davies G, et al. AAGBI: Safer pre-hospital anaesthesia 2017: Association of Anaesthetists of Great Britain and Ireland. Anaesthesia 2017;72(3):379–90.

45. Bernard SA, Nguyen V, Cameron P, et al. Prehospital rapid sequence intubation improves functional outcome for patients with severe traumatic brain injury: a randomized controlled trial. Ann Surg 2010;252(6):959–65.

46. National Highway Traffic Safety Administration. The National EMS Scope of Practice Model. 2007. Available at: https://www.ems.gov/education/EMSScope.pdf. Accessed January 26, 2017.

47. MacKenzie EJ, Rivara FP, Jurkovich GJ, et al. A national evaluation of the effect of trauma-center care on mortality. N Engl J Med 2006;354(4):366–78.

48. Groenestege-Kreb DT, van Maarseveen O, Leenen L, et al. Trauma team. Br J Anaesth 2014;113(2):258–65.

49. Bonjour TJ, Charny G, Thaxton RE. Trauma resuscitation evaluation times and correlating human patient simulation training differences-what is the standard? Mil Med 2016;181(11):e1630–6.

50. MacKenzie EJ, Hoyt DB, Sacra JC. National inventory of hospital trauma centers. JAMA 2003;289(12):1515–22.

51. Hopkins CL, Burk C, Moser S, et al. Implementation of pit crew approach and cardiopulmonary resuscitation metrics for out-of-hospital cardiac arrest improves patient survival and neurological outcome. J Am Heart Assoc 2016;5(1) [pii: e002892].

52. Xiao Y, Schenkel S, Faraj S, et al. What whiteboards in a trauma center operating suite can teach us about emergency department communication. Ann Emerg Med 2007;50(4):387–95.

53. Butler FK, Haymann J, Butler EG. Tactical combat casualty care in special operations. Association of Military Surgeons of the US; 1996.

54. Butler FK. Tactical combat casualty care: update 2009. J Trauma 2010;69(1): S10–3.

55. Drew B, Bennett BL, Littlejohn L. Application of current hemorrhage control techniques for backcountry care: part one, tourniquets and hemorrhage control adjuncts. Wilderness Environ Med 2015;26(2):236–45.

56. Curry N, Hopewell S, Doree C, et al. The acute management of trauma hemorrhage: a systematic review of randomized controlled trials. Crit Care 2011; 15(2):R92.

57. Airwayregistry.org.au. RSI Checklist. Available at: http://www.airwayregistry.org.au/RSI-checklist.html. Accessed December 30, 2016.

58. Buck A. Cliff Reid & the resus room safety officer. Available at: http://resusroom.mx/cliff-reid-the-resus-room-safety-officer. Accessed March 30, 2017.

59. Whitson MR, Mayo PH. Ultrasonography in the emergency department. Crit Care 2016;20(1):227.

60. Montoya J, Stawicki SP, Evans DC, et al. From FAST to E-FAST: an overview of the evolution of ultrasound-based traumatic injury assessment. Eur J Trauma Emerg Surg 2016;42(2):119–26.

61. Levine AR, McCurdy MT, Zubrow MT, et al. Tele-intensivists can instruct non-physicians to acquire high-quality ultrasound images. J Crit Care 2015;30(5):871–5.

62. Adhikari S, Blaivas M, Lyon M, et al. Transfer of real-time ultrasound video of FAST examinations from a simulated disaster scene via a mobile phone. Prehosp Disaster Med 2014;29(3):290–3.

63. Holcomb JB, Tilley BC, Baraniuk S, et al. Transfusion of plasma, platelets, and red blood cells in a 1:1:1 vs a 1:1:2 ratio and mortality in patients with severe trauma: the PROPPR randomized clinical trial. JAMA 2015;313(5):471–82.

64. Shakur H, Roberts I, Bautista R, et al. Effects of tranexamic acid on death, vascular occlusive events, and blood transfusion in trauma patients with significant haemorrhage (CRASH-2): a randomised, placebo-controlled trial. Lancet 2010;376(9734):23–32.

65. Walker AF. The legal duty of physicians and hospitals to provide emergency care. CMAJ 2002;166(4):465–9.

66. Australian and New Zealand College of Anaesthetists. Guidelines for transport of critically ill patients. Available at: http://www.anzca.edu.au/documents/ps52-2015-guidelines-for-transport-of-critically-i.pdf. Accessed March 21, 2017.

67. Centers for Medicare & Medicaid Services. Emergency Medical Treatment & Labor Act (EMTALA). Available at: https://www.cms.gov/Regulations-and-Guidance/Legislation/EMTALA/. Accessed November 25, 2016.

68. Aerosurrance. US HEMS Accident Rates 2006-2015. Available at: http://aerossurance.com/helicopters/us-hems-accident-2006-2015. Accessed March 21, 2017.

69. Nwozuzu A, Fontes ML, Schonberger RB. Mobile extracorporeal membrane oxygenation teams: the North American versus the European experience. J Cardiothorac Vasc Anesth 2016;30(6):1441–8.

70. Garner AA. The role of physician staffing of helicopter emergency medical services in prehospital trauma response. Emerg Med Australas 2005;17(4):387–91.

71. Leeuwenberg T. MedSTAR Emergency Medical Retrieval Service, South Australia. Transfer Checklist. Available at: https://ruraldoctorsdotnet1.files.wordpress.com/2013/04/transfer-abc.pdf. Accessed March 21, 2017.

72. American College of Surgeons. Advanced Trauma Life Support. Available at: https://www.facs.org/quality%20programs/trauma/atls. Accessed January 29, 2017.

73. Emergency Trauma Management Pty Ltd. Emergency Trauma Management course. Available at: etmcourse.com. Accessed January 29, 2017.

The Tragically Hip
Trauma in Elderly Patients

Katrin Hruska, MD[a],*, Toralph Ruge, MD, PhD[a,b,1]

KEYWORDS

- Elderly • Falls • Trauma • Geriatric

KEY POINTS

- Geriatric trauma is different in terms of mechanisms of injury and injuries sustained, which leads to delays in diagnosis and treatment.
- In the geriatric patient, low-impact trauma can be associated with severe injury.
- Elderly trauma patients can have good outcomes with high quality of life, with early interventions and prevention of complications.
- Standard trauma care is based on evidence where the elderly are underrepresented.

WHAT IS GERIATRIC TRAUMA AND WHY DOES IT MATTER?

Trauma is traditionally considered a disease of young men after motor vehicle collisions and interpersonal violence. The acute trauma chain of care has been organized to identify and transport the severely injured patient to high-level trauma centers for life-saving interventions. This strategy has been highly effective, positively impacting the traditional trimodal distribution of mortality (immediate, early, and late) through early recognition and treatment of life-threatening conditions to reflect fewer early and late deaths.[1]

Just as trauma care evolves, so does the population of traumatically injured patients. As life expectancy increases, geriatric patients are more likely to suffer significant injuries later in life. The typical geriatric trauma patient, however, is distinctly different from the typical young and healthy male involved in high risk activities. Geriatric trauma patients are more likely to be female, have multiple comorbidities, and be described as "frail": a biologic syndrome of decreased reserve and resistance to stressors, resulting from cumulative declines across multiple physiologic systems. Frailty is a condition that requires a multidisciplinary team effort to prevent

Neither author has any disclosures or conflicts of interests.
[a] Department of Emergency Medicine, Karolinska University Hospital, Huddinge, Sweden;
[b] Department of Medicine, Solna, Karolinska Institutet, Stockholm, Sweden
[1] Present address: Kyrkvägen 1D, Umeå 903 62, Sweden.
* Corresponding author.
E-mail address: katrin.hruska@sll.se

Emerg Med Clin N Am 36 (2018) 219–235
https://doi.org/10.1016/j.emc.2017.08.014
0733-8627/18/© 2017 Elsevier Inc. All rights reserved.

emed.theclinics.com

deterioration and adverse outcomes after injuries or illnesses that would not otherwise pose serious health threats to nonfrail patients.[2]

The frail geriatric patient who has fallen from standing does not succumb to exsanguination during the golden hour of trauma, but rather dies of pneumonia in the recovery phase or enters the trajectory of rapid functional decline after a hip fracture.

Elderly patients with both low- and high-energy trauma are less likely than younger patients to be sent to a trauma center,[3] despite their higher rates of poor outcomes. New recommendations attempt to address this discrepancy by directing more elderly patients to advanced trauma care. To optimize outcomes, accurate risk stratification, evidence-based treatment options, and clear goals of care are needed. Even among elderly patients, different priorities exist depending on age, frailty, and mechanism of injury. The 94-year-old nursing home patient who fell out of bed is distinctly different from the 67-year-old motorcyclist injured in a crash, even though they both may have sustained life-threatening injuries.

AGE AS A RISK FACTOR IN TRAUMA: WHEN DO YOU GET OLD?

Several studies have shown that trauma in the geriatric population is associated with increased acute and long-term mortality.[4–10]

Advancing age is an independent predictor of mortality after trauma; however, there is no well accepted threshold or cutoff for what constitutes a "geriatric" patient[11] nor is there a definite cutoff that accurately predicts outcome. Various age values have been proposed, ranging between 45 and 80.[11] Adams and colleagues[4] found that age 45 years and older was associated with increased mortality after trauma, whereas Pandya and colleagues[12] found a significant increase in mortality among patients 55 years and older involved in motor vehicle collisions. Other studies found an increased mortality in patients older than 60 years[13,14] and 65 years of age.[15] In a cross-sectional study of 75,658 trauma patients, Caterino and colleagues[16] found a threshold value of 70 to 74 years for mortality rate stratified by Injury Severity Score (ISS). The range of cutoffs are more likely related to study limitations or statistical nuances than inherent differences among the study populations. These studies simply highlight the importance of advanced age on morbidity and mortality after trauma.

Interestingly, Friese and colleagues[17] found that the risk of death after injury is proportional to patient age until 84 years, after which the mortality rates actually decline. This trend may be related to survivor bias, whereby a greater proportion of those living past 84 years of age are in better health, contributing to this somewhat paradoxic finding. A study by Adams and associates[18] suggests that variance in mortality for younger and older trauma patients was minimal (4%–7%) after patients with active do not resuscitate orders were excluded from analysis.

THE ELDERLY ARE NOT JUST OLD ADULTS: FRAILTY AS A RISK FACTOR

Elderly patients have a higher incidence of medical comorbidities and lower physiologic reserves, increasing their susceptibility to even minor trauma.[19,20] In fact, age may be an overly simplistic measure to understand outcomes in geriatric trauma patients and better predictor may be the degree of frailty.[1]

Frailty is composed of both the degree of loss of physiologic reserve and increased incidence and severity of comorbid disease.[21] Biologically, this translates to musculoskeletal, neuroendocrine, nutritional, and immunologic defects that contribute to a physical state of muscular weakness and other functional impairment.[21,22]

Frailty is an independent predictor of postoperative complications, mortality, and hospital duration of stay in elderly patients undergoing emergency general surgery.[23,24] Frail elderly patients not only have higher in-hospital mortality, but also suffer from poorer long-term outcomes compared with their nonfrail counterparts. For example, frail elderly patients have a decreased functional ability 1 year after a fall and an increased mortality risk that persists 3 years after the event.[25] Frailty before hip fracture is associated with greater postfracture pain and deterioration in function[26] and preinjury frailty is the predominant predictor of postinjury functional status and mortality.[27]

The role of frailty and preinjury functional status in predicting outcomes after trauma is profound. Dunham and colleagues[28] concluded that, although frailty was an independent predictor of discharge to a long-term care facility after trauma, dementia and multiple comorbidities were not.

Several instruments have been designed to quantify frailty. The Trauma Specific Frailty Index was derived from the complex, 50-variable Frailty Index, simplified to improve clinical usefulness. The Trauma Specific Frailty Index has been shown to an independent predictor of unfavorable discharge disposition in geriatric trauma patients and in-hospital complications.[29–31]

In a prospective study of 368 consecutive trauma patients admitted to a level 1 trauma center, frailty (as assessed by the Trauma Specific Frailty Index) increased the risk of death from a major complication by almost 3-fold. Nearly 7 in 10 patients who died from a major complication were identified as frail, despite representing only 25% of the study cohort. Frail patients were also less likely to be discharged home (22% vs 72%), suggesting that many survivors suffered significant and permanent functional impairment as a result of their injury.

In summary, there is significant variation in the health status of elderly people that warrants individualized considerations based on frailty rather than age.[11] Frailty is not a treatable condition, but rather a risk factor that needs to be identified to prevent complications, both in the hospital and after discharge.[1] We suggest that all hospitals caring for injured elderly patients ensure that frailty is assessed and managed by a multidisciplinary team of health care providers with expertise in geriatrics.

MECHANISM OF INJURY: HOW DO OLD PEOPLE GET HURT?

Falls are the most common cause of injury in the elderly. When nonelderly patients fall, more than 90% fall on one or both hands outstretched, reducing the impact to the hip and head. In contrast, elderly patients are less likely to protect themselves when falling and only 33% to 50% fall on outstretched hands, with women being less likely to do so than men.[32] Also, the upper extremities of elderly women have nearly one-half the capacity of younger women to absorb the energy generated by a fall.[33]

Motor vehicle collisions are a common cause of serious injury in the elderly population.[34] Elderly patients, especially females, are more susceptible to seatbelt–induced thoracic trauma from low or moderate speed crashes. Thoracic injuries are associated with increased mortality in women age 65 years and older.[34] Patients age 60 and over have a 3-fold risk of blunt thoracic aortic injury when involved in motor vehicle accidents.[35] The presence of multiple rib fractures, even in isolation, has been shown to increase mortality owing to secondary pulmonary and cardiac complications.

The elderly pedestrian is especially vulnerable and overrepresented among fatalities. In the United States, 20% of all pedestrian fatalities are 65 years of age and older[36]; in the European Union, nearly one-half of pedestrian fatalities are in the geriatric population (available: www.erso.eu).

Age-related differences in injury severity are not fully accounted for by mechanism alone. According to Henry and colleagues,[37] pelvic fractures in the elderly are "a different entity" than those typically observed in younger patients. Elderly patients are more likely to suffer lateral compression fractures, an injury pattern often considered less severe than anteroposterior compression fractures. Despite this, elderly patients have higher rates of pelvic bleeding requiring blood transfusions and a greater need for angiographic treatment.[38,39]

In addition to different patterns of injury, the same injury often results in worse outcomes in elderly patients. Clavicle fractures are associated with a surprisingly high mortality rate in patients over 65 years of age who have sustained high-impact trauma.[40] Elderly patients are also more likely to have massive bleeding where the source is not recognized during the primary survey, including retroperitoneal hematoma and stable pelvic ring fractures.[41]

VITAL SIGNS: MAYBE NOT SO VITAL IN THE ELDERLY

In trauma patients, abnormal vital signs correlate positively with patient mortality.[42] Traumatic hemorrhage is associated with decreased systolic blood pressure (SBP), increased heart rate (HR) and an increased Shock Index (HR divided by SBP).[43] However, the role of individual vital signs in predicting mortality and morbidity in geriatric trauma patients is complex, and normal vital signs are not as reassuring as they might be in younger patients.[44–46]

Heffernan and colleagues[47] conducted a retrospective study of 5000 patients, comparing young (17–35 years of age) and elderly (65 years and older) patients with major trauma. They concluded that mortality was significantly higher among elderly patients with HR of greater than 90 bpm. In contrast, only a HR of greater than 130 bpm was associated with increased mortality in young patients. Mortality significantly increased with a SBP of less than 110 mm Hg among geriatric patients, whereas similar outcomes were not observed until the SBP decreased to less than 95 mm Hg in young patients. In addition, a U-shaped association between HR, SBP, and mortality was observed. Discrepant vital sign cutoffs were also observed in patients with occult shock.[44,48] Taken together, the literature highlights the importance of age-adjusted vital sign cutoffs to identify patients in need of aggressive resuscitation. Based on available evidence, we suggest that hypotension be defined as a SBP of less than 110 mm Hg in the geriatric population.

Emergency department triage relies heavily on vital signs upon arrival. The lack of reliable vital sign cutoffs for elderly trauma patients complicates this process. Therefore, elderly trauma patients are at risk for being undertriaged, resulting in delays to injury recognition and management.[49]

Vital signs have been proposed to predict the need for massive transfusion among trauma patients of all ages. The predictive power of HR for massive transfusion among geriatric trauma patients has been questioned.[50] In 1 study, SBP, pulse pressure, diastolic blood pressure, and shock index (SI) were all strongly predictive of massive transfusion, whereas HR was not. This may reflect, in part, the higher rates of cardiac medications among geriatric patients, limiting the expected tachycardic response to massive hemorrhage.[50,51] Similarly, Ohmori and colleagues[52] found that only SI was predictive of the need for massive transfusion, whereas blood pressure, HR, and Glasgow Coma Scale score were not useful.

The need to predict more precisely massive transfusion and mortality among geriatric trauma patients has resulted in the age shock index (age × SI). This has been shown superior to both vital signs alone and unadjusted SI for predicting both mortality and need for massive transfusion among injured elderly patients.[53,54]

WHO IS SICK AND WHO IS NOT: SHOCK IDENTIFICATION AMONG INJURED ELDERLY

In severe traumatic injury, severe hypovolemia can lead to inadequate organ perfusion, ischemic injury, and tissue hypoxia. This in turn creates a metabolic acidosis that manifest as increased base deficit (BD) and elevated serum lactate. Serum lactate is a direct measure of anaerobic metabolism, whereas a BD is a calculated value of the amount of base required to achieve a neutral pH, assuming a normal P_{CO_2}.

The usefulness of BD to characterize the presence and extent of hemorrhagic shock in trauma patients has been studied in younger populations, where BD correlates with transfusion requirements, duration of stay in the intensive care unit (ICU), and all-cause mortality. Contrastingly, only a handful of studies have specifically investigated the use of BD in geriatric trauma. Initial BD measurements performed similarly to serum lactate in mortality prediction; however, lactate was a superior predictor of injury severity and in-hospital mortality.[55–57]

Both BD and serum lactate have important limitations. Lactate levels may be affected by alcohol consumption, and BD may be altered by minute ventilation or intravenous fluids.[58,59] There is no strong evidence that either measure is superior for shock identification or clinical prognostication. Instead, recent guidelines support the use of either measure as a sensitive test to estimate the degree of hemorrhagic shock.[60]

BD and serum lactate can assist in identifying occult shock, a state of hypoperfusion that lacks obvious clinical disturbances or vital sign abnormalities. This "cryptic" form of shock is especially common in geriatric patients, occurring in 16% to 70% of major trauma victims.[61–63] The high incidence of occult hypoperfusion in this patient population can be explained in part by decreased physiologic reserves (or frailty), medical comorbidities, and medications.[64] Occult shock is associated with an increase in trauma-related mortality from 12% to 35% when hypoperfusion persists for more than 12 hours.[65]

Although modified triage and resuscitation guidelines that account for occult shock have been developed, they have not gained widespread use.[66,67]

In summary, current data suggest that both BD and serum lactate represent important biomarkers for shock and occult shock, and should be considered predictors of serious or severe injury in geriatric patients, even when physical examination and vital signs are nonspecific.

TRAUMA CENTERS FOR THE ELDERLY, OR GERIATRIC CARE FOR THE INJURED?

Retrospective cohort studies have shown that elderly patients who are treated at trauma centers fare better than those seen at nontrauma centers.[68] Which elderly patients require transfer remains a considerable challenge, with several studies demonstrating higher rates of undertriage in this population.

New guidelines for field triage of injured patients have attempted to address the issue of undertriage for elderly patients. The 2011 American College of Surgeons Committee on Trauma guidelines included special considerations for older adults, including the following.

1. Risk of injury and death increases with age.
2. SBP of less than 110 mm Hg results in worse outcomes and may represent a shock state.

3. Low-impact mechanisms (eg, ground-level falls) can cause serious injury.
4. Trauma triage instruments have poor discriminatory properties for the elderly. New-gard and colleagues[46] found that using broader cutoffs for vital signs (Glasgow Coma Score $\leq$14, SBP $\leq$110 or $\geq$200, respiratory rate $\leq$10 or $\geq$24 per minute or HR $\leq$60 or $\geq$110 bpm) could increase triage sensitivity for seriously injured geriatric patients at the expense of specificity. Implementation of these criteria pose marked resource and logistical challenges, because an additional 46 patients without serious injuries would need to be transported to a trauma center to identify only 1 with serious injuries (ISS >15).

The adoption of new geriatric trauma center criteria in Ohio[69] (**Box 1**) increased the number of patients aged 70 and over who qualified for trauma center care from 44% to 58%. Despite this, incorporating the revised criteria into the emergency medical services training program only resulted in a 1% increase in initial transportation to a trauma center.

Given the challenges associated with predicting injury severity in the elderly, over-triage is an inevitable outcome of setting low and broad criteria for transporting these patients to a trauma center. A recent analysis of trauma registries in the United States suggests not only an increasing number of elderly patients, but also a high proportion of patients with minor injuries are being preferentially transported to trauma centers. Bradburn and colleagues[38] found that 52% of patients admitted to a regional trauma hospital had an ISS of less than 10, suggesting a trend toward admitting patients with less severe injuries.

Overtriage to trauma centers not only carries a substantial cost,[70] but may result in harm to patients who forgo necessary geriatric care in favor of more focused trauma management. In centers with high volumes of geriatric trauma patients, these risks can be mitigated; however, it requires efforts and investment to centralize geriatric trauma care. Zafar and colleagues[71] found that risk-adjusted death from a complication rates declined from 25% to 20% when going from centers with less than 10% to greater than 50% geriatric trauma. The incidence of major complications did not change significantly, suggesting that reported differences in mortality were not likely to be explained by differences in complication rates. Considering the complexity of trauma triage, clinical pathways for injured elderly patients are needed at all hospitals that see acutely ill patients.

TRAUMA TEAM ACTIVATION

The severity of injuries among elderly patients is consistently underestimated[72] and the elderly benefit from more liberal criteria for trauma team activation (TTA). In 1

Box 1
The Ohio geriatric triage criteria

- Glasgow Coma Scale score of <14 in the presence of known or suspected traumatic brain trauma.
- Systolic blood pressure of <100 mm Hg.
- Fall from any height with evidence of traumatic brain injury.
- Multiple body system injuries.
- Struck by a moving vehicle.
- Presence of any proximal long bone fracture after motor vehicle trauma.

study of 883 elderly trauma patients, only 25% of patients met at least one of the standard TTA criteria.[73] Despite this, mortality was 50% and ICU admission was 39%. More impressively, among severely injured patients (ISS >30), 25% did not meet any TTA criteria. TTA criteria included traditional vital sign abnormalities (SBP <90 mm Hg, HR >120 bpm, respiratory rate <10 or >29 breaths/min, unresponsive to pain, thoracoabdominal gunshot wound). These results highlight how insensitive traditional measures of shock are in the geriatric population, and that more liberal criteria for TTA are warranted. The authors conclude that patients age 70 years and older should be a criterion for TTA, irrespective of physiologic status at the time of assessment. Whether this represents the best use of resources remains to be seen, but suffice it to say that more nuanced considerations of age or frailty should likely be studied.

Rehn et al[74] studied TTA in Norway where patients over 70 years of age were found to be 5 times more likely to be undertriaged. A study of elderly patients by St John and colleagues[75] found that elderly patients with severe injury were less likely to result in TTA, but also that TTA activation in elderly patients over 65 years of age was not significantly associated with a reduced risk of poor outcomes. Younger patients, however, had a clear benefit of TTA (odds ratio, 0.48).

The retrospective design of these studies makes it difficult to assess which elderly patients would benefit from TTA. The patients with poor outcomes who are likely to be missed by current TTA criteria are older and have fewer clinical signs and symptoms, but the optimal management for these patients remains to be established. The Eastern Association for the Surgery of Trauma Flow Diagram for the injured elderly patient offers a systematic approach to initial decision making (**Fig. 1**).

LIFE-THREATENING INJURY FROM MINOR TRAUMA: INTERVENTIONS THAT MATTER

A significant challenge in defining effective trauma management for critically injured geriatric patients is their frequent underrepresentation in clinical trials. Many trauma resuscitation trails exclude patients age 65 years and older. Fortunately, more recently, efforts have been undertaken to promote the inclusion of elderly patients in large clinical studies.

An important question in elderly trauma care is, who requires aggressive intervention and when? Interventions are not without harm, and the benefits and risks must be balanced, especially when directed toward a frail trauma patient susceptible to iatrogenic harms.

For example, the application of a halo vest in elderly patients is an independent predictor of mortality. As such, the risks of prolonged halo immobilization must be carefully weighed against the risks of surgical stabilization.[76] Interestingly, a surgical approach may prove to be appropriate in select elderly populations. Ryang and colleagues[77] found, in a retrospective cohort study of very elderly patients (age 80–89 years) with traumatic odontoid fractures, that operative management had no associated in-hospital mortality and a relatively low 30-day mortality (6%). This suggests that early interventions even in very frail patients, with intense management to prevent complications, can be beneficial. Similar findings are demonstrated among patients with hip fractures, where streamlined processes with adequate pain treatment, early surgery, and early mobilization have been shown to reduce 30-day mortality and duration of stay. Early mobilization seems to be key, making unnecessary restrictions to mobilize for the elderly patient outright harmful.

Patients with isolated hip fractures have a 30-day mortality of up to 10%[78] and a 1-year mortality approaching 20% despite standardized treatment protocols.[79] These

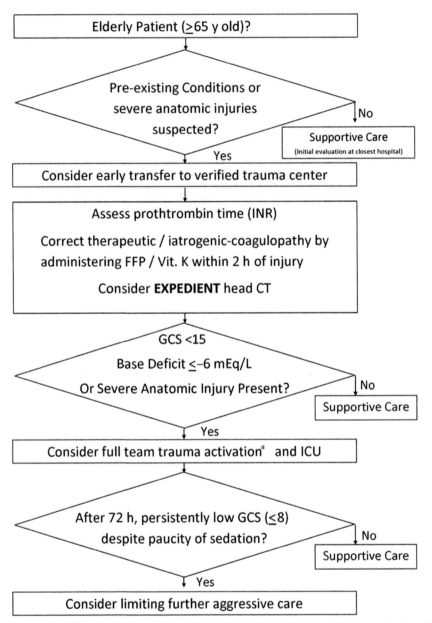

Fig. 1. Care of the injured elder: An evidence-based flow diagram.[a] Evidence for benefit from full team activation derived from study of patients ≥70 years of age. CT, computed tomography; FFP, fresh frozen plasma; GCS, Glasgow Coma Scale; ICU, intensive care unit; INR, International Normalized Ratio.

patients have historically been excluded from trauma registries, even though they have a higher mortality and greater hospital duration of stay than other trauma patients. Whether isolated hip fractures are included in trauma registries varies, and Gomez and colleagues[80] found that these patients constitute from 0% to 31% of all cases at level 1 and 2 trauma centers in the United States, making it difficult to benchmark outcomes for elderly trauma patients.

Traumatic brain injury (TBI) can account for up to 58% of deaths from blunt trauma. Increased mortality among elderly patients with TBI may be due to factors such as comorbid illness, higher rates of intracranial hemorrhage, and rehabilitation-related complications.[81,82] An additional variable relates to unrecognized injuries, which result in delays in clinical management.[81,83–90] Interestingly, although the use of anticoagulation and antiplatelet agents increases the risk of TBI, they were not associated with early neurologic deterioration.[91] The impact of anticoagulation and antiplatelets is uncertain, with conflicting outcomes likely owing to differences in comorbidities. However, it is clear that the risk of traumatic intracranial hemorrhage is greater among patients taking anticoagulants and antiplatelet medications.[92,93]

The survival rate after isolated severe TBI requiring emergent neurosurgical intervention is time dependent. Recent data suggest that early and aggressive treatment of elderly patients with TBI can result in favorable outcomes, similar to younger patients.[94] Identification and timely acute management of patients with TBI in the emergency department is, therefore, essential.[95]

Haller and colleagues[96] found a difference in the trajectory of recovery between older (age >65 years) and younger patients with severe brain injury. Older patients showed no significant functional improvement at the 3- and 12-month follow-ups, but improved health-related quality of life scores, suggesting that elderly might be less burdened by reduced physical abilities.

In CRASH-2 (Clinical Randomization of an Antifibrinolytic in Significant Hemorrhage 2), a study of tranexamic acid (TXA) in trauma, 23% of patients were 44 years or older. Age was not an exclusion criteria, and 4.8% of patients (n = 966) were older than 65 years. Notably, TXA seems to be as efficient in preventing death in elderly patients as in young (Miland J and Roberts I, personal communication, 2017).

TXA has been found to be safe for elderly patients. A systematic review of TXA for patients undergoing surgery for hip fractures found that TXA treatment resulted in a 12% decrease in the risk of postoperative blood transfusion, without increasing the risk of thromboembolic events or stroke.[97]

IMAGING IN GERIATRIC PATIENTS

Dwyer and coworkers studied patients age 65 years and older presenting after ground-level falls who underwent either full body computed tomography scans (ie, the trauma "pan-scan") or injury-focused cross-sectional imaging. No differences in mortality were observed between the 2 groups. However, those who underwent pan-scans had a shorter ICU duration of stay, suggesting that upfront resource use by way of diagnostic imaging might save longer term resource requirements among elderly trauma patients.

Computed tomography scanning has been shown to help reduce mortality in severely injured elderly patients. Maintaining a low threshold for axial imaging in elderly patients should reduce this risk. We suggest a low threshold for pan-scans of elderly patients involved in high-energy trauma, even in the absence of obvious injuries. An early computed tomography pan-scan can also reduce the need for intensive monitoring, which can facilitate early mobilization and shorten periods of fasting, both of which are important for preventing delirium.

GERIATRIC TRAUMA DEATHS: WHY DO OLD PEOPLE DIE?

Elderly patients admitted to trauma centers frequently die from non–trauma-related causes. Kahl and colleagues examined trends in death at a level 1 trauma center: during the study period, the proportion of admitted patients age greater than 65 years increased from 12.1% to 24.6%. The mean age of nonsurvivors increased from 47 years to 56.7 years. More than one-third of deaths were not directly caused by the trauma event, but were due to preexisting medical conditions (16.4%) or traumatic injuries deemed survivable but complicated by preexisting medical conditions (20.9%). The nonsurvivors were also less severely injured, with the ISS decreasing from 35.2 to 28.3.

Elderly patients are less likely to be referred and admitted to the ICU for medical and surgical conditions. If they do undergo surgery, they tend to have a poor prognosis. In a Swedish cohort, 56% of patients who died from organ dysfunction had cervical spine fractures and/or rib fractures that led to respiratory and circulatory compromise and early limitation of medical therapy. Trauma patients of all ages have been shown to have an increased mortality up to 1 year after the initial event, compared with other patients, but this discrepancy is markedly increased in elderly patients.[98] This finding illustrates the need for longer follow-up times for elderly trauma patients, not only focusing on in-hospital mortality.

RECOGNIZING DYING IN THE ELDERLY TRAUMA PATIENT

As more people are reaching advanced age, end-of-life care is changing. A slow decrease in function with multiple hospital admissions precedes death for many elderly individuals. Ground-level falls are part of this process, and even falls without injuries are a risk factor for increased mortality. These patients have high morbidity and mortality, but are unlikely to benefit from TTA. Many of the components of trauma care, including immobilization, prolonged fasting periods, and living in a stressful environment, increase the risk of delirium and poor outcomes for frail patients.

Prognostication is difficult in trauma. The Geriatric Trauma Outcome (GTO) score was developed among a cohort of patients age 65 and older at a level 1 trauma center, and reliably predicts in hospital mortality according to the following formula:

Age + (ISS × 2.5) + 22 (if given packed red blood cells).

The GTO was validated in 18,282 patients from trauma registries at 4 different level 1 centers. A nomogram from the validation sample suggests that a GTO score of 221 translates to a mortality risk of 90% and consequently a nontrivial 10% chance of survival. A representative patient for a score of 221 is a 74 year old with a severe head injury and a life-threatening pelvic fracture who requires blood products during the initial resuscitation. The GTO score's predictive value was confirmed in a Swedish cohort and further improved when patients with limits of care and/or discharge to hospice were excluded. The score could, however, not accurately predict the 1-year mortality. It has been suggested that a frailty index is combined with the GTO score to improve prediction of long-term outcomes, but this has yet to be studied.

Although an estimated mortality risk can be useful information when discussing goals of care, more information is needed about other long term outcomes and preinjury functional status. The patient's own preinjury care preferences are also important particularly because those with preadmission do not resuscitate directives have a 5-fold higher mortality rate when admitted after acute injury.[99] This outcome likely represents a biased approach to resuscitation, whereby interventions are limited because the patient has a preestablished do not resuscitate directive.

FUTURE PERSPECTIVES

Over the past 30 years, the focus of elderly trauma care has shifted. No longer is the question whether severely injured elderly patients benefit from advanced trauma care, but rather how trauma care can best be provided such that it aligns with the specific needs of the elderly patient? It is not surprising that age alone is a poor predictor of outcome, considering the variation in health status for patients 65 years and older. In a Japanese study of trauma victims, 15% of patients older than this cutoff were still working. Although an aging physiology increases the risk of injury from lower severity mechanisms, the initial trauma management should be no less aggressive than it is for younger patients.

Prehospital triage of elderly patients is complex, with high rates of undertriage and overtriage. Overtriage may be necessary to identify the seriously injured, but the potential risks for elderly patients who are erroneously triaged to advanced trauma centers must be addressed. Trauma centers require interprofessional, specialized teams that can meet the needs of frail patients who are at risk of both trauma and non-trauma-related complications.

Geriatric trauma research suffers from a lack of common definitions. Not only is the cutoff age for the definition of elderly different, there is also no consensus on what constitutes a trauma, with some centers including isolated hip fractures and others only severely injured patients with an ISS of greater than 15. The current knowledge about trauma in the elderly is mainly based on retrospective cohort studies from trauma registries and trauma centers. The patient panorama included in those studies ranges from severely injured with high ISS scores, to minor injuries where 1 study reports ISS scores from 0 to 50 with a median of 5. This shows the complexity of geriatric trauma and raises not only the question of when you get old, but also what is a trauma?

The elderly trauma population is heterogenous and needs to be stratified according to known risk factors, including age, gender, injury severity, frailty, and comorbidities. But more than anything, future research needs a shared definition of relevant, patient oriented outcomes.

Top Ten Strategies to Make You a Better Geriatric Trauma Care Provider

1 Engage patients and family members early to establish goals of care after serious injuries.
2 Every elderly trauma patient has at least 1 considerations—injuries sustained, and the medial and frailty-related conditions that precipitated those injuries, complicating management.
3 Frail patients are more likely to die, even if not seriously injured; adequate analgesia, early mobilization, and prevention of complications can have a positive impact on morbidity and mortality.
4 Vital signs are unreliable; calculate the age-adjusted shock index (age × HR/SBP); if it is greater than 50, suspect shock or occult shock. Use age adjusted SI to augment but not replace clinical suspicion; it is not sensitive enough to rule out serious injury.
5 Integrate lactate and/or BD as adjuncts to diagnose occult hypoperfusion; when detected, initiate aggressive resuscitation and follow serial values.
6 Hemodynamically unstable elderly patients need aggressive resuscitation, analogous to nongeriatric patients. Administer TXA if bleeding is suspected and be aware that additional reversal of direct-acting oral anticoagulants might be required in patients with a history of atrial fibrillation or venous thromboembolic disease.
7 TBI is a significant cause of morbidity and mortality among the elderly. A normal Glasgow Coma Scale is common, even among those seriously injured. Maintain a low threshold for obtaining computed tomography scans of the head, particularly when the patient uses anticoagulation or antiplatelet medication.
8 "Stable" pelvic fractures (lateral compression, acetabulum) can result in massive hemorrhage.

9 Even if the patients did not break anything, a fall is a risk factor for bad outcomes. Arrange follow-up care!
10 Elderly are not just old adults. Develop and implement specific trauma treatment protocols for your geriatric patients.

REFERENCES

1. McGwin G Jr, Nunn AM, Mann JC, et al. Reassessment of the tri-modal mortality distribution in the presence of a regional trauma system. J Trauma 2009;66(2): 526–30.
2. Bilotta C, Bergamaschini L, Nicolini P, et al. Frailty syndrome diagnosed according to the Study of Osteoporotic Fractures criteria and mortality in older outpatients suffering from Alzheimer's disease: a one-year prospective cohort study. Aging Ment Health 2012;16(3):273–80.
3. Ryb GE, Dischinger PC. Disparities in trauma center access of older injured motor vehicular crash occupants. J Trauma 2011;71(3):742–7.
4. Adams SD, Cotton BA, McGuire MF, et al. Unique pattern of complications in elderly trauma patients at a Level I trauma center. J Trauma Acute Care Surg 2012;72(1):112–8.
5. Gowing R, Jain MK. Injury patterns and outcomes associated with elderly trauma victims in Kingston, Ontario. Can J Surg 2007;50(6):437–44.
6. Wutzler S, Lefering R, Laurer HL, et al. Changes in geriatric traumatology. An analysis of 14,869 patients from the German Trauma Registry. Unfallchirurg 2008;111(8):592–8 [in German].
7. Zhao FZ, Wolf SE, Nakonezny PA, et al. Estimating geriatric mortality after injury using age, injury severity, and performance of a transfusion: the geriatric trauma outcome score. J Palliat Med 2015;18(8):677–81.
8. Goodmanson NW, Rosengart MR, Barnato AE, et al. Defining geriatric trauma: when does age make a difference? Surgery 2012;152(4):668–74 [discussion: 674–5].
9. McGwin G Jr, George RL, Cross JM, et al. Improving the ability to predict mortality among burn patients. Burns 2008;34(3):320–7.
10. McGwin G Jr, Melton SM, May AK, et al. Long-term survival in the elderly after trauma. J Trauma 2000;49(3):470–6.
11. Jacobs DG, Plaisier BR, Barie PS, et al. Practice management guidelines for geriatric trauma: the EAST Practice Management Guidelines Work Group. J Trauma 2003;54(2):391–416.
12. Pandya SR, Yelon JA, Sullivan TS, et al. Geriatric motor vehicle collision survival: the role of institutional trauma volume. J Trauma 2011;70(6):1326–30.
13. Schiller WR, Knox R, Chleborad W. A five-year experience with severe injuries in elderly patients. Accid Anal Prev 1995;27(2):167–74.
14. van der Sluis CK, Klasen HJ, Eisma WH, et al. Major trauma in young and old: what is the difference? J Trauma 1996;40(1):78–82.
15. Perdue PW, Watts DD, Kaufmann CR, et al. Differences in mortality between elderly and younger adult trauma patients: geriatric status increases risk of delayed death. J Trauma 1998;45(4):805–10.
16. Caterino JM, Valasek T, Werman HA. Identification of an age cutoff for increased mortality in patients with elderly trauma. Am J Emerg Med 2010;28(2):151–8.
17. Friese RS, Wynne J, Joseph B, et al. Age and mortality after injury: is the association linear? Eur J Trauma Emerg Surg 2014;40(5):567–72.

18. Adams SD, Cotton BA, Wade CE, et al. Do not resuscitate status, not age, affects outcomes after injury: an evaluation of 15,227 consecutive trauma patients. J Trauma Acute Care Surg 2013;74(5):1327–30.

19. McGwin G Jr, MacLennan PA, Fife JB, et al. Preexisting conditions and mortality in older trauma patients. J Trauma 2004;56(6):1291–6.

20. Finelli FC, Jonsson J, Champion HR, et al. A case control study for major trauma in geriatric patients. J Trauma 1989;29(5):541–8.

21. Bortz WM 2nd. A conceptual framework of frailty: a review. J Gerontol A Biol Sci Med Sci 2002;57(5):M283–8.

22. Buta BJ, Walston JD, Godino JG, et al. Frailty assessment instruments: systematic characterization of the uses and contexts of highly-cited instruments. Ageing Res Rev 2016;26:53–61.

23. Orouji Jokar T, Ibraheem K, Rhee P, et al. Emergency general surgery specific frailty index: a validation study. J Trauma Acute Care Surg 2016;81(2):254–60.

24. Joseph B, Zangbar B, Pandit V, et al. Emergency general surgery in the elderly: too old or too frail? J Am Coll Surg 2016;222(5):805–13.

25. Tan MP, Kamaruzzaman SB, Zakaria MI, et al. Ten-year mortality in older patients attending the emergency department after a fall. Geriatr Gerontol Int 2016;16(1):111–7.

26. Orive M, Anton-Ladislao A, Garcia-Gutierrez S, et al. Prospective study of predictive factors of changes in pain and hip function after hip fracture among the elderly. Osteoporos Int 2016;27(2):527–36.

27. Maxwell CA, Mion LC, Mukherjee K, et al. Preinjury physical frailty and cognitive impairment among geriatric trauma patients determine postinjury functional recovery and survival. J Trauma Acute Care Surg 2016;80(2):195–203.

28. Dunham CM, Chance EA, Hileman BM, et al. Geriatric preinjury activities of daily living function is associated with glasgow coma score and discharge disposition: a retrospective, consecutive cohort study. J Trauma Nurs 2015;22(1):6–13.

29. Joseph B, Pandit V, Rhee P, et al. Predicting hospital discharge disposition in geriatric trauma patients: is frailty the answer? J Trauma Acute Care Surg 2014;76(1):196–200.

30. Joseph B, Pandit V, Zangbar B, et al. Validating trauma-specific frailty index for geriatric trauma patients: a prospective analysis. J Am Coll Surg 2014;219(1):10–7.e1.

31. Joseph B, Pandit V, Zangbar B, et al. Superiority of frailty over age in predicting outcomes among geriatric trauma patients: a prospective analysis. JAMA Surg 2014;149(8):766–72.

32. Nevitt MC, Cummings SR. Type of fall and risk of hip and wrist fractures: the study of osteoporotic fractures. J Am Geriatr Soc 1994;42(8):909.

33. Sran MM, Stotz PJ, Normandin SC, et al. Age differences in energy absorption in the upper extremity during a descent movement: implications for arresting a fall. J Gerontol A Biol Sci Med Sci 2010;65(3):312–7.

34. Lee WY, Yee WY, Cameron PA, et al. Road traffic injuries in the elderly. Emerg Med J 2006;23(1):42–6.

35. McGwin G Jr, Metzger J, Moran SG, et al. Occupant- and collision-related risk factors for blunt thoracic aorta injury. J Trauma 2003;54(4):655–60 [discussion: 660–2].

36. National Highway Traffic Safety Administration. National Center for Statistics and Analysis. U.S. Department of Transportation. Washington DC. Traffic Safety Facts 2014. 2014.

37. Henry SM, Pollak AN, Jones AL, et al. Pelvic fracture in geriatric patients: a distinct clinical entity. J Trauma 2002;53(1):15–20.
38. Bradburn E, Rogers FB, Krasne M, et al. High-risk geriatric protocol: improving mortality in the elderly. J Trauma Acute Care Surg 2012;73(2):435–40.
39. Kanezaki S, Miyazaki M, Notani N, et al. Clinical presentation of geriatric poly-trauma patients with severe pelvic fractures: comparison with younger adult patients. Eur J Orthop Surg Traumatol 2016;26(8):885–90.
40. Keller JM, Sciadini MF, Sinclair E, et al. Geriatric trauma: demographics, injuries, and mortality. J Orthop Trauma 2012;26(9):e161–5.
41. Ohmori T, Kitamura T, Tanaka K, et al. Bleeding sites in elderly trauma patients who required massive transfusion: a comparison with younger patients. Am J Emerg Med 2016;34(2):123–7.
42. Perel P, Prieto-Merino D, Shakur H, et al. Predicting early death in patients with traumatic bleeding: development and validation of prognostic model. BMJ 2012;345:e5166.
43. Pacagnella RC, Souza JP, Durocher J, et al. A systematic review of the relation-ship between blood loss and clinical signs. PLoS One 2013;8(3):e57594.
44. Martin JT, Alkhoury F, O'Connor JA, et al. 'Normal' vital signs belie occult hypo-perfusion in geriatric trauma patients. Am Surg 2010;76(1):65–9.
45. Brooks SE, Mukherjee K, Gunter OL, et al. Do models incorporating comorbidities outperform those incorporating vital signs and injury pattern for predicting mortal-ity in geriatric trauma? J Am Coll Surg 2014;219(5):1020–7.
46. Newgard CD, Holmes JF, Haukoos JS, et al. Improving early identification of the high-risk elderly trauma patient by emergency medical services. Injury 2016; 47(1):19–25.
47. Heffernan DS, Thakkar RK, Monaghan SF, et al. Normal presenting vital signs are unreliable in geriatric blunt trauma victims. J Trauma 2010;69(4):813–20.
48. Wesley K, Wesley K. TRIAGING GERIATRICS. 110 is the new 90 for systolic blood pressure in elderly patients. JEMS 2015;40(10):29.
49. Phillips S, Rond PC 3rd, Kelly SM, et al. The failure of triage criteria to identify geriatric patients with trauma: results from the Florida Trauma Triage Study. J Trauma 1996;40(2):278–83.
50. Fligor SC, Hamill ME, Love KM, et al. Vital signs strongly predict massive trans-fusion need in geriatric trauma patients. Am Surg 2016;82(7):632–6.
51. Rau CS, Wu SC, Kuo SC, et al. Prediction of massive transfusion in trauma pa-tients with shock index, modified shock index, and age shock index. Int J Environ Res Public Health 2016;13(7) [pii:E683].
52. Ohmori T, Kitamura T, Ishihara J, et al. Early predictors for massive transfusion in older adult severe trauma patients. Injury 2017;48(5):1006–12.
53. Kim SY, Hong KJ, Shin SD, et al. Validation of the shock index, modified shock index, and age shock index for predicting mortality of geriatric trauma patients in emergency departments. J Korean Med Sci 2016;31(12):2026–32.
54. Zarzaur BL, Croce MA, Fischer PE, et al. New vitals after injury: shock index for the young and age x shock index for the old. J Surg Res 2008;147(2):229–36.
55. Callaway DW, Shapiro NI, Donnino MW, et al. Serum lactate and base deficit as predictors of mortality in normotensive elderly blunt trauma patients. J Trauma 2009;66(4):1040–4.
56. Nirula R, Gentilello LM. Futility of resuscitation criteria for the "young" old and the "old" old trauma patient: a national trauma data bank analysis. J Trauma 2004; 57(1):37–41.

57. Zehtabchi S, Baron BJ. Utility of base deficit for identifying major injury in elder trauma patients. Acad Emerg Med 2007;14(9):829–31.

58. Dunne JR, Tracy JK, Scalea TM, et al. Lactate and base deficit in trauma: does alcohol or drug use impair their predictive accuracy? J Trauma 2005;58(5): 959–66.

59. Kaplan LJ, Frangos S. Clinical review: acid-base abnormalities in the intensive care unit – part II. Crit Care 2005;9(2):198–203.

60. Rossaint R, Bouillon B, Cerny V, et al. The European guideline on management of major bleeding and coagulopathy following trauma: fourth edition. Crit Care 2016;20:100.

61. Blow O, Magliore L, Claridge JA, et al. The golden hour and the silver day: detection and correction of occult hypoperfusion within 24 hours improves outcome from major trauma. J Trauma 1999;47(5):964–9.

62. Claridge JA, Crabtree TD, Pelletier SJ, et al. Persistent occult hypoperfusion is associated with a significant increase in infection rate and mortality in major trauma patients. J Trauma 2000;48(1):8–14 [discussion: 14–5].

63. Thom O, Taylor DM, Wolfe RE, et al. Pilot study of the prevalence, outcomes and detection of occult hypoperfusion in trauma patients. Emerg Med J 2010;27(6): 470–2.

64. Salottolo KM, Mains CW, Offner PJ, et al. A retrospective analysis of geriatric trauma patients: venous lactate is a better predictor of mortality than traditional vital signs. Scand J Trauma Resusc Emerg Med 2013;21:7.

65. Schulman AM, Claridge JA, Young JS. Young versus old: factors affecting mortality after blunt traumatic injury. Am Surg 2002;68(11):942–7 [discussion: 947–8].

66. Bourg P, Richey M, Salottolo K, et al. Development of a geriatric resuscitation protocol, utilization compliance, and outcomes. J Trauma Nurs 2012;19(1):50–6.

67. Bar-Or D, Salottolo KM, Orlando A, et al. Association between a geriatric trauma resuscitation protocol using venous lactate measurements and early trauma surgeon involvement and mortality risk. J Am Geriatr Soc 2013;61(8):1358–64.

68. Meldon SW, Reilly M, Drew BL, et al. Trauma in the very elderly: a community-based study of outcomes at trauma and nontrauma centers. J Trauma 2002; 52(1):79–84.

69. Werman HA, Erskine T, Caterino J, et al, Members of the Trauma Committee of the State of Ohio EMSB. Development of statewide geriatric patients trauma triage criteria. Prehosp Disaster Med 2011;26(3):170–9.

70. Newgard CD, Staudenmayer K, Hsia RY, et al. The cost of overtriage: more than one-third of low-risk injured patients were taken to major trauma centers. Health Aff (Millwood) 2013;32(9):1591–9.

71. Zafar SN, Shah AA, Zogg CK, et al. Morbidity or mortality? Variations in trauma centres in the rescue of older injured patients. Injury 2016;47(5):1091–7.

72. Lehmann R, Beekley A, Casey L, et al. The impact of advanced age on trauma triage decisions and outcomes: a statewide analysis. Am J Surg 2009;197(5): 571–4 [discussion: 574–5].

73. Demetriades D, Sava J, Alo K, et al. Old age as a criterion for trauma team activation. J Trauma 2001;51(4):754–6 [discussion: 756–7].

74. Rehn M, Eken T, Krüger AJ, et al. Precision of field triage in patients brought to a trauma centre after introducing trauma team activation guidelines. Scand J Trauma Resusc Emerg Med 2009;17:1.

75. St John AE, Rowhani-Rahbar A, Arbabi S, et al. Role of trauma team activation in poor outcomes of elderly patients. J Surg Res 2016;203(1):95–102.

76. Sharpe JP, Magnotti LJ, Weinberg JA, et al. The old man and the C-spine fracture: impact of halo vest stabilization in patients with blunt cervical spine fractures. J Trauma Acute Care Surg 2016;80(1):76–80.

77. Ryang YM, Török E, Janssen I, et al. Early morbidity and mortality in 50 very elderly patients after posterior atlantoaxial fusion for traumatic odontoid fractures. World Neurosurg 2016;87:381–91.

78. Giannoulis D, Calori GM, Giannoudis PV. Thirty-day mortality after hip fractures: has anything changed? Eur J Orthop Surg Traumatol 2016;26(4):365–70.

79. Schnell S, Friedman SM, Mendelson DA, et al. The 1-year mortality of patients treated in a hip fracture program for elders. Geriatr Orthop Surg Rehabil 2010; 1(1):6–14.

80. Gomez D, Haas B, Hemmila M, et al. Hips can lie: impact of excluding isolated hip fractures on external benchmarking of trauma center performance. J Trauma 2010;69(5):1037–41.

81. Dams-O'Connor K, Cuthbert JP, Whyte J, et al. Traumatic brain injury among older adults at level I and II trauma centers. J Neurotrauma 2013;30(24):2001–13.

82. Brazinova A, Rehorcikova V, Taylor MS, et al. Epidemiology of traumatic brain injury in Europe: a living systematic review. J Neurotrauma 2016. [Epub ahead of print].

83. Faul M, Xu L, Sasser SM. Hospitalized traumatic brain injury: low trauma center utilization and high interfacility transfers among older adults. Prehosp Emerg Care 2016;20(5):594–600.

84. Faul M, Coronado V. Epidemiology of traumatic brain injury. Handb Clin Neurol 2015;127:3–13.

85. Kehoe A, Smith JE, Bouamra O, et al. Older patients with traumatic brain injury present with a higher GCS score than younger patients for a given severity of injury. Emerg Med J 2016;33(6):381–5.

86. Salottolo K, Levy AS, Slone DS, et al. The effect of age on Glasgow Coma Scale score in patients with traumatic brain injury. JAMA Surg 2014;149(7):727–34.

87. Jennett B, Teasdale G, Braakman R, et al. Prognosis of patients with severe head injury. Neurosurgery 1979;4(4):283–9.

88. Kehoe A, Rennie S, Smith JE. Glasgow Coma Scale is unreliable for the prediction of severe head injury in elderly trauma patients. Emerg Med J 2015;32(8): 613–5.

89. Kirkman MA, Jenks T, Bouamra O, et al. Increased mortality associated with cerebral contusions following trauma in the elderly: bad patients or bad management? J Neurotrauma 2013;30(16):1385–90.

90. Bruns J Jr, Hauser WA. The epidemiology of traumatic brain injury: a review. Epilepsia 2003;44(Suppl 10):2–10.

91. Scheetz LJ, Horst MA, Arbour RB. Early neurological deterioration in older adults with traumatic brain injury. Int Emerg Nurs 2017. [Epub ahead of print].

92. Boltz MM, Podany AB, Hollenbeak CS, et al. Injuries and outcomes associated with traumatic falls in the elderly population on oral anticoagulant therapy. Injury 2015;46(9):1765–71.

93. Smith K, Weeks S. The impact of pre-injury anticoagulation therapy in the older adult patient experiencing a traumatic brain injury: a systematic review. JBI Libr Syst Rev 2012;10(58):4610–21.

94. Wutzler S, Lefering R, Wafaisade A, et al. Aggressive operative treatment of isolated blunt traumatic brain injury in the elderly is associated with favourable outcome. Injury 2015;46(9):1706–11.

95. Matsushima K, Inaba K, Siboni S, et al. Emergent operation for isolated severe traumatic brain injury: does time matter? J Trauma Acute Care Surg 2015; 79(5):838–42.

96. Haller CS, Delhumeau C, De Pretto M, et al. Trajectory of disability and quality-of-life in non-geriatric and geriatric survivors after severe traumatic brain injury. Brain Inj 2017;31(3):319–28.

97. Farrow LS, Smith TO, Ashcroft GP, et al. A systematic review of tranexamic acid in hip fracture surgery. Br J Clin Pharmacol 2016;82(6):1458–70.

98. Hwabejire JO, Kaafarani HM, Lee J, et al. Patterns of injury, outcomes, and predictors of in-hospital and 1-year mortality in nonagenarian and centenarian trauma patients. JAMA Surg 2014;149(10):1054–9.

99. Jawa RS, Shapiro MJ, McCormack JE, et al. Preadmission do not resuscitate advanced directive is associated with adverse outcomes following acute traumatic injury. Am J Surg 2015;210(5):814–21.

The Kids Are Alright
Pediatric Trauma Pearls

Angelo Mikrogianakis, MD, FRCPC[a,b,*], Vincent Grant, MD, FRCPC[a,b]

KEYWORDS

- Pediatric trauma • Pediatric primary survey • Pediatric airway • Pediatric C-spine
- Pediatric head trauma • Pediatric trauma diagnostic imaging
- Transport of the pediatric patients with trauma • Pediatric trauma simulation

KEY POINTS

- Initial resuscitation and stabilization of pediatric patients with trauma is of critical importance.
- There are special differences to consider in the ABCs (airway, breathing, circulation) of pediatric trauma care.
- Clinicians should know the goals of pediatric trauma resuscitation.
- Common injury patterns, physiologic differences, and treatment approaches used in pediatric trauma centers may differ from those in adult trauma practices.

INTRODUCTION

Pediatric patients with trauma pose unique challenges, both practical and cognitive, to front-line care providers. Emergency physicians are already skilled at resuscitating and stabilizing patients with trauma. The initial resuscitation of a traumatized child should follow the same Advanced Trauma Life Support (ATLS) principles used with adult trauma resuscitations. Therefore, trained emergency physicians have all the skills and competencies required to manage acutely injured children. What is sometimes lacking is the confidence and experience required to understand the common injury patterns, physiologic differences, and treatment approaches used in pediatric trauma centers, which may differ from adult trauma practices.

Children have anatomic, physiologic, and metabolic differences that are well described in textbooks and the medical literature.[1,2] It is the combination of these factors that leads to unique injury patterns with different approaches and responses to

Disclosure: The authors have nothing to disclose.
[a] Department of Pediatrics, Alberta Children's Hospital, University of Calgary, 2888 Shaganappi Trail Northwest, Calgary, Alberta T3B 6A8, Canada; [b] Department of Emergency Medicine, Cumming School of Medicine, University of Calgary, Calgary, Alberta, Canada
* Corresponding author. Department of Pediatrics, Alberta Children's Hospital, 2888 Shaganappi Trail Northwest, Calgary, Alberta T3B 6A8, Canada.
E-mail address: angelo.mikrogianakis@albertahealthservices.ca

Emerg Med Clin N Am 36 (2018) 237–257
https://doi.org/10.1016/j.emc.2017.08.015
0733-8627/18/© 2017 Elsevier Inc. All rights reserved.

treatment compared with adults. A similar traumatic mechanism can lead to slightly different internal injuries with unique management and treatment strategies between the two groups.

This article is intended for community, nonpediatric trauma center, emergency physicians who are frequently called on to assess, resuscitate, and stabilize injured children before they can be safely transferred to a pediatric trauma center for ongoing definitive care and rehabilitation.

This article focuses on the most common and practical pointers regarding pediatric patients with trauma with a blunt mechanism of injury. It does not focus on penetrating traumatic injuries. Most pediatric patients with blunt trauma are not rushed to the operating room (OR) for emergency surgery. Most pediatric patients with trauma with a blunt mechanism of injury respond and stabilize with an appropriate initial medical resuscitation. Well-resuscitated and stabilized patients are then able to be transported safely to a pediatric trauma center for ongoing definitive care and rehabilitation.

Typical Emergency Medical Services Patch Call

A 5-year-old boy, injured while crossing the street when he was struck by a vehicle at city speeds ($\sim$50 km/h). He is crying and pale, with a hematoma to the left forehead; bruising to the left side of the upper abdomen; and an obvious, closed, deformity of his left tibia and fibula. His vital signs are heart rate (HR), 135 beats/min, respiration rate (RR), 30 breaths/min; blood pressure (BP), 95/65 mm Hg; and O_2 saturations of 91% on room air, which improve to 97% with supplemental O_2.

Key issues to focus on:

- Based on their anatomy, children respond to external forces like bobble-head figurines. They have a large cranium on a short, weak, neck. There is usually some component of head injury (mild, moderate or severe) that needs to be managed. Supportive therapy for traumatic brain injury (TBI) is the mainstay of treatment. Ongoing, active assessment for signs and symptoms of increased intracranial pressure (ICP) is required. Clinical signs of increased ICP necessitate active treatments focused on reducing ICP.
- Cervical spine (C-spine) injuries are rare but C-spine protection and assessment are important. Be concerned about young, nonverbal children who do not move their necks. Be reassured but cautious with young, nonverbal children who freely turn their heads while crying.
- Pulmonary contusions are the most common intrathoracic injuries. Pneumothorax and hemothorax occur less frequently than in adults because of the flexibility of the bones in the rib cage and the transmission of blunt force to the organs and tissues underneath.
- Intra-abdominal injuries most commonly involve bleeding of the large solid organs (ie, spleen and liver).
- Orthopedic injuries and pain management are also common considerations in pediatric patients with multitrauma. Be concerned when children are lying still and not freely moving an extremity. Be reassured when children are spontaneously moving their arms and legs, because they are less likely to have a significant fracture in that limb. Pain and hypovolemia are both common causes of tachycardia, so they need to be addressed in the initial approach to the patient.

PRIMARY SURVEY

ATLS principles for initial assessment are the same in pediatric patients as in adult patients with trauma. The ABCDE (airway, breathing, circulation, disability, expose) cognitive model is organized to identify and treat life-threatening issues as soon as possible.[3] A Broselow tape and color-coded pediatric resuscitation equipment system (eg, cart, bags) should be readily available so that unnecessary challenges and delays in locating the proper-sized equipment can be minimized. Continuous monitoring of vital signs is essential for ongoing assessment of response to interventions. A vigilant algorithm of assess, reassess, and reassess again must be maintained to accurately follow a patient's positive trajectory toward improvement and stabilization, or to quickly recognize and respond to a patient's deterioration, which would require more aggressive resuscitation and treatment. Call for assistance as early as necessary. Mobilize transport teams and obtain clinical support and advice from pediatric experts as early as possible. There is no shame in calling for advice. Pediatric experts are always willing to assist, advise, and accept patients in transfer. Pediatric trauma centers do not put up obstacles to patient transfer and should always be there to assist their community partners.

Pediatric Primary Survey: Airway, Breathing, Circulation, Disability, Exposure

A talking or crying child has a patent airway, is breathing spontaneously, and has sufficient BP to maintain cerebral perfusion and could be considered stable initially.[4] In contrast, a quiet, nonvocalizing child with an altered level of consciousness (LOC) likely has severe, multisystem injuries.[4] Emergency departments (EDs) should be equipped with a quick and accessible reference for age-specific vital signs as well as tips for key numbers to remember or cutoffs to keep in mind. Check vital signs, temperature, and glucose level immediately. On initiating assessment of the ABCDEs, make sure to oxygenate, start intravenous lines, and begin fluid resuscitation.

- Airway with C-spine protection:
  - Clear secretions, and assess patency and need for immediate tracheal intubation
    - Indications for early intubation include[5,6]:
    - Airway obstruction, unrelieved by simple maneuvers.
    - Apnea.
    - Cardiac arrest.
    - Decreasing LOC (airway protection and control of CO_2).
    - Severe maxillofacial trauma.
    - Inhalation injury.
  - Focus on oxygenation. Always be prepared to support pediatric patients with good quality bag-valve-mask (BVM) ventilation. BVM maintains oxygenation and compensates for poor respiratory effort while providing time to smoothly and properly prepare for a pediatric intubation in the adult ED (**Fig. 1**).
  - Most pediatric patients can be oxygenated using O_2 or BVM initially until the primary survey can be completed and intubation equipment and drugs can be prepared. BVM is the key airway skill for non–pediatric emergency medicine physicians. The ability to properly maintain a mask fit, provide continuous positive airway pressure (CPAP), and bag-mask ventilate is a more valuable skill than being able to intubate the trachea.[5]
  - For successful BVM, ensure a tight seal and use high-flow oxygen. Be sure to apply CPAP as well as a jaw thrust and chin lift. If tolerated, an oral airway may assist by lifting an obtunded child's large tongue off the posterior pharyngeal wall. Use a 2-handed mask support technique if having difficulties in achieving an adequate seal and fit.[5]

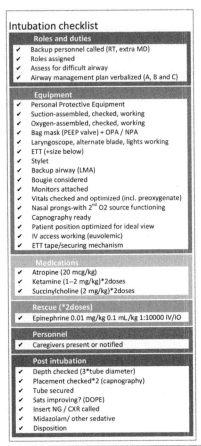

Intubation checklist

Roles and duties
- ✓ Backup personnel called (RT, extra MD)
- ✓ Roles assigned
- ✓ Assess for difficult airway
- ✓ Airway management plan verbalized (A, B and C)

Equipment
- ✓ Personal Protective Equipment
- ✓ Suction-assembled, checked, working
- ✓ Oxygen-assembled, checked, working
- ✓ Bag mask (PEEP valve) + OPA / NPA
- ✓ Laryngoscope, alternate blade, lights working
- ✓ ETT (+size below)
- ✓ Stylet
- ✓ Backup airway (LMA)
- ✓ Bougie considered
- ✓ Monitors attached
- ✓ Vitals checked and optimized (incl. preoxygenate)
- ✓ Nasal prongs-with 2nd O2 source functioning
- ✓ Capnography ready
- ✓ Patient position optimized for ideal view
- ✓ IV access working (euvolemic)
- ✓ ETT tape/securing mechanism

Medications
- ✓ Atropine (20 mcg/kg)
- ✓ Ketamine (1–2 mg/kg)*2doses
- ✓ Succinylcholine (2 mg/kg)*2doses

Rescue (*2doses)
- ✓ Epinephrine 0.01 mg/kg 0.1 mL/kg 1:10000 IV/IO

Personnel
- ✓ Caregivers present or notified

Post intubation
- ✓ Depth checked (3*tube diameter)
- ✓ Placement checked*2 (capnography)
- ✓ Tube secured
- ✓ Sats improving? (DOPE)
- ✓ Insert NG / CXR called
- ✓ Midazolam/ other sedative
- ✓ Disposition

Age	Wgt kg	Uncuff ETT	Cuffed ETT	Blade (MAC)	Straight Blade	Depth cm	LMA	AirQ LMA	OPA	NPA
Prem	<3	2.5 – 3		0	0 or 1	7–8	0 to 1		Pink	12F
Term	>3	3 – 3.5	2.5 – 3	0	0 or 1	8–9	0 to 1	1.0	Blue	14F
6 – 12mo	6	3.5 – 4	3 – 3.5	1	1	10	1 to 1.5			14–16F
1	11	4	3.5	1 or 2	1 or 2	11	1.5	1.5	Black	18F
2	13	4.5	4	2	2	12	2			20F
3	15			2	2					22F
4	17	5	4.5	2	2	13		1.5 – 2		22F
5	19			2	2				White	24F
6	21	5.5	5	2	2	14	2.5	2		
7	23			2	3					
8		6	5.5	3	3	16			Green	26F
9				3	3					
10		6.5	6	3	3	18	3	2.5		

All sizes to be confirmed clinically before use. Drs. Michelle McTimoney, Dominique Eustace and Martin Gauthier. Last updated March 2015

Fig. 1. Intubation checklist (front and back). *, times; ETT, endotracheal tube; LMA, laryngeal mask airway; MD, doctor of medicine; NPA, nasopharyngeal airway; OPA, oropharyngeal airway; PEEP, positive end-expiratory pressure; RT, respiratory therapist.

○ Ensure adequate C-spine protection, particularly when moving the patient. A collar should be on all school-aged and adolescent children. Rolls and tape should be used for infants and toddlers.

- Breathing:
  - Assess for adequacy of respirations (spontaneous effort, breath sounds, and oxygen saturation levels).
  - Apply supplemental oxygen to all pediatric patients with trauma. Children desaturate quickly. It is important to prevent hypoxia.
    - O_2 by face mask in older patients. O_2 flow rate of 6 to 10 L/min.
    - O_2 by nasal prongs or mask in infants. O_2 flow rate of 2 L/min in infants/children less than 2 years of age. Flow rate of 4 L/min for children more than 2 years of age.
  - If the patient is intubated in the field, always reassess respirations bilaterally and confirm endotracheal tube (ETT) position after arriving in the ED.
    - Because of the short length of the trachea, right mainstem intubations are common in children. Always consider this if there are decreased breath sounds from the right chest.
    - Monitor the patient's end-tidal CO_2 continuously.
  - Insert a nasogastric (NG) tube to decompress the stomach; this is especially important if the child is difficult to ventilate or the child's stomach is becoming distended from BVM. A distended stomach interferes with ventilation.
- Circulation with control of external hemorrhage:
  - The accurate assessment of circulation and the adequate resuscitation of shock are ongoing challenges for those health care providers who do not treat pediatric trauma on a regular basis.
  - The most common cause of shock in pediatric patients with trauma is hypovolemia caused by bleeding.
  - Some of the most common bleeding sites are spleen, liver, pelvis, scalp, long bone fractures, and hemothorax.
  - The circulating blood volume in a child is only 80 mL/kg. Therefore, in smaller children, even a small amount of blood loss can have a significant impact on hemodynamics and perfusion.
  - Start 1 to 2 intravenous (IV) lines and draw trauma blood work while the ABCDEs are being assessed.
    - Order crossmatch or type and screen.
  - If unable to establish rapid intravenous access in an unstable patient, then insert an intraosseous (IO) line to begin the resuscitation.
  - When first intravenous/intraosseous access is established, give 20 mL/kg normal saline (NS) crystalloid bolus to start treatment while completing the assessment. Monitor HR (tachycardia), check capillary refill, and assess for sites of bleeding (abdomen, pelvis, long bone fractures). Hypotension is a late sign of decompensated shock.
  - Use warmed solutions if the patient is already cold. Prevent hypothermia.
  - Use a rapid infuser if a patient is unstable or decompensating and it is necessary to deliver volume support more quickly. Young children may require the push-pull method of fluid delivery by a syringe. Regular intravenous infusion pumps are too slow and should not be used in the initial stabilization of patients with trauma.
  - Be wary of tachycardia and signs of peripheral vasoconstriction (delayed capillary refill, cool extremities, weak peripheral pulses). Do not wait for BP to decrease. Compensated shock can quickly lead to rapid decompensation and arrest.
  - If the patient has not stabilized after the second 20-mL/kg bolus of NS crystalloid, then prepare to give 10 to 20 mL/kg of blood (uncrossmatched or type specific).

- o Assess for and control obvious sources of bleeding (eg, blood-soaked clothing).
  - Internal bleeding (bulging abdomen, hemothorax) requires aggressive resuscitation toward definitive management.
  - If there is a suspicion of an obvious open-book pelvic fracture, wrap or splint the pelvis to decrease blood loss.
- o Most pediatric patients with trauma do not require an urgent trauma laparotomy or thoracotomy in the OR and stabilize when resuscitated properly.
- Disability:
  - o Conduct a brief neurologic examination and check neurologic responses.
  - o Spontaneous movement.
  - o Sensation or complaints of pain.
  - o Responsiveness to voice.
  - o Assess Glasgow Coma Scale (GCS) score (Pediatric GCS). The AVPU (alert, voice, pain, unresponsive) test can be a useful surrogate for GCS. In general, patients who are either P or U have a GCS less than 8 and cannot protect their own airways.
- Expose patient:
  - o Assess all surface areas (including diaper) while preventing risk of hypothermia by keeping the trauma room warm and covering the patient with warm blankets after the assessment.
  - o Quickly conduct a musculoskeletal assessment for obvious limb deformities (**Box 1**).

Recently Published Innovations That May Affect the Primary Survey

Acker and colleagues[7] recently attempted to improve on shock recognition and treatment. A novel look at the shock index, pediatric age adjusted (SIPA) may be able to predict severity more accurately than BP alone. Hypotension alone (systolic BP [SBP] <90 mm Hg for ages 4–6 years; SBP <100 mm Hg for ages 7–16 years) predicted need for the OR (13%), ETT (17%), and transfusion (22%). SIPA score (defined as HR divided by systolic BP) predicts the need for OR (30%), ETT (40%), and transfusion (53%).[7] Because tachycardia is an early but nonspecific indicator of hypovolemia and SBP is a specific but late marker of hypovolemia, it makes sense that combining the two measures into the SIPA may improve the ability to predict the need for important interventions such as OR, intubation, or blood transfusion.

Golden and colleagues[8] studied whether or not admission hematocrit could predict the need for transfusion secondary to hemorrhage in pediatric patients with blunt trauma. They found a significant decrease in admission hematocrit for patients requiring a transfusion. Cutoff admission hematocrit of 35% or less had a sensitivity of 94% and negative predictive value of 99.9% in identifying children who needed a transfusion after blunt trauma.[8]

Obtaining trauma laboratory tests in pediatric patients can be a challenge. The future may involve noninvasive methods of assessment. Ryan and colleagues[9] studied a novel, noninvasive hemoglobin measurement device. The pulse co-oximeter (Pronto device) was studied in 114 patients. There was good correlation between hemoglobin levels across various methods of measurement, including noninvasive strategies.[9]

Diagnostic Imaging for Blunt Pediatric Trauma at Referring Center Before Transport

The ninth edition of ATLS recommends only chest and pelvic radiographs for patients with blunt trauma at the referring center before transport.[3] For children whose C-spines cannot be clinically cleared, a lateral neck radiograph may be used as a screening tool

---

Box 1
Back to the case: summary of airway, breathing, circulation, disability, exposure survey and initial actions

Airway

- Patent; no obvious injury or obstruction

Breathing

- Good, spontaneous effort, mildly tachypneic at 30 breaths/min
- O_2 saturation is good at 97% on 10 L/min by face mask
- Decreased breath sounds to LLL with bruising
- Trachea midline

Circulation

- Tachycardic at 135 beats/min
- Abdomen tender in LUQ with bruising
- Pelvis stable and nontender
- Capillary refill 3 seconds centrally and 4 seconds peripherally

Disability

- Eyes closed, opens to speech, confused, obeys commands
- Patient is verbal (V in AVPU score); GCS = 13

Exposure

- Closed deformity of left tibia/fibula, good pulses
- No other obvious injuries

Actions

- Maintain O_2 saturation with supplemental oxygen
- Start intravenous line and give 20 mL/kg of NS
- Draw trauma laboratory tests
- Maintain C-spine precautions

Abbreviations: LLL, left lower lobe; LUQ, left upper quadrant.

---

but is not mandatory as long as the C-spine remains immobilized and protected. Pelvic radiographs on pediatric patients may be omitted in children at low risk for fracture with a normal GCS and normal hemodynamic status without any signs of abdominal trauma, abnormalities on pelvic examination, or an associated femur fracture or hematuria.[10]

- C-spine radiograph: may be done if unable to clinically clear or may be deferred if child is left in cervical collar for transport
- Chest radiograph: yes
- Pelvic radiograph: yes, if suspicion of pelvic fracture or hemodynamic instability
- Computed tomography (CT) imaging: should not delay transport; usually best decision is to allow the pediatric trauma center to perform CT imaging

Puckett and colleagues[11] recently studied advanced imaging at referral centers before transfer to designated pediatric trauma centers and concluded that advanced imaging at referral centers exposes children to excess radiation. Overall, the mean radiation dosing was 54% lower at pediatric trauma centers (51% lower for CT abdomen and pelvis and 62% lower for CT head). These findings support the ATLS recommendation for prompt transfer without delay for advanced imaging.[11] Therefore, do not delay transfer to definitive treatment with investigations that are likely to need to be repeated and will not aid the immediate clinical management (**Box 2**).

HEAD INJURY

Many pediatric patients with trauma present with a component of TBI, which can be mild, moderate, or severe. Resuscitative efforts must preserve cerebral perfusion pressure (CPP) without increasing ICP. Remember that the CPP is the difference between the mean arterial pressure and the ICP (CPP = MAP − ICP). Initial principles of TBI management are the same in adult and pediatric patients with similar goals of therapy. First, do no harm. Provide the necessary supportive therapies of the primary survey and initial resuscitation. Avoid secondary neuronal injury by preventing hypoxia and hypotension. Further ICP spikes are preventable with appropriate administration of analgesics and anxiolytic agents before noxious stimuli.[12]

In children, most TBI involves closed, intracranial injury without signs of increased ICP and should be managed supportively. Protect the airway if there is a low GCS, oxygenate, ventilate to normal Pco_2 (35–40 mm Hg), and resuscitate with fluid and/or blood as needed to prevent hypotension and maintain CPP.[3]

Less frequently, children have closed, intracranial injuries with signs of increased ICP (depressed LOC plus asymmetric pupils or bradycardia, hypertension, and/or irregular respirations). This situation requires recognition and aggressive medical treatment by raising the head of the bed, moderate hyperventilation (Pco_2 30–35 mm Hg) and medical treatment with 3% hypertonic saline (5 mL/kg), which is preferred by pediatric centers, or mannitol (1 g/kg) if hypertonic saline is not readily available. Transfer as soon as possible for definitive neurosurgical assessment and care.[3]

A statewide study by Gross and colleagues[13] assessed patients 15 to 17 years old with severe TBI and found no significant difference in mortality (adjusted odds ratio [AOR], 0.82; $P = .754$), functional status at discharge ($P = .136$), or total complication rate (AOR, 1.21; $P = .714$) between adult and pediatric trauma centers. Clearly, the principles and goals of TBI management are similar for adults and children. Adolescents with TBI receive similar care and may have comparable outcomes. The challenges for front-line emergency care providers is the resuscitation and stabilization of young infants and children with TBI (**Box 3**).

CERVICAL SPINE

Children can be a challenge to treat, especially based on their age and developmental level. Restraining them can be problematic and those with C-spine injuries are no exception. It can also be difficult for children to communicate where their pain or neurologic symptoms are coming from. A key adage is to protect the cord and investigate later. Trauma teams must always have a high suspicion index for spinal cord

---

Box 2
Back to the case: next steps in management

Actions
- Call for lateral C-spine and chest radiograph
- Obtain focused abdominal sonography in trauma (FAST) when able

---

Box 3
Back to the case

Assess

- GCS remains 13
- No signs of increased ICP
- No signs of skull fracture or hemotympanum

Actions

- Patient has closed head injury without signs of increased ICP
- Supportive therapy
- Prevent hypoxia and hypotension
- GCS adequate, does not require intubation for airway protection

---

injuries, especially when there are multiple injuries. This high suspicion-index is maintained by ensuring proper resuscitation, protecting the spinal column, and avoiding excessive spinal manipulation. Most children do not require sedation to remain properly immobilized. Sometimes pain control, removal of the uncomfortable backboard, a parent's presence, or distraction techniques may be all that are required to immobilize the child.[14] If a patient is unstable but immobilized, spinal column evaluation can be deferred until stabilization. It is estimated that spinal cord injury occurs in 1% to 2% of pediatric patients with trauma.[15,16] The most common location of the injury (60%–80%) is in the C-spine.[17]

Note that investigating cord injuries in children requires knowing the distinct differences between the adult and pediatric spine with respect to injury patterns, anatomic variances, and radiographic characteristics.[14]

By 8 years of age, children's spines are anatomically similar to those of adults, with the important difference being that children's spines do not take on adult-type fracture patterns until early adolescence.[14,15,17] Children less than 14 years old tend to have higher C-spine injuries (C1–C4) because the immature spine's fulcrum is at the C2 to C3 level. Patients more than 14 year old tend to have lower C-spine injures (C5–C7)[17,18] because the adolescent/adult fulcrum is lower at the C5 to C6 level.[14,19,20]

The patterns of C-spine injury in children less than 10 years old tend to be dislocations and spinal cord injuries without radiographic abnormalities (SCIWORA).[17,18]

Clinically, patients with SCIWORA injuries have obvious neurologic deficits consistent with spinal cord injury on physical examination, but their routine radiographs do not show a fracture. Higher levels of imaging, such as MRI, are needed to define the exact injury.

The main reason why children are prone to dislocation and SCIWORA injuries is because of the pediatric spine's increased mobility.[17,19] The injury patterns in children more than 10 years of age tend to be fractures and are more easily identifiable on routine radiographs or CT scans.[14,17]

The trauma literature reveals conflicting recommendations on optimal C-spine imaging and questions persist as to whether radiographs or CT is a better approach. In adults, there is literature and local practice patterns that support early and aggressive CT use for patients with trauma. Pediatrics is different. The rate of C-spine injury is low. There are also potential long-term side effects of increasing doses of radiation to the entire body and the thyroid gland in C-spine imaging specifically. In light of that, pediatric algorithms are generally less aggressive. The available evidence for pediatric

C-spine clearance is limited and some is extrapolated from adult studies. The authors advocate an organized, stepwise approach to investigation and CT radiation minimization.[21] In the absence of conclusive evidence, the Trauma Association of Canada (TAC) Pediatric Subcommittee National Pediatric Cervical Spine Evaluation Pathway: Consensus Guidelines provide a logical and safe approach to the pediatric C-spine in traumatized patients (**Figs. 2** and **3**).[21]

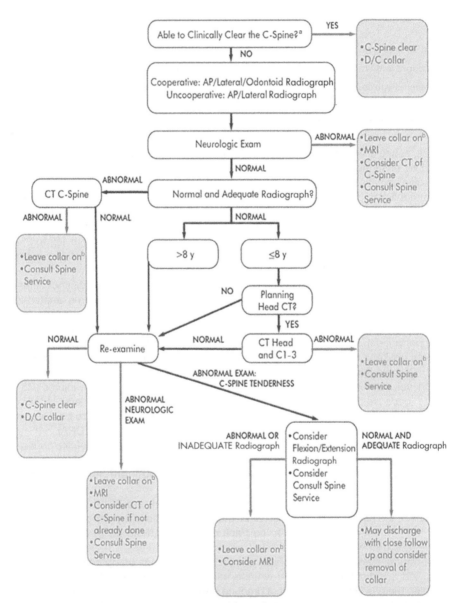

Fig. 2. TAC national pediatric C-spine evaluation pathway: reliable (Awake and alert with GCS = 15) clinical examination. [a] Meets NEXUS (National Emergency X-Radiography Utilization Study) criteria and moves head in flexion/extension and 45° to both sides with no pain. [b] Change to long-term C-spine collar as soon as appropriate.

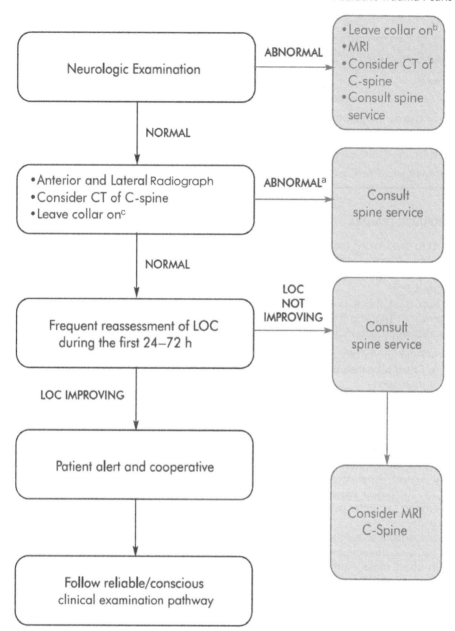

Fig. 3. TAC national pediatric C-spine evaluation pathway: unreliable (Unconscious or decreased LOC with GCS less than 15) clinical examination. [a] Consider thoracic/lumbar spine injury in patients with a documented C-spine injury. [b] Change to long-term C-spine collar as soon as appropriate.

Connelly and colleagues[22] studied limiting C-spine CT use in pediatric patients with trauma. Implementation of an institutional performance and patient safety program around C-spine imaging decreased CT rates 30% to 13% (*P*<.001), whereas radiographs increased 7% to 25% (*P*<.001). Based on these changes, they estimated a 22% (male) and 38% (female) decrease in lifetime attributable risk for any cancer (**Box 4**).[22]

Box 4
Back to the case

Assess

• Patient has some neck pain but no numbness or tingling

• Grossly normal peripheral neurologic examination

Actions

• Maintain C-spine protection

• Await lateral neck radiograph

THORACIC TRAUMA

Next to head injury, thoracic trauma is the second most common cause of mortality in pediatric trauma.[23] In multi-injured children, thoracic trauma increases mortality 20-fold. It accounts for between 4.5% and 8% of the patients cared for in pediatric trauma centers.[24,25]

Note that thoracic trauma patterns of injury differ between infants and teenagers.[24,25] Thoracic trauma injuries often result in abnormal ABCs (airway, breathing, circulation), which may require:

• Fluid and/or blood administration
• Chest tube insertion
• Intubation

Less than 10% need emergency surgery to control bleeding or air leak from the lung.[26]

A compliant and pliable chest wall results in more forces transmitted to internal organs, rather than rib fractures, meaning significant contusion and respiratory compromise in infants and children, but rarely rib fractures or externally visible chest wall signs.[23] Therefore, pulmonary contusions are the most common intrathoracic injury. Increased tissue elasticity results in increased mediastinal mobility, which seems to be protective because vascular injuries to the heart or great vessels are rare.[26,27]

Golden and colleagues[28] studied the role and influence of CT chest in the evaluation of pediatric thoracic trauma and advocate limiting its use. They studied 139 patients with chest radiograph (CXR) and CT for blunt thoracic trauma. Chest CT versus CXR increased diagnosis of contusion/atelectasis (30.3% vs 60.4%), pneumothorax (7.2% vs 18.7%), and fractures (4.3% vs 10.8%). Most importantly, chest CT only changed the management of 4 patients in their series (**Box 5**).[28]

ABDOMINAL TRAUMA

Approximately 8% to 12% of all patients with blunt trauma have intra-abdominal injuries. Although more common than thoracic injuries, abdominal injuries are 40% less fatal.[29] Mortality from solid organ injuries is typically determined by the degree of injury.[30–32]

Important anatomic differences between children and adults include[30]:

• Children are smaller, transferring kinetic energy over a smaller area.[33]
• Ribs are less calcified and more pliable, resulting in more force transmitted to thoracic and upper abdominal organs.[33]

Box 5
Back to the case

Assess

- Respiration rate, 28 breaths/min; O_2 saturation, 98% on face mask
- Trachea midline
- Respiratory effort not labored
- Review CXR
- No pneumothorax or hemothorax
- Pulmonary contusions in left lung

Actions

- Continue as doing
- Assess circulation with plan to reassess breathing

- Thinner abdominal wall and weaker musculature provide less protection to intra-abdominal organs.[33]
- Infants and young children are at higher risk for multiple organ injuries because of the close proximity of intra-abdominal organs.[33,34]

Be particularly suspicious of intra-abdominal injuries with high-risk mechanisms, including lap belts (hollow viscus injury), handle bars (pancreatic injury), snowboarding, and all-terrain vehicle incidents (liver and spleen lacerations).[30,33]

Front-line care providers must understand the most common injury patterns and use physical examination, laboratory investigations, and focused abdominal sonography in trauma (FAST) and CT to diagnose abdominal injuries in children. Most solid organ abdominal injuries are treated nonoperatively. Nonoperative treatment requires a high index of suspicion, appropriate fluid and blood resuscitation, as well as accurate diagnosis and evaluation of injuries. Contact and refer pediatric patients early for definitive care at a pediatric trauma center because most solid organ injuries in children can be managed through nonoperative treatment in experienced centers.[33] For example, nonoperative management of splenic injuries is successful in 97% of cases, with the highest success rates in pediatric trauma centers compared with adult centers. Effective nonoperative management depends on aggressive and adequate fluid and blood resuscitation. Larger volumes of blood loss may require activation of massive transfusion protocols (**Fig. 4**). Remember to insert an NG tube and indwelling urinary catheter in children with abdominal injury before transfer in order to increase the sensitivity of serial physical examinations. Although less common, hollow viscus injuries do not cause immediate hemodynamic instability and instead require performance of serial examinations to detect an evolving peritonitis.

Focused Abdominal Sonography in Trauma in Children

Intra-abdominal free fluid detected on FAST examination is not necessarily an indication for emergent laparotomy in children, as it might be in adult patients with trauma.[10] A positive FAST is useful in highlighting potential intra-abdominal bleeding and stressing the importance of appropriate and aggressive fluid and blood resuscitation. FAST examinations are not adequate to rule out intra-abdominal injuries.[10] Sola and colleagues[35] support FAST in combination with physical examination and laboratory markers to possibly forego the use of abdominal CT scans in low-risk children.

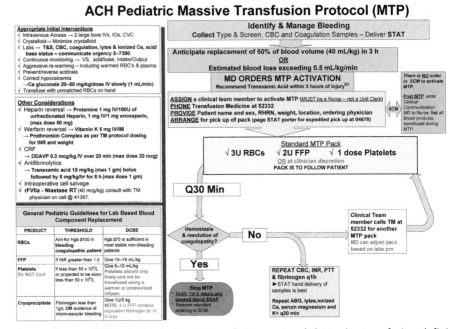

ACH Pediatric Massive Transfusion Protocol (MTP)

Appropriate Initial Interventions
- √ Intravenous Access → 2 large bore IVs, IOs, CVC
- √ Crystalloid → Minimize crystalloid
- √ Labs → T&S, CBC, coagulation, lytes & ionized Ca, acid/ base status – communicate urgency 5–7390
- √ Continuous monitoring → VS, acid/base, Intake/Output
- √ Aggressive re-warming – including warmed RBC's & plasma
- √ Prevent/reverse acidosis
- √ Correct hypocalcemia
  →Ca gluconate 20–50 mg/kg/dose IV slowly (1 mL/min)
- √ Transfuse with unmatched RBCs on hand

Other Considerations
- √ Heparin reversal → Protamine 1 mg IV/100U of unfractionated Heparin, 1 mg IV/1 mg enoxaparin, (max dose 50 mg)
- √ Warfarin reversal → Vitamin K 5 mg IV/IM
  → Prothrombin Complex as per TM protocol dosing for INR and weight
- √ CRF
  → DDAVP 0.3 mcg/kg IV over 20 min (max dose 20 mcg)
- √ Antifibrinolytics:
  → Tranexamic acid 15 mg/kg (max 1 gm) bolus followed by 5 mg/kg/hr for 8 h (max dose 1 gm)
- √ Intraoperative cell salvage
- √ rFVIIa - Niastase RT (40 mcg/kg) consult with TM physician on call @ 41367.

Identify & Manage Bleeding
Collect Type & Screen, CBC and Coagulation Samples – Deliver **STAT**

Anticipate replacement of 50% of blood volume (40 mL/kg) in 3 h
OR
Estimated blood loss exceeding 0.5 mL/kg/min

MD ORDERS MTP ACTIVATION
Recommend Tranexamic Acid within 3 hours of injury[b,c]

ASSIGN a clinical team member to activate MTP (MUST be a Nurse – not a Unit Clerk)
PHONE Transfusion Medicine at 52332
PROVIDE Patient name and sex, RHRN, weight, location, ordering physician
ARRANGE for pick up of pack (page STAT porter for expedited pick up at 04678)

There is NO order in SCM to activate MTP.

Post MTP: enter Clinical Communication: MD to Nurse, list all Blood products transfused during MTP.

Standard MTP Pack
√ 3U RBCs   √ 2U FFP   √ 1 dose Platelets
OR at clinician discretion
PACK IS TO FOLLOW PATIENT

Q30 Min

General Pediatric Guidelines for Lab Based Blood Component Replacement		
PRODUCT	THRESHOLD	DOSE
RBCs	Aim for Hgb ≥100 in bleeding coagulopathic patient	Hgb ≥70 is sufficient in most stable non-bleeding patients
FFP	If INR greater than 1.5	Give 10–15 mL/kg
Platelets Do NOT Cool	If less than 50 x 10⁹/L or projected to be soon less than 50 x 10⁹/L	Give 5–10 mL/kg Platelets should drip freely and not be transfused using a warmer or pressurized infuser.
Cryoprecipitate	Fibrinogen less than 1g/L OR evidence of microvascular bleeding	Give 1U/5 kg NOTE: 4 U FFP contains equivalent fibrinogen to 10 U cryo

Hemostasis & resolution of coagulopathy?   **No**

Yes

Stop MTP
* Notify TM & return any unused blood ASAP
* Resume standard ordering in SCM

REPEAT CBC, INR, PTT & fibrinogen q1h
► STAT hand delivery of samples is best

Repeat ABG, lytes,ionized Ca, serum magnesium and K+ q30 min

Clinical Team member calls TM at 52332 for another MTP pack
MD can adjust pack based on labs prn

Fig. 4. Alberta Children's Hospital mass transfusion protocol. [a] Massive transfusion definitions: replacement of 50% of blood volume in 3 hours (40 mL/kg) or blood loss greater than 2 mL/kg/min or replacement of a blood volume (80 mL/kg) in 24 hours. [b] Royal College of Paediatrics and Child Health evidence statement: major trauma and the use of tranexamic acid in children, November 2012. [c] CRASH-2 trial collaborators. Effects of tranexamic acid on death, vascular occlusive events, and blood transfusion in trauma patients with significant haemorrhage (CRASH-2): a randomised, placebo-controlled trial. Lancet 2010;376:23.

FAST combined with aspartate transaminase or alanine transaminase levels greater than 100 IU/L is an effective screening tool for intra-abdominal injury in children following blunt abdominal trauma. Pediatric patients with negative FAST and liver transaminase levels less than 100 IU/L may be observed rather than subjected to the radiation risk of CT.[35]

The role and indications for point-of-care ultrasonography (POCUS) in pediatric trauma is a growing area of research. POCUS is being studied for its usefulness in detecting pneumothorax and as an adjunct to physical examination in assessment of volume status. A complete review of the current state of POCUS for pediatric trauma is beyond the scope of this article (**Boxes 6** and **7**).

Use of Angiography

Fenton and colleagues[36] studied angiography use in pediatric patients with blunt abdominal trauma. They studied 12,044 patients who were evaluated for blunt abdominal trauma. A total of 8% of all patients had abdominopelvic injuries. Only 3% (n = 26 patients) underwent angiography (29 procedures: 21 abdomen, 8 pelvic, 3 both). Eleven patients underwent embolization of the spleen. No hepatic, renal, or pelvic vessels were embolized. Median time to interventional radiology (IR) was 7.3 hours. These findings suggest that it may be unnecessary for pediatric trauma centers to have access to IR within 30 minutes.[36]

Box 6
Back to the case

Assess

- After first bolus of 20 mL/kg of NS patient remains HR 130 beats/min, capillary refill of 3.5 seconds
- Tenderness and bruising to LUQ with LLL pulmonary contusion
- Clinical suspicion for an acute splenic injury

Actions

- Start second bolus of 20 mL/kg of NS
- FAST study positive for free fluid in abdomen
- Call for packed red blood cells (PRBCs) or massive transfusion protocol (MTP)

Assess

- Patient remains tachycardic, pale, and poorly perfused after second NS bolus

Action

- Transfuse 10 mL/kg of PRBCs
- Call pediatric trauma center for advice, support, and transport

---

Box 7
Back to the case

Assess

- Repeat primary survey

A

- Patent, no concerns

B

- Stable, no change with good O_2 saturation on face mask

C

- HR, 100 beats/min; BP, 98/65 mm Hg; capillary refill, 2 seconds; warm extremities

Actions

- Continue intravenous hydration
- Have further PRBCs plus or minus MTP available and ready
- Splint left tibia/fibula
- Give 1 μg/kg of fentanyl if needed for pain
- Speak with pediatric trauma center
- Complete secondary survey
- Complete trauma transport checklist
- Continue to support hemodynamics as needed with fluids and blood
- Prepare patient for transport

A recent systematic review of pediatric blunt renal trauma management by LeeVan and colleagues[37] supports current conservative management protocols. Short-term and long-term outcomes are favorable in grade IV and V renal injuries. Interventions based on CT findings alone are not recommended. The review supports emergent operative management only for persistent hemodynamic instability, and minimally invasive interventions should be used when indicated (angioembolization, stenting, percutaneous drainage).[37]

Pelvic Fractures

Swaid and colleagues[38] conducted a comparison study of pelvic fractures and associated abdominal injuries between pediatric and adult patients with blunt trauma. They found a 0.8% incidence of pelvic fractures in pediatric patients compared with 4.3% in adults ($P<.0001$). Overall mortality was similar between the two groups (5.4% vs 5.2%). The only statistically significant difference in injury between pediatric patients and adults was rectal injury (1.2% pediatric vs 0.2% adult; $P<.0001$). In pediatric patients, they found no correlation between severity of pelvic fractures and severity of concomitant splenic/hepatic injuries.[38]

TRANSPORT

Pediatric patients with trauma are best cared for in centers that are prepared to treat sustained injuries.[39,40] Critically ill children have better clinical outcomes when they are treated in tertiary pediatric intensive care units (PICU).[40] The centralization of PICUs has increased the need for interhospital transport and therefore many countries have developed specialized pediatric retrieval teams that undertake the stabilization and safe transfer of critically ill children. There is good evidence that, when specialized transport teams are matched correctly, the incidence of complications is decreased.[41]

Preparing for Transport: Before Leaving the Sending Facility

Once a decision has been made to move the patient, as long as the patient is deemed safe for transport, then avoid undue delay,[39,40] especially if the patient requires definitive care or emergent surgery at a tertiary care hospital. A few details that must be taken into account are:

- Optimizing the patient's condition before transport.
- Ensuring that the patient has received a full primary and secondary survey before departure.
- Communicating with the receiving hospital before the patient's departure. Clinicians must be able to anticipate patient care needs during transport and be prepared to manage those needs (**Box 8**).

Pediatric Trauma Training Using Simulation-Based Education

Severe pediatric blunt trauma is a high-acuity, low-frequency situation that requires both clinical competence and team confidence. The authors highly support and advocate multi-disciplinary, simulation-based training in pediatric trauma resuscitation.

Two reports published by the Institute of Medicine report the importance of collaborative practice and interdisciplinary training in the coordination of health care.[42] Pediatric trauma resuscitation is a complex and time-sensitive procedure. Effective teamwork is essential to better outcomes.[43] Teamwork does not occur spontaneously, so, simulation-based practice is essential. Focus groups of various trauma team members (physicians, nurses, respiratory therapists). Four key areas of

---

Box 8
Pediatric trauma transport checklist

- Ensure the airway is patent and/or secure before transport
- If there is a risk of losing airway on the transport, then intubate before departure
- If intubated, mechanical ventilation is preferred to hand bagging
- Confirm ETT placement before departure with chest radiograph and end-tidal CO_2 detection
- Secure the ETT
- Consider a predeparture blood gas measurement to assess adequacy of ventilation and oxygenation
- Ensure suction is working and available
- Assess the need for chest tube before transport
- If there is the potential for free air, consider pressurizing the cabin or limiting altitude
- Adequately fluid resuscitate the patient before transport
- Control hemorrhage by direct pressure, staples, or suturing (if necessary)
- Consider ongoing fluid losses in fluid calculations
- Aim for at least 2 large-bore intravenous lines (or equivalent) for transport
- Secure and protect all intravenous lines; ensure there is no kinking or blockage
- Use intraosseous access if you are unable to obtain intravenous access
- Secure intraosseous needle with tape and gauze to prevent its dislodgement during transport
- For fluid-refractory shock, bring blood products on the transport if clinically indicated
- Assess the need for analgesia, sedation, and neuromuscular blockade before departure
- Ensure proper and sufficient medications are available and on board
- Consider continuous infusions of sedatives/analgesics, rather than intermittent boluses, especially for longer transports

Data from Cheng A. Transport of the pediatric trauma patient. In: Mikrogianakis A, Valani R, Cheng A, editors. The hospital for sick children manual of pediatric trauma. Philadelphia: LWW; 2008. p. 277–8.

---

improvement identified through participation in simulation are leadership, communication, cooperation/teamwork, and roles.[44] In situ trauma simulations are highly recommended so that teams are practicing in the authentic patient care environment with the same equipment that they will use during a real trauma care situation. Training in the in situ environment also allows the evaluation of space, systems, and equipment in an attempt to identify latent safety threats and maximize safe and high-quality care.[44]

SUMMARY

Caring for pediatric patients with trauma requires all elements of the health care system to work together by appreciating how best to assess children, understanding the most common injuries incurred, and knowing how to treat those injuries most efficiently and effectively. Front-line emergency physicians have the necessary knowledge and competencies through ATLS. Pediatric experts are keen to provide advice and to support front-line colleagues requiring assistance (**Box 9**).

Box 9
Top 10 pediatric trauma pearls

1. Follow general ATLS principles
   - A systematic approach avoids missing key findings in both the primary and secondary surveys
   - Almost all pediatric trauma cases result from a blunt mechanism and rely on an effective trauma resuscitation (ABCDEs) and very rarely on an emergent operation

2. Call for patient transport/advice/support as soon as possible
   - Helps to maintain situational awareness and avoid fixation errors
   - Obtain radiographs when they will be helpful
   - Do not delay transfer for advanced imaging (CT scanning) unless it will change management acutely or change decision to transport

3. Maintain oxygenation at all times
   - Most pediatric arrests are from prolonged hypoxemia

4. Beware of persistent tachycardia
   - Cardiac output completely HR dependent
   - Treat hypovolemia aggressively
   - Hypotension is a late sign of uncompensated shock
   - Goal of trauma resuscitation is to normalize vital signs

5. Be mindful of atypical spaces for significant hemorrhage in children
   - Difficult to diagnose because of compensation
   - Pelvis, long bones, subgaleal space

6. Do not be afraid of transfusion of blood components
   - Pediatric blood volume is estimated to be only 80 mL/kg, and 25% blood volume loss is predicted to cause hypotension
   - A 1-year-old patient weighing 10 kg would only have to lose 200 mL (<1 cup) of blood to reach this level
   - A 6 year old patient weighing 20 kg only has to lose 400 mL (<2 cups) of blood to reach this level

7. Avoid hypothermia if possible
   - Children prone to hypothermia with large surface area to volume ratio (especially the heads of infants and toddlers)
   - Remove all wet clothing
   - Use warm intravenous fluids and a warming blanket
   - Hypothermia significantly affects volume status and, along with acidosis, leads to coagulopathy

8. Be mindful of using analgesia to treat pain
   - Treatment of pain is often an afterthought
   - Splint all fractures
   - Ensure adequate volume resuscitation before giving medications that may compromise hemodynamics

9. Allow parents to be present whenever possible
   - The trauma room is an unfamiliar/fearful/anxiety-provoking environment
   - History taking and cooperation can be challenging
   - Children on a backboard with spine protection cannot see their parents in the trauma room (allow parents to make eye contact and touch their children whenever appropriate)

10. Be mindful of the possibility of nonaccidental trauma
    - Do the injuries match the mechanism?
    - Maintain an appropriate index of suspicion

REFERENCES

1. Kenefake ME, Swarm M, Walthall J. Nuances in pediatric trauma. Emerg Med Clin North Am 2013;31(3):627–52.
2. Kissoon N, Dreyer J, Walia M. Pediatric trauma: differences in pathophysiology, injury patterns and treatment compared with adult trauma. CMAJ 1990;142(1): 27–34.
3. ATLS Subcommittee, American College of Surgeons' Committee on Trauma; International ATLS working group. Advanced Trauma Life Support (ATLS®): the ninth edition. J Trauma Acute Care Surg 2013;74(5):1363–6.
4. Chiu P. Primary survey, secondary survey and adjuncts. In: Mikrogianakis A, Valani R, Cheng A, editors. The hospital for sick children manual of pediatric trauma. Philadelphia: Lippincott Williams & Wilkins; 2008. p. 9–20.
5. Karsli C. Airway management. In: Mikrogianakis A, Valani R, Cheng A, editors. The hospital for sick children manual of pediatric trauma. Philadelphia: Lippincott Williams & Wilkins; 2008. p. 21–30.
6. The Pediatric Airway Course. Calgary (Canada): The Alberta Children's Hospital; 2015.
7. Acker SN, Bredbeck B, Partrick DA, et al. Shock index, pediatric age-adjusted (SIPA) is more accurate than age-adjusted hypotension for trauma team activation. Surgery 2017;161(3):803–7.
8. Golden J, Dossa A, Goodhue CJ, et al. Admission hematocrit predicts the need for transfusion secondary to hemorrhage in pediatric blunt trauma patients. J Trauma Acute Care Surg 2015;79(4):555–62.
9. Ryan ML, Maxwell AC, Manning L, et al. Noninvasive hemoglobin measurement in pediatric trauma patients. J Trauma Acute Care Surg 2016;81(6):1162–6.
10. Beno S. Translating Emergency Knowledge for Kids (TREKK) bottom line recommendations for multisystem trauma. 2015. Available at: https/trekk.ca.
11. Puckett Y, Bonacorsi L, Caley M, et al. Imaging before transfer to designated pediatric trauma centers exposes children to excess radiation. J Trauma Acute Care Surg 2016;81(2):229–35.
12. Kochanek PM, Carney N, Adelson PD, et al. Guidelines for the acute medical management of severe traumatic brain injury in infants, children, and adolescents–second edition. Pediatr Crit Care Med 2012;13(Suppl 1):S1–82.
13. Gross BW, Edavettal MM, Cook AD, et al. Big children or little adults? A statewide analysis of adolescent isolated severe traumatic brain injury outcomes at pediatric versus adult trauma centers. J Trauma Acute Care Surg 2017;82(2):368–73.
14. Jain S. Pediatric cervical spine injuries. In: Mikrogianakis A, Valani R, Cheng A, editors. The hospital for sick children manual of pediatric trauma. Philadelphia: Lippincott Williams & Wilkins; 2008. p. 115–29.
15. Brown RL, Brunn MA, Garcia VF. Cervical spine injuries in children: a review of 103 patients treated consecutively at a level 1 pediatric trauma center. J Pediatr Surg 2001;36(8):1107–14.
16. Brown GJ, CN, McCaskill ME, et al. An approach to pediatric cervical spine injury. In: Pediatric emergency medicine database. The Children's Hospital at Westmead.
17. Kokoska ER, Keller MS, Rallo MC, et al. Characteristics of pediatric cervical spine injuries. J Pediatr Surg 2001;36(1):100–5.
18. Patel JC, Tepas JJ 3rd, Mollitt DL, et al. Pediatric cervical spine injuries: defining the disease. J Pediatr Surg 2001;36(2):373–6.
19. Roche C, Carty H. Spinal trauma in children. Pediatr Radiol 2001;31(10):677–700.

20. Proctor MR. Spinal cord injury. Crit Care Med 2002;30(11 Suppl):S489–99.
21. Chung S, Mikrogianakis A, Wales PW, et al. Trauma Association of Canada Pediatric Subcommittee national pediatric cervical spine evaluation pathway: consensus guidelines. J Trauma 2011;70(4):873–84.
22. Connelly CR, Yonge JD, Eastes LE, et al. Performance improvement and patient safety program-guided quality improvement initiatives can significantly reduce computed tomography imaging in pediatric trauma patients. J Trauma Acute Care Surg 2016;81(2):278–84.
23. Sartorelli KH, Vane DW. The diagnosis and management of children with blunt injury of the chest. Semin Pediatr Surg 2004;13(2):98–105.
24. Eichelberger M. Pediatric trauma prevention, acute care, rehabilitation. Mosby Year Book; 1993.
25. Holmes JF, Sokolove PE, Brant WE, et al. A clinical decision rule for identifying children with thoracic injuries after blunt torso trauma. Ann Emerg Med 2002; 39(5):492–9.
26. Herrera P, Langer JC. Thoracic trauma in children. In: Mikrogianakis A, Valani R, Cheng A, editors. The hospital for sick children manual of pediatric trauma. Philadelphia: Lippincott Williams & Wilkins; 2008. p. 131.
27. Bliss D, Silen M. Pediatric thoracic trauma. Crit Care Med 2002;30(11 Suppl): S409–15.
28. Golden J, Isani M, Bowling J, et al. Limiting chest computed tomography in the evaluation of pediatric thoracic trauma. J Trauma Acute Care Surg 2016;81(2): 271–7.
29. Cooper A, Barlow B, DiScala C, et al. Mortality and truncal injury: the pediatric perspective. J Pediatr Surg 1994;29(1):33–8.
30. Zamakhshary M, Wales P. Abdominal and pelvic trauma. In: Mikrogianakis A, Valani R, Cheng A, editors. The hospital for sick children manual of pediatric trauma. Philadelphia: Lippincott Williams & Wilkins; 2008. p. 145–60.
31. Fact Sheet #2. The National Pediatric Trauma Registry. October, 1993.
32. C.E.a.I.R.C.N.P.S.R. Institute, editor. Childhood Injury. Cost and Prevention Facts. 1996.
33. Wegner S, Colletti JE, Van Wie D. Pediatric blunt abdominal trauma. Pediatr Clin North Am 2006;53(2):243–56.
34. Gaines BA, Ford HR. Abdominal and pelvic trauma in children. Crit Care Med 2002;30(11 Suppl):S416–23.
35. Sola JE, Cheung MC, Yang R, et al. Pediatric FAST and elevated liver transaminases: an effective screening tool in blunt abdominal trauma. J Surg Res 2009; 157(1):103–7.
36. Fenton SJ, Sandoval KN, Stevens AM, et al. The use of angiography in pediatric blunt abdominal trauma patients. J Trauma Acute Care Surg 2016;81(2):261–5.
37. LeeVan E, Zmora O, Cazzulino F, et al. Management of pediatric blunt renal trauma: a systematic review. J Trauma Acute Care Surg 2016;80(3):519–28.
38. Swaid F, Peleg K, Alfici R, et al. A comparison study of pelvic fractures and associated abdominal injuries between pediatric and adult blunt trauma patients. J Pediatr Surg 2017;52(3):386–9.
39. Cheng A. Transport of the pediatric trauma patient. In: Mikrogianakis A, Valani R, Cheng A, editors. The hospital for sick children manual of pediatric trauma. Philadelphia: Lippincott Williams & Wilkins; 2008. p. 275–80.
40. Graneto JW, Soglin DF. Transport and stabilization of the pediatric trauma patient. Pediatr Clin North Am 1993;40(2):365–80.

41. Woodward GA, Insoft RM, Pearson-Shaver AL, et al. The state of pediatric inter-facility transport: consensus of the second National Pediatric and Neonatal Inter-facility Transport Medicine Leadership Conference. Pediatr Emerg Care 2002; 18(1):38–43.
42. Committee on Quality Health Care in America, Institute of Medicine. Crossing the quality chasm; a new health system for the 21st century. Washington, DC: National Academy Press; 2001.
43. Capella J, Smith S, Philp A, et al. Teamwork training improves the clinical care of trauma patients. J Surg Educ 2010;67(6):439–43.
44. Burke RV, Demeter NE, Goodhue CJ, et al. Qualitative assessment of simulation-based training for pediatric trauma resuscitation. Surgery 2017;161(5):1357–66.

Moving?

Make sure your subscription moves with you!

To notify us of your new address, find your **Clinics Account Number** (located on your mailing label above your name), and contact customer service at:

Email: journalscustomerservice-usa@elsevier.com

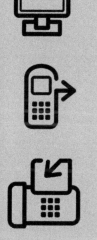

800-654-2452 (subscribers in the U.S. & Canada)
314-447-8871 (subscribers outside of the U.S. & Canada)

Fax number: 314-447-8029

Elsevier Health Sciences Division
Subscription Customer Service
3251 Riverport Lane
Maryland Heights, MO 63043

*To ensure uninterrupted delivery of your subscription, please notify us at least 4 weeks in advance of move.

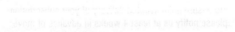

Printed and bound by CPI Group (UK) Ltd, Croydon, CR0 4YY

08/05/2025

01864706-0001